SimChart® for the medical office

LEARNING THE MEDICAL OFFICE WORKFLOW

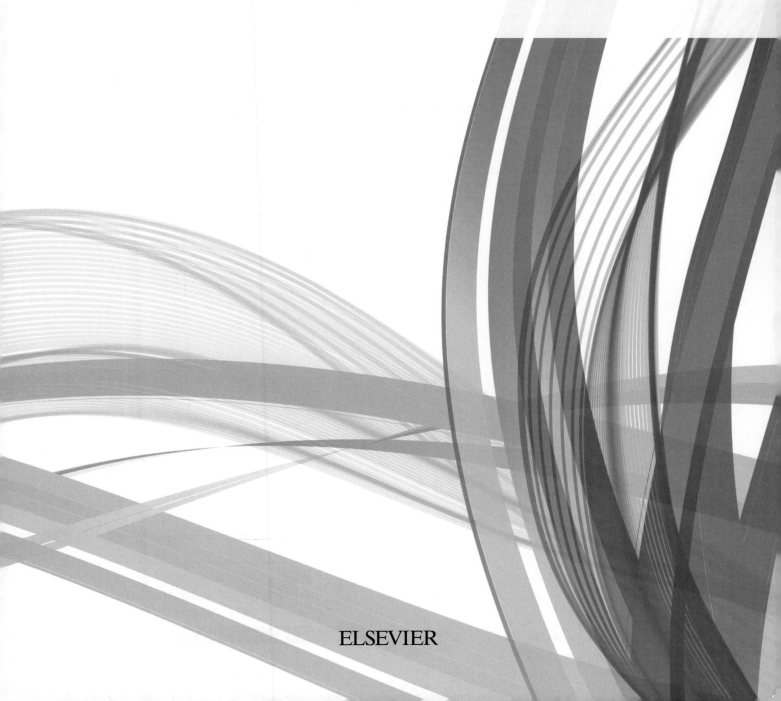

ELSEVIER

ELSEVIER

3251 Riverport Lane
St. Louis, Missouri 63043

Notices

Practitioners and researchers must always rely on their own experience and knowledge in evaluating and using any information, methods, compounds or experiments described herein. Because of rapid advances in the medical sciences, in particular, independent verification of diagnoses and drug dosages should be made. To the fullest extent of the law, no responsibility is assumed by Elsevier, authors, editors or contributors for any injury and/or damage to persons or property as a matter of products liability, negligence or otherwise, or from any use or operation of any methods, products, instructions, or ideas contained in the material herein.

International Standard Book Number: 978-0-323-64197-5

Publishing Director, Education Content: Kristin Wilhelm
Senior Content Development Specialist: Becky Leenhouts
Director of Clinical Solutions: Heidi Pohlman
Publishing Services Manager: Deepthi Unni
Project Manager: Bharat Narang

Printed in Canada

Last digit is the print number: 9 8 7 6 5 4 3 2

Working together
to grow libraries in
developing countries

www.elsevier.com • www.bookaid.org

Reviewers

Amy DeVore, MSTD, CPC, CMA (AAMA)
Program Advisor and Associate Professor
Medical Assisting Program
Butler County Community College
Chicora, Pennsylvania

Jeanne Lawo, RN MSN
Clinical Nurse Manager
SLUCare Ambulatory Practices
St. Louis, Missouri

Julie Pepper, CMA (AAMA)
Instructor
Medical Assisting Program
Chippewa Valley Technical College
Eau Claire, Wisconsin

Nikki Marhefka, M Ed, MT(ASCP), CMA (AAMA)
Program Director
Medical Assisting Program
Central Penn College
Summerdale, Pennsylvania

Beverly Philpott, CMA (AAMA), CPhT
Adjunct Faculty
Medical Assisting Program
Kirkwood Community College

Kim Smith Norris, CPC, MBA
Program Director
Medical Billing and Coding
Carrington College
Tucson, Arizona

To the Instructor

SimChart for the Medical Office: Learning the Medical Office Workflow was developed to provide step by step guidance in utilizing all of the features of SimChart for the Medical Office. Utilizing all of the helpful materials provided within the program, this text will walk you and your students through the three modules of the product as well as provide practice with the TruCode encoder feature.

Organization

The text is organized into four units:
1. **Navigating SimChart for the Medical Office.** This unit introduces the student to the product and provides background on the three modules, the simulation playground, the encoder, and some of the typical workflow steps that medical assistants will encounter.
2. **Front Office.** This unit introduces students to the front office module of the product and concludes with 20 related assignments for students to complete in SimChart for the Medical Office.
3. **Clinical Care.** This unit introduces students to the clinical care module of the product and concludes with 41 related assignments for students to complete in SimChart for the Medical Office.
4. **Coding & Billing.** This unit introduces students to the coding & billing module of the product and concludes with 49 related assignments for students to complete in SimChart for the Medical Office.

Quick Tips

The following are some tips that will help you to utilize SimChart for the Medical Office to the fullest.

Familiarize Yourself with Instructor Resources

Access Instructor Resources as often as needed; whenever you have a question regarding a process or where to locate a particular feature. Watch *A Guided Tour of SimChart for the Medical Office* before logging in to SimChart for the Medical Office for the first time.

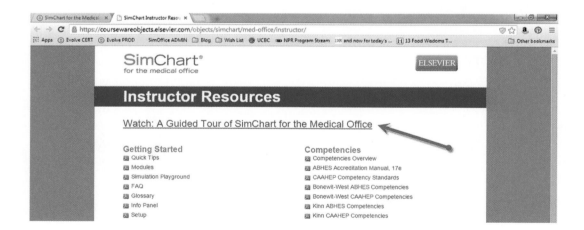

Refer to the Lesson Plan Index

The *Lesson Plan Index* in the Implementation and Lesson Plan folders provides suggested activities to incorporate SimChart for the Medical Office in lectures and labs. *The Lesson Plan Index* is organized by week with details on the level of activity, the forum for delivery, and the use of setting.

Review the Assignments and Grading Features

The instructor view is comprised of Assignments and Grading. When you log in to SimChart for the Medical Office, you land within the **Assignments** module.

- Select a Course Name from the Course List to review selected assignments. Within the **Grading** module, follow the same path to review the auto-graded questions and simulation work for an assignment.

Release Assignments to Your Course

Elsevier provides 110 pre-built, peer-reviewed assignments. In the **Assignments** module, you can **Assign All** or **Review & Select** assignments. Keep in mind that assignments cannot be retracted once assigned to the class.

- **Assign All** is a quick and easy way to give students access to all of the assignments for practice and completion. Daily or weekly assignments can be provided to students by way of syllabus or in-class discussion to keep students on task.
- **Review & Select** gives you the ability to time your assignment releases using the selection assignment function.

Create Your Own Folder Structure

- After selecting a course in the Assignments module, select the Organize tab to review and organize assignments into folders. For example, categorize assignments by the week you wish to release them to students or archive any assignments not needed. Refer to *Assigning Assignments* in the Assignments folder for more information.

Review a Graded Assignment

Students cannot make additional changes after submitting an assignment. The application automatically generates a preliminary grade based on a student's quiz performance. Once a student clicks the Submit Assignment button, the assignment moves from the Open Assignments tab to the Graded Assignments tab in the student view and the quiz results are immediately available for student review. An instructor can then manually review a student's simulation work, enter a grade for the simulation work, and use the Grading Rubric to approve or adjust the automatically generated grade.

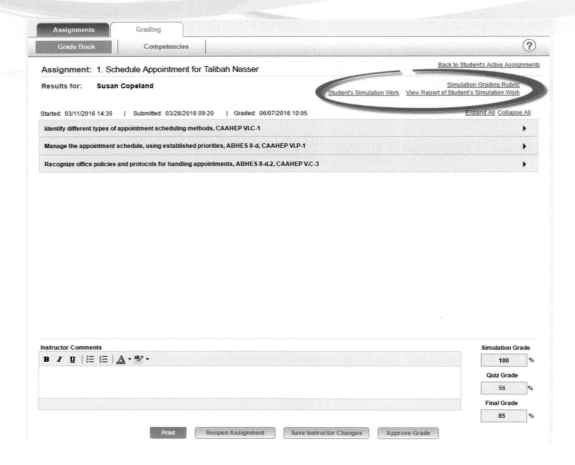

Allow Students to Reattempt an Assignment

Clicking the **Reopen Assignment** button sends a student's assignment back to the Open Assignments tab in the student view and labels it as **REOPENED**. This allows a student to continue the simulation exercise of an assignment and make changes to the post-case quiz. The student can resubmit the assignment for grading when finished.

Students Review and Print Graded Assignments

Once a student submits an assignment, the assignment moves from the Open Assignments tab to the Graded Assignments tab in the student view and the automatic grade displays. If an instructor changes a grade based on a student's simulation work, the Grade column in the Graded Assignments grid displays the percentage for that assignment in bold. Students can print assignments and add them to a portfolio.

10 Ways to Implement SimChart for the Medical Office

1. Register a Patient and Schedule an Appointment

Conduct contests to see which student can register a patient and schedule a new patient appointment the quickest, ensuring that all information is entered correctly.

2. Correspondence

Have students create appointments and then complete Appointment Reminder letters to confirm upcoming patient appointments. As students progress through the modules, have them complete additional communication using the templates in Correspondence.

3. Review Legal Documents

When discussing advance directives, have students access and complete the document in the simulation. Although most forms are electronic, some forms such as the Advance Directive must be printed and completed by hand in order to demonstrate office workflow. In a medical office, a medical assistant would hand an Advance Directive to a patient for them to fill out by hand. The medical assistant would then upload the completed form to the patient record

4. Document Vital Signs

Instruct students to take each other's vital signs and document that information in the patient record.

5. Differentiate Between Medication Types

Give students a list of various medication types, including prescriptions, over-the-counter products, and herbal supplements. Have students document each medication in the patient record.

6. Request Orders and Lab Requisitions

Role-play scenarios in which one student acts as the medical assistant and the other acts as a patient who needs a procedure.

7. Code Diagnoses and Procedures

Give students a list of ICD and CPT codes and have them determine which codes are correct for a patient encounter.

8. Explain How a Superbill is Connected to a Claim

Group students into pairs. Have each student complete a Superbill, then have them switch patients to complete the Claim.

9. Discuss Accounts Receivable Principles

Have each student complete a Superbill and Ledger for a different patient. Then, complete the Day Sheet as a class using each student's patient information.

10. Complete a Patient Visit from Beginning to End

Demonstrate how medical assisting is connected to an electronic health record by walking students through a patient visit. Begin with scheduling an appointment, then move to documenting clinical care, and end by submitting a Superbill and Claim.

To the Student

SimChart for the Medical Office: Learning the Medical Office Workflow will provide you with unique, hands-on learning of the simulated medical office. The assignments in this text provide realistic practice of all of the tasks you will encounter in a real medical office—from front office (administrative) skills to clinical skills to practice management skills (billing, coding, and insurance).

Completing a medical assistant program is a rigorous undertaking. The medical assistant profession is complex and requires a student to gain a complete understanding of how a medical office functions, from the time the patient makes an appointment until the insurance carrier pays for the services provided in the encounter. Follow these tips to become a successful medical assistant student.

Quick Tips

Familiarize Yourself With Student Resources

Review all of the resource materials before class and refer to them whenever you have a question regarding a particular process or feature in SimChart for the Medical Office.

Review the Assignments

The student homepage is comprised of an **Open Assignments** tab and a **Graded Assignments** tab. All available assignments appear in the Open Assignments tab. As you complete and submit assignments, they move to the Graded Assignments tab for review.

Although student performance within the **Quiz** of an assignment generates a grade that is automatically visible, an instructor can still modify this grade based on simulation work. The grade is not final until your instructor approves the automatically generated score and the Grade column in the grid displays the percentage for that assignment in bold.

Follow Your Instructor's Lead

Instructors can incorporate SimChart for the Medical Office into the classroom several ways. Follow instructions regarding how and when to use the application.

Access the Simulation

The **Simulation Playground** button above the list of assignments directs you to a practice version of the medical office. Within this environment, you can practice common medical office tasks such as registering patients, scheduling appointments, documenting patient care, and completing the coding and billing for a patient encounter.

Information documented in the Simulation Playground remains saved but is not submitted for grading. However, your instructor can access your Simulation Playground in order to review your practice.

If desired, you can erase your work in the Simulation Playground and begin a new session by selecting the 'Start new simulation session and clear all previously saved patient information' radio button upon entry.

Save Your Work

Almost every screen has a **Save** button. Be sure to save your work in all screens before progressing or exiting. You can even save work within an assignment before submitting, making it easy to return and continue.

Review Assignment Details and Complete Simulation

- Click the **Open Assignments** tab and then click the title of the assignment to complete. Review the assignment description, objectives, and competencies before clicking the **Start Assignment** button in the **Description** tab to enter the simulation. After completing the simulation, click the **Back to Assignment** link and the **Quiz** tab to answer the questions tied to the assignment.

Answer All Quiz Questions to Submit Assignment

All assignments include questions tied to a specific competency that is reinforced by the simulation tasks. Answer all questions before submitting an assignment.

Check Your Work

- An assignment cannot be edited once it is submitted, so check all answers to quiz questions and ensure that your simulation work is accurate and complete before clicking the **Submit Assignment** button.

Review Graded Assignment Upon Completion

The system automatically grades quiz questions upon submission and moves the assignment from the **Open Assignments** tab to the **Graded Assignments** tab.
- Select the title of the graded assignment to review the automatically generated grade. Once you submit an assignment, your instructor can evaluate the simulation work manually.

After reviewing the simulation portion of an assignment, your instructor can provide comments and approve or adjust the automatically generated grade. After your instructor approves a grade, the Grade column in the Graded Assignments grid displays the percentage for that assignment in bold. You can then print the graded assignment.

Use Available Resources

Instructors are the best resource, but they can't answer questions if students don't ask them. If one student has a question, another student probably does too, so you will be doing everyone a favor by asking.
- Ask your instructor questions after class or during office hours if you are uncomfortable asking during class.
- Email your instructor if questions arise outside of class.

Fellow students are another great resource. Social networking sites can also be a great way to stay in contact outside of class.
- Form study groups to review content on an ongoing basis or prepare for exams.
- Create a Facebook group for a specific class and post questions and/or study tools for everyone to access.

Textbooks are the basis for most class content. Glossaries, indexes, and online resources can provide additional details about unfamiliar terms and topics.
- List questions from the chapter before class and ask the instructor if your questions are not answered during class.
- Make notes and highlight important content.

Teamwork

The ability to work well with others is an invaluable tool in the workforce. Group projects are a great opportunity to develop interpersonal skills that will make you an asset to any team.
- Volunteer to be the leader of the group or use your people skills to bring out the quiet one in the group.
- If you are typically the quiet member of a group, offer at least one suggestion during every group meeting.

- Practice active listening and do not interrupt. Avoid distractions. Give the person you are speaking with your undivided attention so you process the message.
- Body language can sometimes convey more than words. Observing the body language of others while you are delivering a message will help you to determine if they are receiving the intended message.
- Respect diversity. Understanding that people come from different backgrounds will facilitate collaboration. Team players are respectful of everyone's opinion.
- Gossiping is destructive to a productive learning and work environment. The impact of gossiping can hurt feelings and induce anger, neither of which help to create a positive environment.

Be Considerate

Group projects can also serve as an opportunity to develop skills that help you cooperate with all types of personalities. Remember that practicing consideration will not go unnoticed. Your instructor will remember the example you set, which will come in handy when you ask them to provide a referral letter.

- Be considerate of all classmates in and out of class.
- Do not interrupt your teacher or your classmates as this is rude and disruptive.
- Remember that everyone comes from different backgrounds, so keep an open mind and learn from what others share in class.
- Do not gossip. Gossip damages relationships and is unprofessional.

Be Professional

Approaching school as if it were a job allows you to start developing your professionalism skills the moment you start your medical assistant program. Consistent attendance helps you retain more information, participating in class demonstrates that you are engaged in class discussion, balancing priorities helps you to be prepared for any unexpected scheduling complications, and adhering to established policies will all help you succeed.

- Participate in class. You do not have to raise your hand to answer every question, but you should always be engaged in class discussion.
- Determine daycare details in advance and establish a backup plan in case your transportation falls through.
- Keep a calendar to track all of your commitments and be realistic about how long activities really take.
- Contact your instructor immediately if absence is unavoidable.
- Follow the dress code. If you are not already required to follow a dress code while in school, you will certainly have a dress code for practicum.
- Make sure scrubs are in good condition. Pants should not drag on the floor, and tops should be an appropriate length.
- Cover tattoos and remove visible body piercings.
- Always behave professionally when dressed in scrubs and avoid going out socially in scrubs because it could reflect poorly upon healthcare professions.

Work Ethic

Taking responsibility for your education and seeking clarification when you don't understand something in class will help you develop the habit of ensuring comprehension in the workplace. This will ultimately help you to provide the best patient care possible.

- Do your own work and credit your sources. Understand plagiarism and its consequences. Allowing others to use your work is still considered cheating.
- Complete all assignments before the due date and remember that you receive the grade you earn; instructors do not "give" grades.
- Always clean up after yourself. Whether you are in the lab or in a lecture, make sure that your workspace is as clean as or cleaner than when you sat down.

Many of the skills needed to obtain and maintain a job can be developed while a student is still in a Medical Assistant program.

Positive Mental Attitude

Nobody wants to work with someone who always has a negative outlook. Those who tend to see the worst should use this time as an opportunity to start changing their mindset.
- Keep your self-talk positive. When presented with a difficult situation, identify an aspect of the situation that will benefit the patient, organization, or staff.
- Smile, even when you don't feel like it. Smiling can help create positive interactions which contribute to a positive environment overall.
- Embrace change. Change is inevitable, especially in healthcare. Viewing change as an opportunity to learn and improve rather than a chore can also contribute to a positive environment. Try to identify how change can benefit the patient, organization, and staff.

Time Management

Time management is a skill needed for school as well as work. Figuring out how to balance priorities while in school can carry over to your work.
- Determine daycare details in advance. Having a plan in place when your child or daycare provider is sick can help to minimize schedule complications. Investigate the options available in your area. Is there a center that accepts sick children? Can a close friend or family member care for your child?
- Secure reliable transportation or establish a backup plan if you have car trouble. Know the bus routes and ask other students or co-workers about carpooling.
- Keep a calendar to track all of your commitments and prevent double-booking. Most cellular phones provide a calendar function and paper agendas are also available. Whichever version you prefer, keep it current with your work schedule, personal activities, and family activities.
- Be realistic about how long activities really take. For example, if you don't have more than one hour available for a dentist appointment and you know that traffic is always hectic, you should choose another day for the appointment.

Lifelong Learning

Change occurs frequently in healthcare and developing tools to help with staying current in your field will make you a better medical assistant.
- Join your national and local professional organization.
- The American Association of Medical Assistants (CMA (AAMA)) provides continuing education opportunities including an annual national convention, CMA Today magazine, membership in the state organization that provides opportunities at a more local level, and online and paper-based CEUs.
- The American Medical Technologists (RMA) provides an annual national meeting, AMT State Society meetings, and online and paper-based CEUs.
- Find workshops and seminars that promote new skill development or update existing skills. For example, diagnostic and procedural coding manuals are updated every year. Attending a workshop regarding this topic will ensure that you are using current coding criteria. Requesting information and demonstrations from manufacturers when they release laboratory tests or equipment is another good way to remain current.

Dressing for Success

Since healthcare is a conservative field, follow the dress code policy at all times.
- Cover tattoos and remove visible body piercings. Some dress code policies even go so far as to state that there can only be one earring in each ear.

- If scrubs are required, make sure they are in good condition. Pants should not drag on the floor and tops should be an appropriate length.
- Some positions require business casual attire. If unsure as to what clothes are allowed, be sure to ask. Business casual is not the same as casual clothing worn at home. Sweatpants, yoga pants, shorts, midriff baring tops, flip flops, shirts with logos or statements, and halter tops are not appropriate.

Resume Building

All of the skills obtained in school help to build a resume that will attract potential employers. Welcome every opportunity to learn a new skill and showcase these skills in your resume.
- Create a portfolio with examples of different skills learned, such as a business letter written using Microsoft Word, a project organized using Microsoft Excel, samples of EHR documentation using an application such as SimChart for the Medical Office, and a checklist of clinical and administrative skills gained during practicum. Refer *Appendix A* for more information.
- List experience using software programs such as SimChart for the Medical Office, Microsoft Word, Microsoft Excel, Microsoft PowerPoint, or Microsoft Access. Include extracurricular activities such as tutoring or involvement in any student or professional organizations. This type of background demonstrates a willingness to expand beyond the basics required in school.

Contents

Unit 1 | Navigating SimChart for the Medical Office

Objectives

- Understand the three modules that make up SimChart for the Medical Office.
- Know how the Simulation Playground and Encoder features work.
- Understand the info panel for each of the modules in SimChart for the Medical Office.
- Explain what an assignment is and how to access and complete reopened assignments.
- Comprehend the basic workflow steps associated with each of the modules in SimChart for the Medical Office.

About SimChart for the Medical Office

Modules

SimChart for the Medical Office is organized within three modules which contain the main aspects of the medical office workflow: Front Office, Clinical Care, and Coding & Billing (Figure 1-1). The default landing page upon entering the simulation is the Front Office Calendar to represent opening the medical office for the day. From that point, users can navigate freely throughout all of the modules of the medical office workflow in order to practice or accomplish the specific tasks of an assignment.

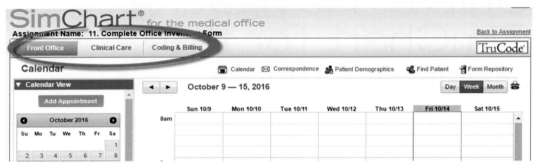

Figure 1-1 The three modules of SimChart for the Medical Office: Front Office, Clinical Care, and Coding & Billing.

- The **Front Office** module features the Calendar, which is the most frequently referenced aspect of daily medical office workflow. (See workflow items 1- 6 at the end of this unit for some typical front office tasks.)
- The **Clinical Care** module features all of the clinical charting for a patient record. (See workflow items 7-20 at the end of this unit for some typical clinical care tasks.)
- The **Coding & Billing** module contains all practice management functionality necessary to complete an encounter. (See workflow items 21-24 at the end of this unit for some typical coding & billing tasks.)

Simulation Playground

The Simulation Playground is the practice environment of SimChart for the Medical Office. Although the same functionality is available in assignments, the Simulation Playground is meant to serve as an opportunity for students to familiarize themselves with simulation features prior to completing assignments.

Simulation Playground Access for Students

In the Simulation Playground, students can practice aspects of clinical documentation, office workflow, and practice management. Encourage students to collaborate by registering each other as new patients, documenting vital signs, and coding Superbills. Students can even review an assignment description and practice the assignment in the Simulation Playground before beginning the graded assignment. This practice can help students become familiar with identifying the steps necessary to complete an assignment.

- Upon entry, continue work or clear previous work to begin a new session. Select the first radio button, unless you want to clear your work (Figure 1-2).

Simulation Playground Access for Instructors

- Instructors can access the simulation by clicking the **Simulation Playground** button within the Assignments tab (Figure 1-3).

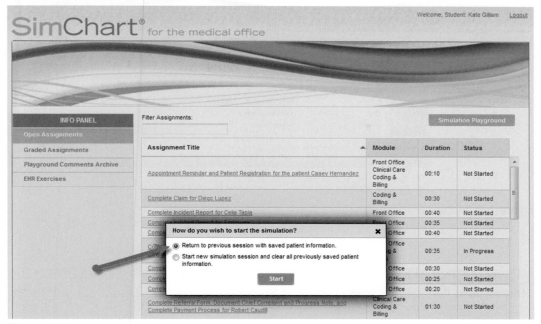

Figure 1-2 Simulation Playground radio buttons: return to previous session or start new simulation session.

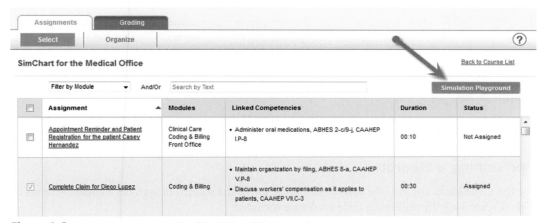

Figure 1-3 Instructor access to the Simulation Playground.

- To review a student's Simulation Playground, click the **Student's Playground** link at the top of an individual student's Active Assignments screen.

Encoder

The TruCode Encoder tool is an electronic medical coding resource to use when documenting diagnoses or procedures in SimChart for the Medical Office. Since SimChart for the Medical Office is intended for educational use, a limited set of CPT codes are available within the tool. There are two ways to access the encoder:

1. Clicking the TruCode button in the top right corner opens the tool in a new tab to use as reference while navigating throughout the application. This button is always visible throughout the application (Figure 1-4).
2. Placing a cursor in a field that requires coding will reveal an additional TruCode button. Accessing the tool this way will auto-populate the selected code where the cursor is placed in the simulation (Figure 1-5).

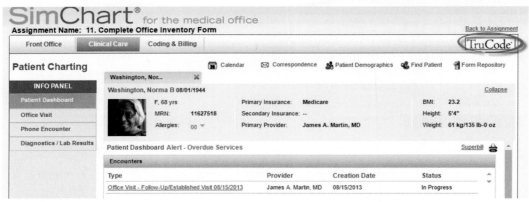

Figure 1-4 TruCode Encoder.

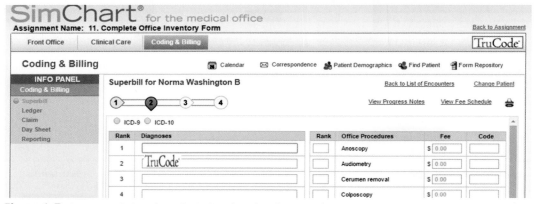

Figure 1-5 Auto-populating the selected code using the encoder.

Performing a Search

Use the CodeBooks control (the search field at the top of the screen) to search for codes by terms or code (Figure 1-6). The following code books are included:
- **ICD-10-CM Diagnosis** and **External Cause** – These books consist of an alphabetic index where you can look up terms and a tabular of codes, which includes all instructional notes.
- **ICD-10-PCS Procedure** – This book consists of an alphabetic index where you can look up terms and a table where you choose the specifics of the procedure to construct the ICD-10-PCS procedure code.
- **ICD-9-CM Diagnosis**, **E Code**, and **Procedure** – These books consist of an alphabetic index where you can look up terms and a tabular of codes, including all instructional notes.
- **CPT** and **HCPCS** – In these books, both the index and tabular are searched simultaneously and tabular results are displayed based upon the search.

Search Results

When searching a code book by terms (except for CPT and HCPCS), the alphabetic index appears in the control. The Search Results pane displays all index entries from the alphabetic index that match the search terms (Figure 1-7).

If a code has an instructional note, the **I** symbol appears to the left of the code when the code is highlighted. Instructional notes contain Includes, Excludes, and Notes from the chapter, section, and category levels.
- To view the note, click the symbol (Figure 1-8).

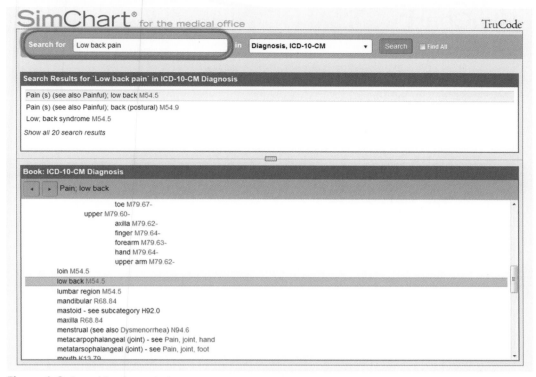

Figure 1-6 Searching by code type.

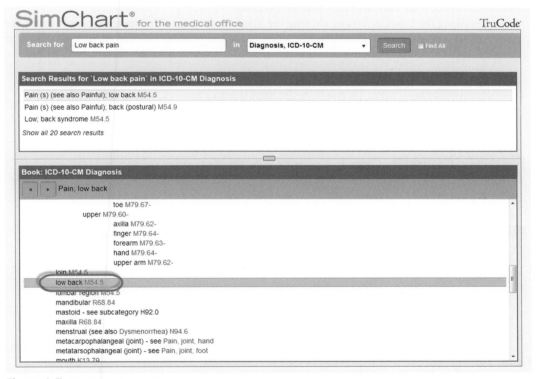

Figure 1-7 The Search Results pane.

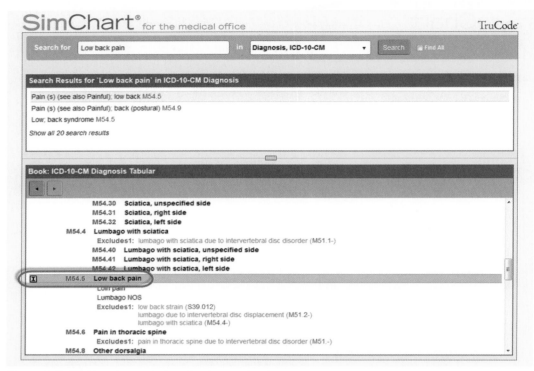

Figure 1-8 Clicking the symbol to view instructional notes.

Documentation

Documentation options vary depending on access point.

- Accessing the Encoder tool by clicking the TruCode button in the top right corner opens the tool in a new tab to use as reference while navigating throughout the application. In order to document this way, copy the desired code and paste it into the correct field within the simulation.
- Accessing the Encoder tool by placing a cursor in a field requiring coding reveals an additional TruCode button and will auto-populate the selected code where the cursor is placed in the simulation (Figure 1-9).

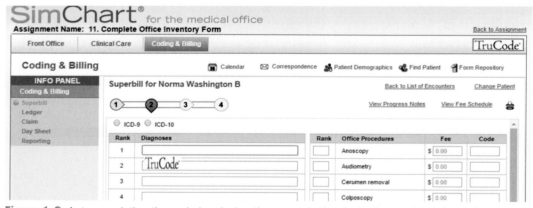

Figure 1-9 Auto-populating the code by placing the cursor in the desired area of the simulation.

- Expand the list of codes beneath the desired code by clicking the code associated with a diagnosis (Figure 1-10).
- After expanding a diagnosis to confirm that it is the most specific code available, click the code that appears in red in order to auto-populate it within the simulation and continue documenting (Figures 1-11 and 1-12).

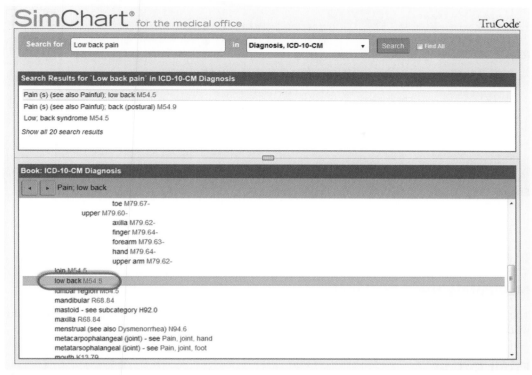

Figure 1-10 Expanding the list of codes.

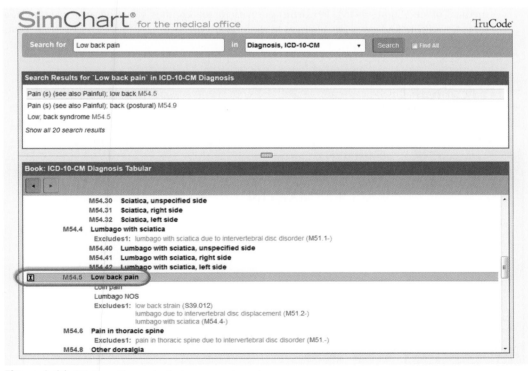

Figure 1-11 Click on the code that appears in red.

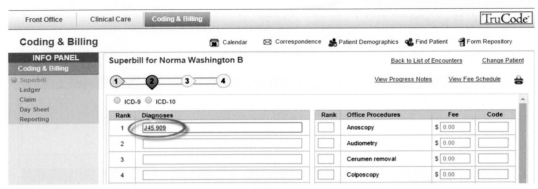

Figure 1-12 The code auto-populated in the simulation.

Info Panel

Navigating the Info Panel

The Info Panel is visible on the left side of the screen in all modules and contains tasks specific to the workflow of that particular module.

Front Office

The Front Office module defaults to the calendar view. Form Repository or Correspondence sections can be selected by clicking on the icons at the top of the screen.

- Selecting the **Form Repository** icon displays patient and office form templates to use in the medical office (Figure 1-13). Performing a patient search after selecting a form unlocks a form for editing and saves any changes to that patient's record.

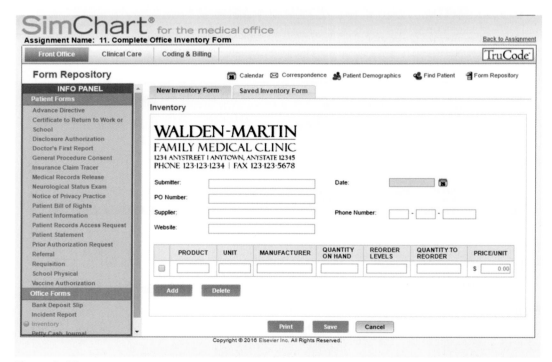

Figure 1-13 Templates in the Form Repository.

- Selecting the **Correspondence** icon displays the email, letter, and phone communication templates available for use in the medical office.

Clinical Care

The Info Panel in the Clinical Care module displays patient visit options. Selecting a patient displays the Patient Dashboard for that patient. Before documenting in the patient record, a student must create a patient encounter in order to tie documentation to a specific date and time (Figure 1-14).

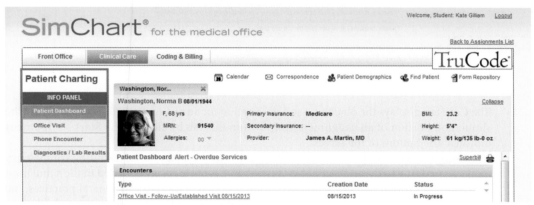

Figure 1-14 The Info Panel in the Clinical Care module.

Coding & Billing

The Info Panel in the Coding & Billing module displays the **Superbill**, **Ledger**, **Claim**, **Day Sheet Reporting** and **Auditing** (Figure 1-15). You must perform a patient search and select an encounter before coding a Superbill. After submitting a Superbill, you may progress to the Claim.

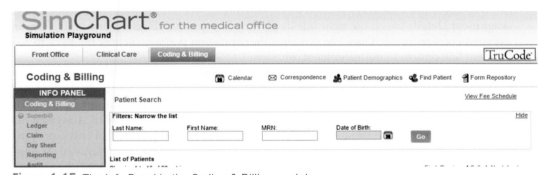

Figure 1-15 The Info Panel in the Coding & Billing module.

Assignment Overview

Assignment Components

The assignments available in SimChart for the Medical Office have been authored and peer-reviewed by medical assisting instructors. An assignment is comprised of a description, objectives, competencies, a simulation exercise, and quiz questions.

- Access assignments after logging in to SimChart for the Medical Office. All assignments are located in the **Open Assignments** tab of the Info Panel. Click the assignment title to enter and view the components of an assignment (Figure 1-16).

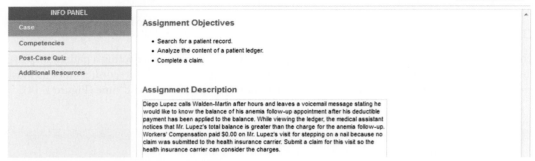

Figure 1-16 Click the assignment title to enter and view the components of an assignment.

- The **Case** tab displays the objectives and description for an assignment. You can also enter the simulation portion of an assignment from within this tab by clicking the **Start Assignment** button at the bottom of the screen.
- The **Competencies** tab lists the competencies tied to the assignment, including competency name, accrediting body, and competency number. Competencies addressed in the simulation are reinforced with quiz questions. Since some competencies speak to general practices, the application incorporates quiz questions that address general best practices any medical office should adopt.
- The **Post-Case Quiz** tab contains review questions that complement the concepts addressed in the simulation exercise. As mentioned above, quiz questions address general best practices any medical office should adopt.
- The **Additional Resources** tab lists additional content such as texts or articles to refer to when completing an assignment. If there are no resources listed, none have been provided.

Student Workflow

- Students should review the **Case** and **Competency** tabs before clicking the **Start Assignment** button to begin the simulation portion of an assignment. Within the simulation, clicking the **Assignment Details** tab on the right side displays the assignment objectives and description in case you need a reminder. Once you complete the simulation portion, clicking the **Back to As-signment** link returns to the assignment overview.
- Next, answer the quiz questions before clicking the **Submit Assignment** button. Review questions for each assignment generate an automatic initial grade an instructor can ap-prove or adjust after reviewing a student's simulation work. Although the auto-graded as-signment is immediately available for your review from within the **Graded Assignments** tab, an instructor can still modify this grade, so you should understand that this automati-cally generated grade is not final. Final grades are displayed in bold in the **Graded Assign-ments** tab.

Reopened Assignments

If you are disappointed with your simulation work and your instructor lets you make changes to your assignment, or your instructor believes that retaking a quiz would benefit your development, your instructor can reopen a submitted assignment.

If an instructor has reopened an assignment, that assignment moves back to the Open Assign-ments tab with a status of REOPEN.

- When your instructor reopens an assignment, you may continue working on the simula-tion as well as make changes to your post-case quiz. Review the **Description** and **Compe-tencies** tabs to ensure that you understand what tasks you are expected to perform within the assignment.

- Click the Reopen Assignment button to continue working. Comments from your instructor can be viewed by clicking the Instructor Comments link in the top right corner.
- When you finish documenting in the EHR, click the **Back to Assignment** link. Click the Post-Case Quiz tab to modify any quiz questions. Click the **Resubmit Assignment** button when finished.

The resubmitted assignment moves back to the **Graded Assignments** tab. Your grade will remain the same as your previous attempt until your instructor reviews your reattempted simulation work and adjusts your grade. Final grades appear in bold within the Grade column.

Workflow Steps

1. Review Case and Competencies tabs.
2. Click the Start Assignment button within the Case tab.
3. Complete the simulation work.
4. Click the Back to Assignment button.
5. Complete the review questions within the Post-Case Quiz tab.
6. Click the Submit Assignment button within the Post-Case Quiz tab.
7. Review the auto-graded assignment within the Graded Assignments tab.

Medical Office Workflow Tasks

SimChart for the Medical Office assignments enforce workflows medical assistants will encounter in most medical offices. The general steps required to complete assignment tasks are provided in this guide. These steps, along with information provided in the Assignment Description or simulation, provide students with all of the information necessary to successfully complete assignments.

The amount of information provided within the simulation is determined by the purpose of the assignment. For example, the Assignment Description for an assignment titled, *Document the Patient Visit and Submit the Superbill for Celia Tapia,* should contain all of the information necessary to complete that assignment. On the other hand, the simulation for an assignment titled, *Submit the Superbill for Celia Tapia,* should contain all of the information necessary to complete that assignment. Students must determine where to navigate within the simulation to locate the necessary information in this case. Following, you will find 24 workflow steps that are typical to the medical assistant workflow.

1. Register a Patient

1. Click the **Patient Demographics** icon.
2. Perform a patient search to confirm that a record does not already exist.
3. Click the **Add Patient** button.
4. Using the patient information form provided with an assignment as reference, complete the required fields (*) within the **Patient, Guarantor,** and **Insurance** tabs. Click the **Save Patient** button before moving to a different tab.
5. After providing information in all three tabs, click the **Save Patient** button to save the demographic information.
6. Click the X to close out of the Patient Demographics. You can click on the Find Patient link and conduct a search to open the new patient record. Select your new patient record to create an encounter and begin documenting patient care.

2. Schedule an Appointment

1. Click the **Add Appointment** button or anywhere within the calendar to open the New Appointment window.
2. Select the appointment type using the **Appointment Type** radio buttons.
3. Select the visit type using the **Visit Type** dropdown.
4. Document the reason for the patient visit in the **Chief Complaint** text box.

5. Select the **Search Existing Patients** radio button to determine if the patient requesting the appointment is an established patient. If the patient is not an established patient, select the **Create New Patient** radio button to gather necessary patient data prior to the patient's first office visit.

6. If the patient is an established patient, confirm the patient's date of birth to ensure you have located the correct patient record. Select the radio button next to the patient name and click the **Select** button. Confirm the auto-populated details.

7. Select the correct provider by using the Provider dropdown menu.

8. Use the calendar picker to confirm or select the appointment day in the **Date** field.

9. Select a start and end time for the appointment using the **Start Time** and **End Time** dropdown menus.

10. Click the **Save** button. The patient's appointment will display in the calendar.

3. Prepare Patient and Office Communication

1. Click the **Correspondence** icon to access email, letter, and phone message templates.

2. Select the correct template from the Correspondence Info Panel.

3. For patient communication, click the **Patient Search** button to perform a patient search and save the communication to the patient record. Performing a patient search before preparing a letter will help to ensure accurate documentation in the patient record.

4. Using the Patient Search fields, locate the correct patient record. Once you locate the correct patient in the List of Patients, confirm the date of birth to ensure you have located the correct patient record.

5. Select the radio button next to the patient name and click the **Select** button. Confirm the auto-populated details and provide any additional details needed.

6. Click the **Send** button.

7. All patient correspondence is saved in the Correspondence section of the Patient Dashboard. Within the Clinical Care module, select the letter from the **Correspondence** section of the Patient Dashboard. The letter will open in a new browser tab for reference or printing.

4. Prepare Patient and Office Forms

1. Click the **Form Repository** icon to access patient and office form templates.

2. Select the correct template from the Form Repository Info Panel.

3. For patient forms, click the **Patient Search** button to perform a patient search to auto-populate patient demographic information and save the form to the patient record. Performing a patient search before preparing a form will help to ensure accurate documentation in the patient record. Confirm the auto-populated details and enter any additional information needed.

4. Using the Patient Search fields, locate the correct patient record. Once you locate the correct patient in the List of Patients, confirm the date of birth to ensure you have located the correct patient record.

5. Select the radio button next to the patient name and click the **Select** button. Confirm the auto-populated details and provide any additional details needed.

6. Complete the necessary information and click the **Save to Patient Record** button.

7. Within the Clinical Care module, select the form from the **Forms** section of the Patient Dashboard. The letter will open in a new browser tab for reference or printing.

 HELPFUL HINT

Although most forms are electronic, some forms such as the Inventory form and the Advance Directive must be printed and completed by hand in order to demonstrate office workflow. For example, a medical assistant would give an Advance Directive to a patient for them to fill out by hand. The medical assistant would then upload the completed form to the patient record.

5. Create a Phone Encounter

1. Click the **Find Patient** icon.
2. Using the Patient Search fields, locate the correct patient record. Once you locate the correct patient in the List of Patients, confirm the date of birth to ensure you have located the correct patient record.
3. Select the radio button next to the patient name and click the **Select** button. Confirm the auto-populated details and provide any additional details needed.
4. Create a phone encounter for the patient by clicking **Phone Encounter** in the Info Panel.
5. In the Create New Encounter window, document the name of the caller in the **Caller** field. The patient's provider will auto-populate.
6. Document the reason for the call in the **Message** field.
7. Click the **Save** button and begin documenting within the encounter. The **Record** dropdown is expanded upon entering an encounter in order to communicate the record sections available for documentation. Refer to the following pages for instructions regarding the sections of Clinical Care.

6. Create a New Office Visit

Create a new office visit encounter to document patient care on a new day.
1. After performing a patient search and locating the correct patient, create an encounter by clicking **Office Visit** in the Clinical Care Info Panel.
2. Select the correct visit type from the **Visit Type** dropdown.
3. Select the correct provider from the **Provider** Dropdown.
4. Click the **Save** button and begin documenting within the encounter. The **Record** dropdown is expanded upon entering an encounter in order to communicate the record sections available for documentation. Refer to the following pages for instructions regarding the sections of Clinical Care.

7. Document in an Existing Office Visit

Document patient care for the same day within an existing encounter.
1. After performing a patient search and locating the correct patient, select the existing encounter from the Encounters section of the Patient Dashboard to begin documenting within the encounter.

8. Document an Allergy

1. Click the **Find Patient** icon.
2. Using the Patient Search fields, locate the correct patient record. Once you locate the correct patient in the List of Patients, confirm the date of birth to ensure you have located the correct patient record.
3. Select the radio button next to the patient name and click the **Select** button. Confirm the auto-populated details and provide any additional details needed. Create a new encounter or select an existing encounter to begin documenting. The Allergies section automatically appears upon entering the encounter.
4. Click the **Add Allergy** button to document patient allergies. An Add Allergy window will appear.
5. Select the correct radio button in the **Allergy Type** field. The Allergen dropdown options change based on the Allergen Type selected.
6. Complete all fields and click the **Save** button.
7. Use the icons in the Action column to edit or delete your documentation.

9. Document a Chief Complaint

1. Click the **Find Patient** icon.
2. Using the Patient Search fields, locate the correct patient record. Once you locate the correct patient in the List of Patients, confirm the date of birth to ensure you have located the correct patient record.
3. Select the radio button next to the patient name and click the **Select** button. Confirm the auto-populated details and provide any additional details needed. Create a new encounter or select an existing encounter to begin documenting.
4. Select **Chief Complaint** from the **Record** dropdown menu.
5. Document the reason for the patient visit in the **Chief Complaint** field. Use the patient's exact words if possible.
6. Document the site of the complaint (e.g., "near wrist") in the **Location** field.
7. Document symptom characteristics (e.g., "swollen") in the **Quality** field.
8. Document pain intensity in the **Severity** field. You may use a 0-10 scale with 0 being no pain (e.g., "6/10").
9. Document the length of time the complaint has been occurring (e.g., "four days") in the **Duration** field.
10. Document when the complaint occurs (e.g., "when walking") in the **Timing** field.
11. Document the circumstances of when the patient experiences symptoms (e.g., "with movement of the hand") in the **Context** field.
12. Document circumstances that change the nature of the complaint (e.g., "immobilizing wrist and applying ice") in the **Modifying Factors** field.
13. Document any additional symptoms (e.g., "numbness in fingers") in the **Associated Signs and Symptoms** field.
14. Click the **Save** button.

10. Document a Health History

1. Click the **Find Patient** icon.
2. Using the Patient Search fields, locate the correct patient record. Once you locate the correct patient in the List of Patients, confirm the date of birth to ensure you have located the correct patient record.
3. Select the radio button next to the patient name and click the **Select** button. Confirm the auto-populated details and provide any additional details needed. Create a new encounter or select an existing encounter to begin documenting.
4. Select **Health History** from the **Record** dropdown menu. Note the four tabs on the top of the screen: Medical History, Social and Family History, Pregnancy History (for a female patient), and Dental History.
5. Beginning within the **Medical History** tab, click the **Add New** button to document past medical history, past hospitalizations, or surgeries.
6. Use the icons in the Action column to edit or delete your documentation.
7. Continue to enter the rest of the history and click the **Save** button.

11. Document an Immunization

1. Click the **Find Patient** icon.
2. Using the Patient Search fields, locate the correct patient record. Once you locate the correct patient in the List of Patients, confirm the date of birth to ensure you have located the correct patient record.
3. Select the radio button next to the patient name and click the **Select** button. Confirm the auto-populated details and provide any additional details needed. Create a new encounter or select an existing encounter to begin documenting.
4. Select **Immunizations** from the **Record** dropdown menu.

5. Locate the row for the correct immunization in the **Vaccine** column and click on the green plus sign to the far right of that row. That row will become active to document an immunization.
6. Document the specific vaccine administered in the **Type** column.
7. Document the amount administered in the **Dose** column.
8. Document the date administered in the **Date** column.
9. Document the physician ordering the immunization in the **Provider** column.
10. Document how the immunization is administered (e.g., "SubQ, IM") and where the immunization is administered (e.g., "right deltoid") in the **Route/Site** column.
11. Document the manufacturer and lot number of the immunization in the **Mfr/Lot#** column.
12. Document the expiration date of the immunization in the **Exp** column.
13. Document any reactions to the immunization in the **Reaction** column.
14. Complete all fields and click the **Save** button.

12. Document a Medication

1. Click the **Find Patient** icon.
2. Using the Patient Search fields, locate the correct patient record. Once you locate the correct patient in the List of Patients, confirm the date of birth to ensure you have located the correct patient record.
3. Select the radio button next to the patient name and click the **Select** button. Confirm the auto-populated details and provide any additional details needed. Create a new encounter or select an existing encounter to begin documenting.
4. Select **Medications** from the **Record** dropdown menu. Note the three tabs on the top of the screen: Prescription Medications, Over-the-Counter Products, and Herbal and Natural Remedy Products. It is important to document all three types.
5. Within the tab of the type of medication you wish to document, click the **Add** button below the medication grid. An Add Medication window will appear.
6. Select the correct medication from the **Medication** dropdown menu or start typing the medication in the field.
7. Document the strength of the medication (e.g., "20 mg") in the **Strength** field.
8. Document the structure of the medication when consumed (e.g., "tablet") in the **Form** field.
9. Document how the medication is consumed (e.g., "oral") in the **Route** field.
10. Document how often the medication should be taken (e.g., "daily") in the **Frequency** field.
11. Document the reason for the medication in the **Indication** field.
12. Document the amount of the medication in the **Dose** field.
13. Document a Start Date for the medication in the **Start Date** field.
14. Indicate if a medication is current using the **Active** radio button, or if a patient has stopped taking the medication, using the **Discontinued** radio button.
15. Continue to document the rest of the medications and click the **Save** button.

13. Document an Out-of-Office Order

1. Click the **Find Patient** icon.
2. Using the Patient Search fields, locate the correct patient record. Once you locate the correct patient in the List of Patients, confirm the date of birth to ensure you have located the correct patient record.
3. Select the radio button next to the patient name and click the **Select** button. Confirm the auto-populated details and provide any additional details needed. Create a new encounter or select an existing encounter to begin documenting.
4. Select **Order Entry** from the **Record** dropdown menu.
5. Click the **Add** button below the Out-of-Office table to add an order.
6. Select the correct procedure from the **Order** dropdown and document any additional information needed. Fields vary based on the ordered procedure selected.
7. Click the **Save** button.

14. Prepare a Medication Prescription

If a patient calls for a medication refill, create a phone encounter. Refer to *Create a Phone Encounter* for more information.

1. Click the **Find Patient** icon. Using the Patient Search fields, locate the correct patient record. Once you locate the correct patient in the List of Patients, confirm the date of birth to ensure you have located the correct patient record.
2. Select the radio button next to the patient name and click the **Select** button. Confirm the auto-populated details and provide any additional details needed. Create a new encounter or select an existing encounter to begin documenting.
3. Select **Order Entry** from the **Record** dropdown menu and click the **Add** button below the Out-of-Office table to add an order.
4. Select **Medication Prescription** from the **Order** dropdown.
5. Document the disease the medication is treating in the **Diagnosis** field.
6. Document the complete name of the drug in the **Drug** field. Check the **Refill** checkbox if needed and provide the refill details.
7. Document the amount of the medication in the **Dose** field, the structure when consumed (e.g., "tablet") in the **Form** field, and how the medication is consumed (e.g., "oral") in the **Route** field.
8. Document physician directions to be printed on the label in the **Directions** field.
9. Document the amount of the medication in the **Quantity** field.
10. Document the timespan the medication should be taken (e.g., "10 days") in the **Days Supply** field.
11. Select the issue method using the **Electronic transfer** and **Paper** radio buttons.
12. Provide any additional information needed and click the **Save** button. Only a credentialed medical assistant can send the medication order.
13. Use the icons in the Action column to edit or delete documentation. To print, click the edit icon in the Action column of the order and click the **Print** button.

15. Order a Requisition

1. Click the **Find Patient** icon.
2. Using the Patient Search fields, locate the correct patient record. Once you locate the correct patient in the List of Patients, confirm the date of birth to ensure you have located the correct patient record.
3. Select the radio button next to the patient name and click the **Select** button. Confirm the auto-populated details and provide any additional details needed. Create a new encounter or select an existing encounter to begin documenting.
4. Select **Order Entry** from the **Record** dropdown menu and click the **Add** button below the Out-of-Office table to add an order.
5. Select **Requisition** from the **Order** dropdown. Select the correct department from the **Requisition Type** field and complete any additional fields needed.
6. Click the **Save** button. Use the icons in the Action column to edit or delete your documentation.
7. Select the correct requisition type in the **Requisition** form of the Front Office **Form Repository**, then select the requisition from the **Requisition Type** dropdown menu. Click the **Patient Search** button and select the correct patient to auto-populate patient demographic information and save the form to the patient record.
8. Place the cursor in the **Diagnosis Code** field and click **TruCode** to access the encoder. The selected code will auto-populate where the cursor is placed in the simulation.
9. Enter the search terms in the Search field and select the source (**Diagnosis, ICD-10-CM**) from the dropdown menu. Click the **Search** button.
10. Click the code that appears in red next to the desired search result to expand this code and confirm that this is the most specific code available (Figure 1-17). Click the code that appears in the tree for the desired search result (Figure 1-18). This code will auto-populate in the **Diagnosis Code** field.
11. Complete any additional fields needed and click the **Save to Patient Record** button. The saved form will appear in the Forms section of the Patient Dashboard for reference and printing.

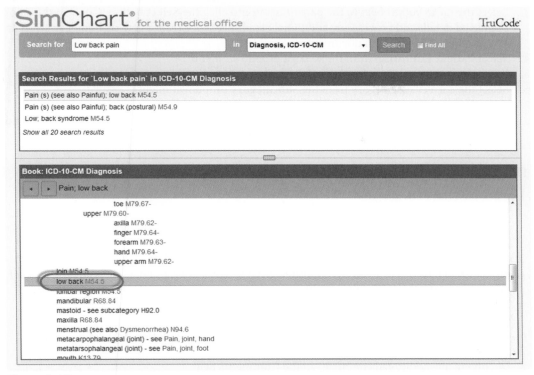

Figure 1-17 Select the most specific code possible.

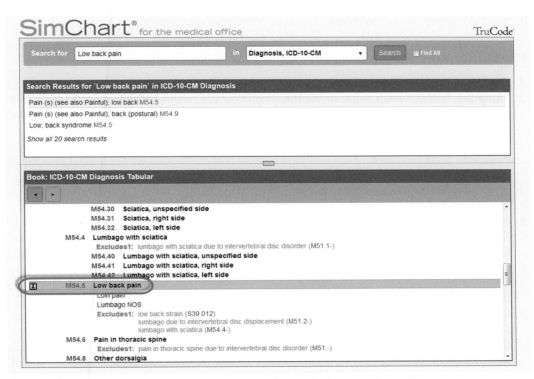

Figure 1-18 Click the code that appears in the tree for the desired search result.

16. Document Patient Education

1. Click the **Find Patient** icon.
2. Using the Patient Search fields, locate the correct patient record. Once you locate the correct patient in the List of Patients, confirm the date of birth to ensure you have located the correct patient record.

3. Select the radio button next to the patient name and click the **Select** button. Confirm the auto-populated details and provide any additional details needed. Create a new encounter or select an existing encounter to begin documenting.
4. Select **Patient Education** from the **Record** dropdown menu.
5. Select the correct category from the **Category** dropdown menu.
6. Select the correct subcategory from the **Subcategory** dropdown menu.
7. Select the teaching topic checkbox in the **Teaching Topics** field.
8. Click the **Save** button. This teaching topic will move from the **New** tab to the **Saved** tab. Expand the accordion of the saved patient education category to view and print the handout.

17. Document Preventative Services

1. Click the **Find Patient** icon.
2. Using the Patient Search fields, locate the correct patient record. Once you locate the correct patient in the List of Patients, confirm the date of birth to ensure you have located the correct patient record.
3. Select the radio button next to the patient name and click the **Select** button. Confirm the auto-populated details and provide any additional details needed. Create a new encounter or select an existing encounter to begin documenting.
4. Select **Preventative Services** from the **Record** dropdown menu.
5. Click the **Add** button below the grid of the correct category.
6. Select the correct recommendation from the **Health Recommendation** dropdown menu.
7. Document the date using the calendar picker.
8. Document any additional comments in the **Comments** field.
9. Click the **Save** button. The preventative service you added will display in the Preventative Services table.
10. Use the icons in the Action column to edit or delete your documentation.

18. Document Problem List

1. Click the **Find Patient** icon.
2. Using the Patient Search fields, locate the correct patient record. Once you locate the correct patient in the List of Patients, confirm the date of birth to ensure you have located the correct patient record.
3. Select the radio button next to the patient name and click the **Select** button. Confirm the auto-populated details and provide any additional details needed. Create a new encounter or select an existing encounter to begin documenting.
4. Select **Problem List** from the **Record** dropdown menu.
5. Click the **Add** button to add the correct problem as specified by the assignment.
6. In the Add Problem window, document the correct diagnosis in the **Diagnosis** field.
7. Select the ICD-10 radio button. Place the cursor in the corresponding text field and click **Tru-Code** to access the encoder. The selected code will auto-populate where the cursor is placed in the simulation.
8. Enter the search terms in the Search field and select the source (**Diagnosis, ICD-10-CM**) from the dropdown menu. Click the **Search** button.
9. Click the code that appears in red next to the desired search result to expand this code and confirm that this is the most specific code available (see Figure 1-17).
10. Click the code that appears in the tree for the desired search result (see Figure 1-18). This code will auto-populate in the Add Problem window. Review the *Using the Encoder* resource for additional information regarding the encoder.
11. Document the correct date in the Date Identified field.
12. Select the **Active** radio button in the Status field.
13. Click the **Save** button. The Problem List table will display the new problem.
14. Use the icons in the Action column to edit or delete your documentation.

19. Document Progress Notes

1. Click the **Find Patient** icon.
2. Using the Patient Search fields, locate the correct patient record. Once you locate the correct patient in the List of Patients, confirm the date of birth to ensure you have located the correct patient record.
3. Select the radio button next to the patient name and click the **Select** button. Confirm the auto-populated details and provide any additional details needed. Create a new encounter or select an existing encounter to begin documenting.
4. Select **Progress Note** from the **Record** dropdown menu.
5. Document the encounter date in the **Date of Service** field.
6. Document how the patient describes his or her symptoms in the **Subjective** field.
7. The physician completes documentation in the **Objective** field based on observations and completes documentation in the Assessment field based on the data provided in the Subjective and Objective fields. The physician then documents strategies for addressing the patient's symptoms in the Plan field and the effectiveness of the Plan in the Evaluation field.
8. Click the **Save** button.
9. Print the Progress Note by clicking the print icon in the top right corner.

20. Document Vital Signs

1. Click the **Find Patient** icon.
2. Using the Patient Search fields, locate the correct patient record. Once you locate the correct patient in the List of Patients, confirm the date of birth to ensure you have located the correct patient record.
3. Select the radio button next to the patient name and click the **Select** button. Confirm the auto-populated details and provide any additional details needed. Create a new encounter or select an existing encounter to begin documenting.
4. Select **Vital Signs** from the **Record** dropdown menu. Note the two tabs on the top of the screen: Vital Signs and Height/Weight. It is important to document in both tabs.
5. In the **Vital Signs** tab, click the **Add** button to document the patient's vital signs. The Position field below the Blood Pressure heading refers to the position of the patient.
6. Click the **Save** button. The table will display the vital signs documented.
7. In the **Height/Weight** tab, click the Add button to document height and weight.
8. Click the **Save** button. The table will display the height and weight documented.
9. Use the icons in the Action column to edit or delete your documentation.

21. Complete a Superbill

1. Click the **Find Patient** icon.
2. Using the Patient Search fields, locate the correct patient record. Once you locate the correct patient in the List of Patients, confirm the date of birth to ensure you have located the correct patient record.
3. After reviewing the patient encounter, click the **Superbill** link below the Patient Header. Select the correct encounter from the Encounters Not Coded table and confirm the auto-populated details. The View Progress Notes and View Fee Schedule links in the top right corner of the Superbill provide information necessary in completing the Superbill.
4. On page 1, select the ICD-9 or ICD-10 radio button (as specified by the instructor or assignment) and document the code.
5. Place the cursor in the Rank 1 **Diagnosis** field and click **TruCode** to access the encoder.
6. Enter the search terms in the Search field and select the source (**Diagnosis, ICD-10-CM**) from the dropdown menu. Click the **Search** button.
7. Click the code that appears in red next to the desired search result to expand this code and confirm it is the most specific code available (see Figure 1-17). Click the code that appears in the tree for the desired search result (see Figure 1-18). This code will auto-populate in the Diagnosis field and you can then document the associated diagnosis. Review the *Using the Encoder* resource for additional information regarding the encoder.

8. Document "1" in the Rank column for the correct service with the corresponding ICD-10 code. Follow the steps outlined above to complete coding. Click the **Save** button. Then, click the **Next** button to progress through the Superbill.

9. On Page 4, document the copayment amount in the **Copay** field. The charges for today's visit will autopoulate in the **Today's Charges** field. Document the amount the patient owes in the Balance **Due field**.

10. Document any additional information needed and click the **Save** button.

11. Select the "I am ready to submit the Superbill" checkbox at the bottom of the screen. Select the **Yes** radio button to indicate that the signature is on file. Document the correct date in the Date field and click the **Submit Superbill** button.

22. Submit a Claim

1. Select **Claim** from the left Info Panel and perform a patient search to locate the claim.

2. Select the correct encounter and click the Edit button in the Action column. Confirm the auto-populated details. Seven tabs appear: Patient Info, Provider Info, Payer Info, Encounter Notes, Claim Info, Charge Capture, and Submission. Certain patient demographic and encounter information is auto-populated in the claim.

3. Review any auto-populated information in the **Patient Info**, **Provider Info**, and **Payer Info** tabs. Document any additional information needed and click the **Save** button.

4. Click the **Encounter Notes** tab. Review the auto-populated information and document additional information needed. Select the **Yes** radio button to indicate the HIPAA form is on file and provide the date. Document any additional information needed and click the **Save** button.

5. Click the **Claim Info** tab. Review the auto-populated information and document any additional information needed. Click the **Save** button.

6. Click the **Charge Capture** tab. Document the encounter date in the **DOS From** and **DOS To** columns. Place the cursor in the **CPT/HCPCS** column field and click **TruCode** to access the encoder. Enter the search terms in the Search field and select the source from the dropdown menu. Click the **Search** button.

7. Click the code that appears in red next to the desired search result to expand this code and confirm it is the most specific code (see Figure 1-17). Click the code that appears in the tree for the desired search result (see Figure 1-18). This code will auto-populate in the CPT/HCPCS field. Review the *Using the Encoder* resource for additional information regarding the encoder.

8. Document the place of service in the **POS** column. Click on the **Place of Service** link at the top of the screen for reference.

9. Document the diagnosis pointer from the Encounter Notes tab in the **DX** column and any modifiers needed in the **M1**, **M2**, and **M3** columns. Document the correct charge in the **Fee** column. Document the quantity used, if applicable, in the **Units** column. Click **Save**.

10. Click the **Submission** tab. Select the "I am ready to submit the Claim" checkbox. Select the Yes button to indicate the signature is on file and select the date. Click the **Save** button. Click the **Submit Claim** button.

23. Update a Ledger

1. Within the Coding & Billing tab, select **Ledger** from the left Info Panel.

2. Perform a patient search to locate the ledger for the correct guarantor.

3. Select the radio button for the correct patient and click the **Select** button. Confirm the auto-populated details in the header.

4. Select the arrow to the right of the patient's name to expand the ledger.

5. Document the correct date in the **Transaction Date** column using the calendar picker. Document the Date of Service in the **DOS** field.

6. Document the correct provider name using the dropdown in the **Provider** column.

7. Place the cursor in the Service column field and click **TruCode** to access the encoder. The **Service** column can also be used to enter a form of payment if only a payment is made.

8. Enter the search terms in the Search field and select the source (**Diagnosis, ICD-9-CM or Diagnosis, ICD-10-CM**) from the dropdown menu. Click the **Search** button.

9. Click the code that appears in red next to the desired search result to expand this code and confirm it is the most specific code available (see Figure 1-17). Click the code that appears in the tree for the desired search result (see Figure 1-18). This code will auto-populate in the Diagnosis field and you can then document the associated diagnosis. Review the *Using the Encoder* resource for additional information regarding the encoder.
10. Document the total charges in the **Charges** column.
11. Document the amount the patient paid in the **Payment** column.
12. Document the amount paid by insurance in the **Adjustment** column. The balance will auto-populate in the Balance column and the total will auto-populate in the **Total Ledger Balance** field below the table.
13. Click the **Save** button.

24. Complete a Day Sheet

1. Within the Coding & Billing tab, select **Day Sheet** from the left Info Panel.
2. Document the current date in the **Date** column using the calendar picker.
3. Document the correct patient name in the **Patient Name** column.
4. Document the correct provider in the **Provider** column.
5. Place the cursor in the **Service** column field and click **TruCode** to access the encoder. Enter the search terms in the Search field and select the source from the dropdown menu. Click the **Search** button.
6. Click the code that appears in red next to the desired search result to expand this code and confirm it is the most specific code (see Figure 1-17). Click the code that appears in the tree for the desired search result (see Figure 1-18). This code will auto-populate in the Service field. Review the *Using the Encoder* resource for additional information regarding the encoder.
7. Document the total charges in the **Charges** column.
8. Document the amount the patient paid in the **Payment** column.
9. Document the amount of any adjustments in the **Adjustment** column.
10. Document the new balance in the **New Balance** column.
11. Document the old balance in the **Old Balance** column.
12. Click the **Save** button.

Unit 2 | Front Office

Objectives

- Register a patient.
- Search for a patient record.
- Schedule an appointment.
- Prepare patient paperwork.
- Accurately update patient information and demographics.
- Prepare a scheduling matrix according to established guidelines.
- Schedule an appointment and create an appointment reminder letter.
- Compose professional communication for patients and medical assistant staff.
- Access and complete all forms necessary for the front office workflow.
- Complete an Incident Report for a patient-related incident, an employee-related incident, and an emergency.

Module Overview

The Front Office module features the Calendar, which is the most frequently referenced aspect of daily medical office workflow. The Calendar is also the default landing page upon entering the simulation. From here, students must determine where to navigate in order to complete an assignment or exercise. Students can manage patient appointments using the Calendar View; the Exam Room View and Provider View are read-only.

The Form Repository, accessed by clicking the Form Repository icon at the top of the screen, contains frequently used patient and office forms. Although most forms are electronic, some forms such as the Inventory form and the Advance Directive must be printed and completed by hand in order to demonstrate office workflow. For example, a medical assistant would give an Advance Directive to a patient for them to fill out by hand. The medical assistant would then upload the completed form to the patient record.

Additionally, students can create patient and office communication using letter and email templates in Correspondence, accessed by clicking the Correspondence icon at the top of the screen.

 HELPFUL HINT

Select the desired correspondence or form template and then perform a patient search to assign the document to a patient and auto-populate demographic information. These documents can be printed and/or saved to a patient record.

See the following pages for assignments related to the Front Office module.

1. Schedule Appointment for Talibah Nasser

▪ Objectives

- Search for a patient record.
- Schedule an appointment.

▪ Overview

Talibah Nasser is calling the Walden-Martin office to request a post-operative follow-up appointment with Jean Burke, NP in approximately two weeks. She recently had a laparoscopic cholecystectomy and states that she is doing fine. Tuesday afternoons work well for her and the appointment should last 30 minutes.

▪ Competencies

- Display sensitivity when managing appointments, CAAHEP VI.A-1, ABHES 5-h, 7-e, 10-b
- Identify different types of appointment scheduling methods, CAAHEP VI.C-1, ABHES 7-e
- Manage appointment schedule, using established priorities, CAAHEP VI.P-1, ABHES 7-e

Estimated completion time: 20 minutes

Measurable Steps

1. Within the Calendar of the Front Office module, click the Add Appointment button or anywhere within the calendar to open the New Appointment window (Figure 2-1).

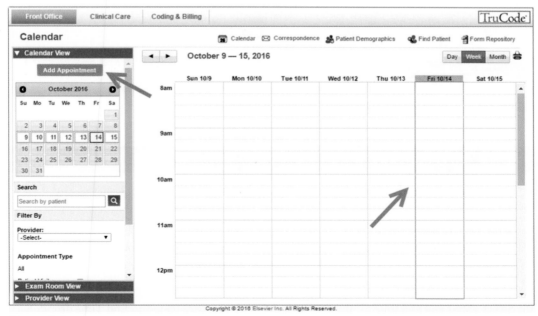

Figure 2-1 Add Appointment.

2. Select the Patient Visit radio button as the Appointment Type.
3. Select Follow-Up/Established Visit from the Visit Type dropdown.
4. Document "Cholecystectomy follow-up" in the Chief Complaint text box.
5. Select the Search Existing Patients radio button.
6. Using the Patient Search fields, search for Talibah Nasser's patient record. Once you locate Talibah Nasser in the List of Patients, confirm her date of birth (Figure 2-2).

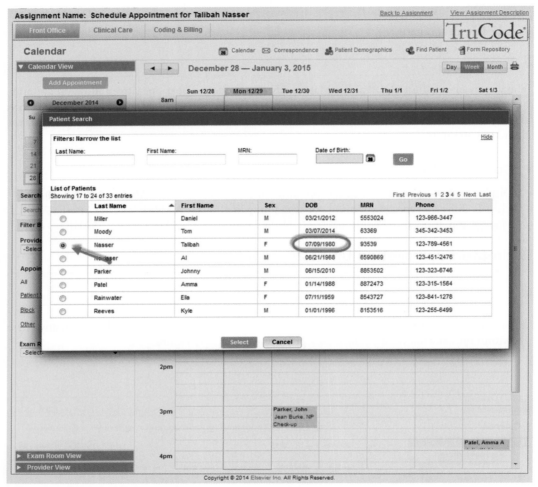

Figure 2-2 Using the Patient Search fields to find Talibah Nasser.

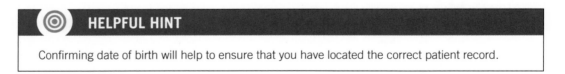

> **HELPFUL HINT**
>
> Confirming date of birth will help to ensure that you have located the correct patient record.

7. Select the radio button for Talibah Nasser and click the Select button. Confirm the auto-populated details.
8. Confirm that Jean Burke, NP is selected as the Provider in the Provider dropdown.
9. Use the calendar picker to confirm or select the appointment day.
10. Select a start and end time for the appointment using the Start Time and End Time dropdowns.
11. Click the Save button.
12. Talibah Nasser's appointment will appear on the calendar (Figure 2-3).

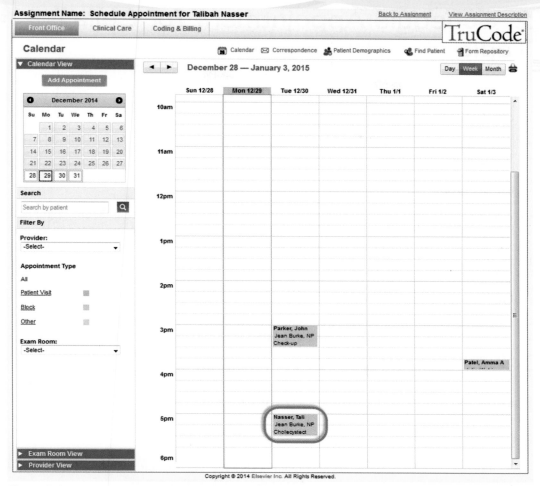

Figure 2-3 Talibah Nasser's appointment in the calendar.

⭐ Now use the Back to Assignment link to complete the Post-Case Quiz found on the Info Panel for this assignment!

2. Schedule Appointment for Celia Tapia

■ Objectives

- Search for a patient record.
- Schedule an appointment.

■ Overview

Celia Tapia would like to schedule an appointment with Dr. Martin. She thinks she might have a bladder infection because she feels like she has to urinate constantly and experiences pain during urination. Dr. Martin has an opening at 1:15 pm today. Schedule the urgent appointment for 30 minutes.

■ Competencies

- Display sensitivity when managing appointments, CAAHEP VI.A-1, ABHES 5-h, 10-b
- Identify different types of appointment scheduling methods, CAAHEP VI.C-1, ABHES 7-e
- Manage appointment schedule, using established priorities, CAAHEP VI.P-1, ABHES 7-e
- Measure and record vital signs, CAAHEP I.P-1, ABHES 8-b

Estimated completion time: 20 minutes

Measurable Steps

1. Within the Calendar of the Front Office module, click the Add Appointment button or anywhere within the calendar to open the New Appointment window (Figure 2-4).

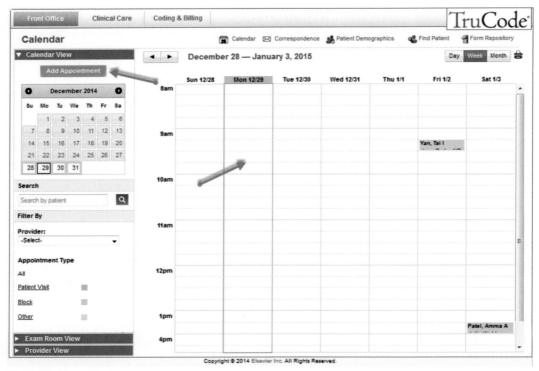

Figure 2-4 Add Appointment.

2. Select the Patient Visit radio button as the Appointment Type.
3. Select Urgent Visit from the Visit Type dropdown.
4. Document "Dysuria, urinary frequency" in the Chief Complaint text box.
5. Select the Search Existing Patients radio button.
6. Using the Patient Search fields, search for Celia Tapia's patient record. Once you locate Celia Tapia in the List of Patients, confirm her date of birth (Figure 2-5).

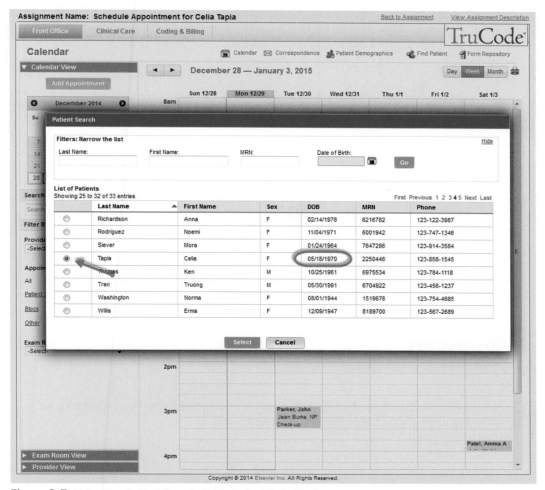

Figure 2-5 Using the Patient Search fields to find Celia Tapia.

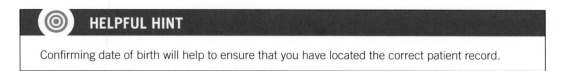

HELPFUL HINT

Confirming date of birth will help to ensure that you have located the correct patient record.

7. Select the radio button for Celia Tapia and click the Select button. Confirm the auto-populated details.
8. Confirm that James A. Martin, MD is selected as the Provider in the Provider dropdown.
9. Use the calendar picker to confirm or select the appointment day.
10. Select a start and end time for the appointment using the Start Time and End Time dropdowns.
11. Click the Save button.
12. Celia Tapia's appointment will appear on the calendar (Figure 2-6).

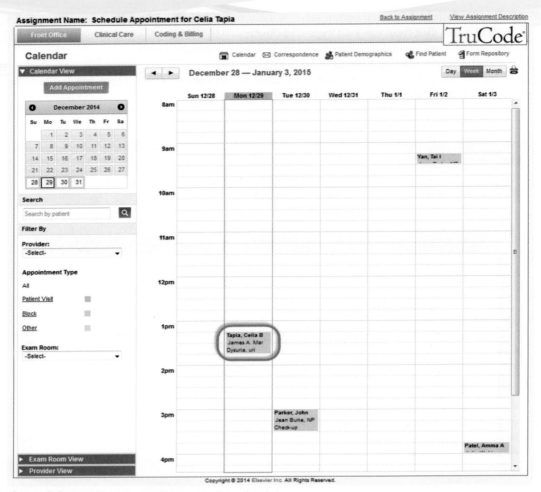

Figure 2-6 Celia Tapia's appointment in the calendar.

Now use the Back to Assignment link to complete the Post-Case Quiz found on the Info Panel for this assignment!

3. Prepare Scheduling Matrix

■ Objectives

- Prepare a scheduling matrix according to established guidelines.

■ Overview

The Walden-Martin medical office just implemented an electronic health record system with a scheduling feature. Dr. Walden would like to block time every day for a 30-minute lunch break at 11:30 am. Dr. Martin would like to block time every day for a 30-minute lunch break at 12:00 pm and rounds from 8:00 am to 9:00 am. Jean Burke, NP would like to block time every day for a 30-minute lunch break at 12:30 pm and next Wednesday for an out-of-office meeting from 2:00 pm to 4:00 pm. Block the schedule for lunch breaks, rounds, and meetings for the next month.

■ Competencies

- Display sensitivity when managing appointments, CAAHEP VI.A-1, ABHES 5-h, 10-b
- Identify different types of appointment scheduling methods, CAAHEP VI.C-1, ABHES 7-e
- Discuss applications of electronic technology in professional communication, CAAHEP V.C-8, ABHES 7-b, 7-g, 7-h
- Utilize an EMR, CAAHEP VI.P-6, ABHES 7-b
- Manage appointment schedule, using established priorities, CAAHEP VI.P-1, ABHES 7-e

Estimated completion time: 25 minutes

Measurable Steps

1. Within the Calendar of the Front Office module, click the Add Appointment button or anywhere within the calendar to open the New Appointment window (Figure 2-7).

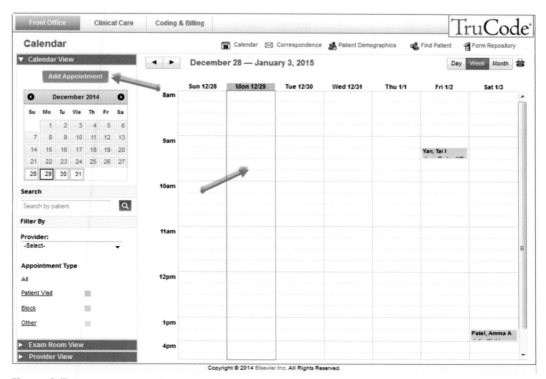

Figure 2-7 Add Appointment.

2. Select the Block radio button as the Appointment Type.
3. Select Lunch from the Block Type dropdown.
4. Select Julie Walden, MD from the For dropdown.
5. Using the calendar picker, select a date.
6. Select 11:30 AM from the Start Time dropdown.
7. Select 12:00 PM from the End Time dropdown.
8. Check the Recurrence checkbox.
9. Check the Daily radio button in the Recurrence Pattern field.
10. Check the End By radio button in the Recurrence Duration field and use the calendar picker to select an end date (Figure 2-8).

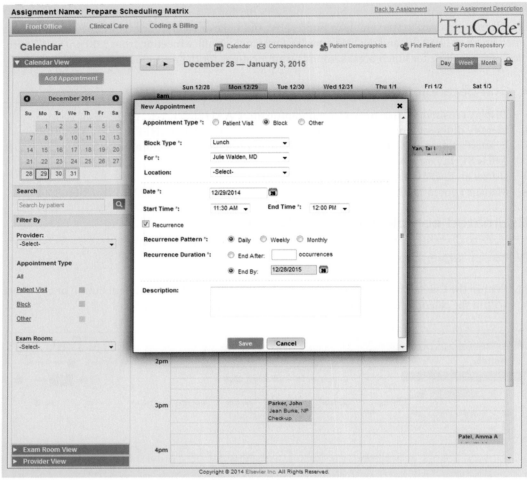

Figure 2-8 Use the calendar picker to select an end date.

11. Click the Save button.
12. The calendar will display Dr. Walden's lunch break.
13. Click the Add Appointment button or anywhere within the calendar to open the New Appointment window. Select the Block radio button as the Appointment Type.
14. Select Other from the Block Type dropdown and document "Rounds" in the Other field.
15. Select James A. Martin, MD from the For dropdown.
16. Using the calendar picker, select a date.
17. Select 8:00 AM from the Start Time dropdown.
18. Select 9:00 AM from the End Time dropdown.
19. Check the Recurrence checkbox.

20. Check the Daily radio button in the Recurrence Pattern field.
21. Check the End By radio button in the Recurrence Duration field and use the calendar picker to select an end date.
22. Click the Save button. The calendar will display Dr. Martin's blocked time.
23. Click the Add Appointment button or anywhere within the calendar to open the New Appointment window. Select the Block radio button as the Appointment Type.
24. Select Lunch from the Block Type dropdown.
25. Select James A. Martin, MD from the For dropdown.
26. Using the calendar picker, select a date.
27. Select 12:00 PM from the Start Time dropdown.
28. Select 12:30 PM from the End Time dropdown.
29. Check the Recurrence checkbox.
30. Check the Daily radio button in the Recurrence Pattern field.
31. Check the End By radio button in the Recurrence Duration field and use the calendar picker to select an end date.
32. Click the Save button.
33. The calendar will display Dr. Martin's lunch break.
34. Click the Add Appointment button or anywhere within the calendar to open the New Appointment window.
35. Select the Block radio button as the Appointment Type.
36. Select Lunch from the Block Type dropdown.
37. Select Jean Burke, NP from the For dropdown.
38. Using the calendar picker, select a date.
39. Select 12:30 PM from the Start Time dropdown.
40. Select 1:00 PM from the End Time dropdown.
41. Check the Recurrence checkbox.
42. Check the Daily radio button in the Recurrence Pattern field.
43. Check the End By radio button in the Recurrence Duration field and use the calendar picker to select an end date.
44. Click the Save button.
45. The calendar will display Jean Burke's lunch break.
46. Click the Add Appointment button or anywhere within the calendar to open the New Appointment window.
47. Select the Block radio button as the Appointment Type.
48. Select Out-of-office from the Block Type.
49. Select Jean Burke, NP from the For dropdown.
50. Using the calendar picker, select next Wednesday as the date.
51. Select 2:00 PM from the Start Time dropdown.
52. Select 4:00 PM from the End Time dropdown.
53. Click the Save button.
54. The calendar will display Jean Burke's blocked time (Figure 2-9).

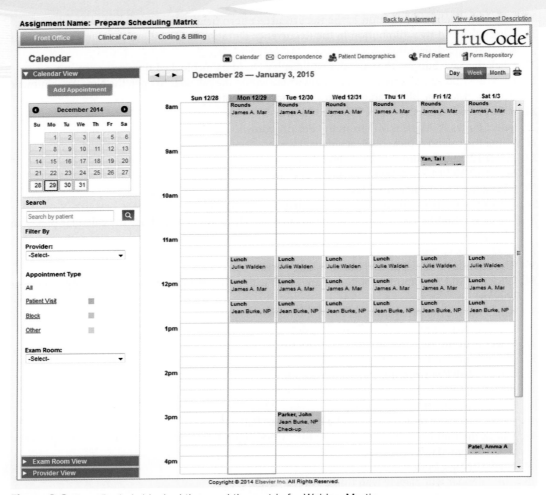

Figure 2-9 Jean Burke's blocked time and the matrix for Walden-Martin.

⭐ Now use the Back to Assignment link to complete the Post-Case Quiz found on the Info Panel for this assignment!

4. Schedule Appointment and Prepare Appointment Reminder Letter for Amma Patel

■ Objectives

- Search for a patient record.
- Create an Appointment Reminder letter.
- Compose professional communication.

■ Overview

Amma Patel is calling the Walden-Martin office to schedule a post-operative follow-up appointment with Dr. Walden in 3 weeks. Thursday mornings work well for her and the appointment should last 30 minutes. It is Walden-Martin policy to send appointment reminder letters to patients. Schedule the appointment and prepare an Appointment Reminder letter for Amma Patel.

■ Competencies

- Compose professional correspondence utilizing electronic technology, CAAHEP V.P-8, ABHES 7-g, 7-h
- Utilize Electronic Medical Records (EMR) and Practice Management Systems, CAAHEP VI.P-6, ABHES 7-b
- Input patient data utilizing a practice management system, CAAHEP VI.P-7
- Protect the integrity of the medical record, CAAHEP X.A-2

Estimated completion time: 20 minutes

Measurable Steps

1. Within the Calendar of the Front Office module, click the Add Appointment button or anywhere within the calendar to open the New Appointment window.
2. Select the Patient Visit radio button as the Appointment Type.
3. Select Follow-up/Established from the Visit Type dropdown.
4. Document "post-operative follow-up" in the Chief Complaint text box.
5. Select the Search Existing Patients radio button.
6. Using the Patient Search fields, search for Amma Patel's patient record. Once you locate Amma Patel in the List of Patients, confirm her date of birth.
7. Select the radio button for Amma Patel and click the Select button. Confirm the auto-populated details.
8. Confirm that Julie Walden, MD is selected as the Provider in the Provider dropdown.
9. Use the calendar picker to confirm or select the appointment day.
10. Select a start and end time for the appointment using the Start Time and End Time dropdowns.
11. Click the Save button.
12. Amma Patel's appointment will appear on the calendar.

13. Click on the Correspondence icon (Figure 2-10).

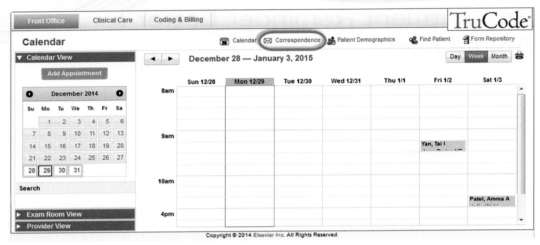

Figure 2-10 Correspondence icon.

14. Select the Appointment Reminder template from the Letters section of the left Info Panel.
15. Click the Patient Search button to perform a patient search and assign the letter to Amma Patel (Figure 2-11).

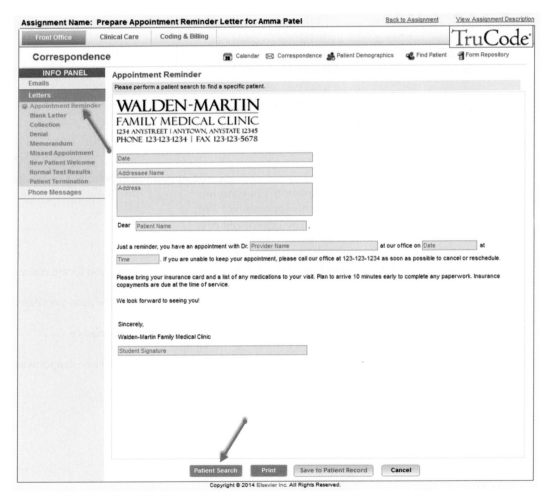

Figure 2-11 Using the Patient Search fields to find Amma Patel.

16. Confirm the auto-populated details. Select the upcoming appointment from the Select Appointments column on the left. Document any additional information needed.
17. Click the Save to Patient Record button.
18. In the Date Selection box, select today's date. Click the OK button.
19. Click on the Find Patient icon.
20. Using the Patient Search fields, search for Amma Patel's patient record. Once you locate her in the List of Patients, confirm her date of birth.

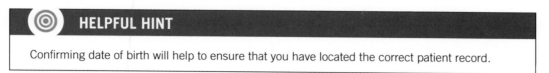

HELPFUL HINT

Confirming date of birth will help to ensure that you have located the correct patient record.

21. Select the radio button for Amma Patel and click the Select button. Confirm the auto-populated details.
22. Scroll down to view the Correspondence section of the Patient Dashboard (Figure 2-12).

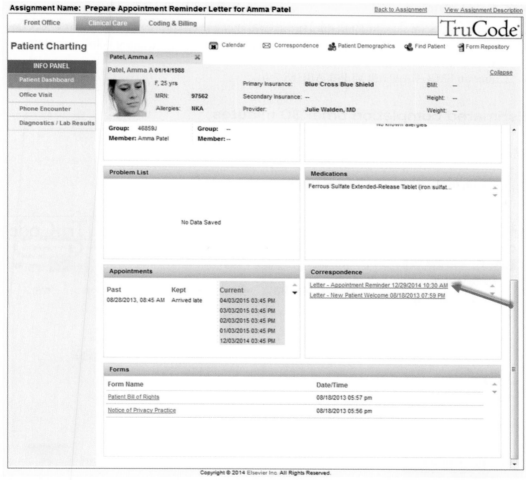

Figure 2-12 The Correspondence section of the Patient Dashboard.

23. Select the letter you prepared. The letter will open in a new window, allowing you to print.

✦ Now use the Back to Assignment link to complete the Post-Case Quiz found on the Info Panel for this assignment!

5. Prepare Certificate to Return to Work for Diego Lupez

■ Objectives

- Search for a patient record.
- Access patient forms.
- Update patient information using the correct form.

■ Overview

Diego Lupez stepped on a nail at work one week ago and has now been cleared to return to work without restrictions. Prepare a Certificate to Return to Work form for Diego Lupez. Assume the signature of the physician is on file.

■ Competencies

- Identify information required to file a third party claim, CAAHEP VIII.C-1b, ABHES 7-a, 7-d
- Describe components of the Health Information Portability & Accountability Act (HIPAA), CAAHEP X.C-3, ABHES 4-h
- Utilize an EMR, CAAHEP VI.P-6, ABHES 7-b

Estimated completion time: 30 minutes

Measurable Steps

1. Click on the Form Repository icon (Figure 2-13).

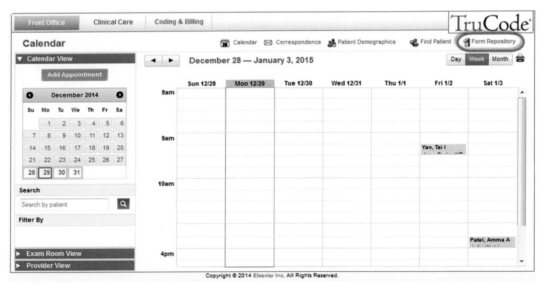

Figure 2-13 Form Repository icon.

2. Select Certificate to Return to Work or School from the Patient Forms section of the left Info Panel (Figure 2-14).
3. Click the Patient Search button to perform a patient search and assign the form to Diego Lupez.

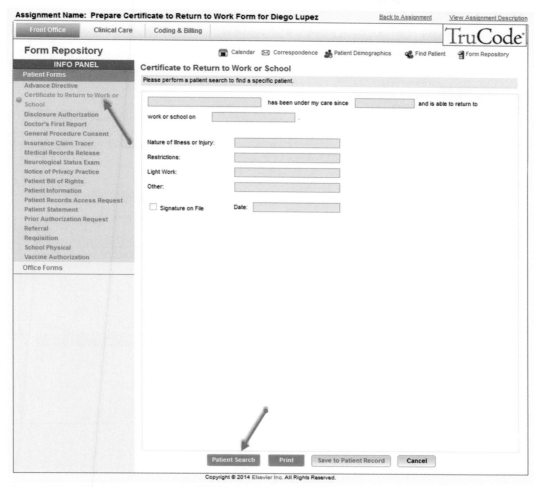

Figure 2-14 Perform a patient search to assign the form to Diego Lupez.

4. Confirm the auto-populated details and document any additional information needed (including clicking the box for Signature on File).
5. Click the Save to Patient Record button. In the Date Selection box, select today's date. Click the OK button.
6. Click on the Find Patient icon.
7. Using the Patient Search fields, search for Diego Lupez's patient record. Once you locate him in the List of Patients, confirm his date of birth.

8. Select the radio button for Diego Lupez and click the Select button. Confirm the auto-populated details.
9. Scroll down to view the Forms section of the Patient Dashboard (Figure 2-15).
10. Select the form you prepared. The form will open in a new window, allowing you to print.

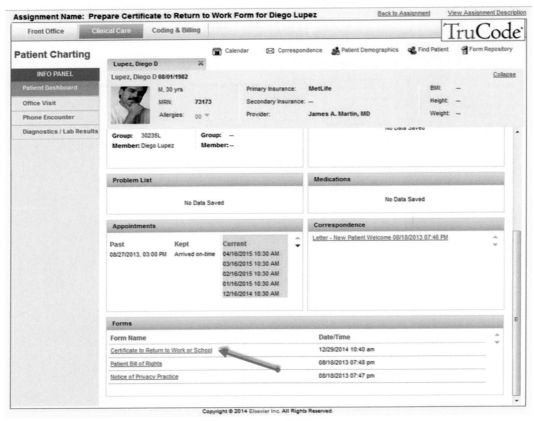

Figure 2-15 The Forms section of the Patient Dashboard.

⭐ Now use the Back to Assignment link to complete the Post-Case Quiz found on the Info Panel for this assignment!

6. Prepare Medical Records Release Form for Daniel Miller

■ **Objectives**

- Search for a patient record.
- Access patient forms.
- Update patient information using the correct form.

■ **Overview**

Daniel Miller will be attending a new daycare that requires copies of immunization records before his first day. Daniel's mother, Tracy Miller, stopped by the office to request these records. Prepare a Medical Records Release form with an expiration of one year to Laura Wasser's attention at the following address:

Tiny Tots Watch
4531 Anystreet
Anytown, AL 12345

■ **Competencies**

- Apply HIPAA rules in regard to privacy and the release of information, CAAHEP X.P-2, ABHES 4-h
- Apply the Patient's Bill of Rights as it relates to choice of treatment, consent for treatment, and refusal of treatment, CAAHEP X.P-4, ABHES 4-b, 4-g
- Demonstrate sensitivity to patient rights, CAAHEP X.A-1, ABHES 4-g, 5-h, 10-b
- Describe components of the Health Information Portability & Accountability Act (HIPAA), CAAHEP X.C-3, ABHES 4-h
- Measure and record vital signs, CAAHEP I.P-1, ABHES 8-b
- Protect the integrity of the medical record, CAAHEP X.A-2, ABHES 4-a
- Utilize an EMR, CAAHEP VI.P-6, ABHES 7-b

Estimated completion time: 25 minutes

Measurable Steps

1. Click on the Form Repository icon (Figure 2-16).
2. Select Medical Records Release from the Patient Forms section of the left Info Panel (Figure 2-17).
3. Click the Patient Search button to perform a patient search and assign the form to Daniel Miller.

 HELPFUL HINT

Performing a patient search before completing a form helps to ensure accurate documentation.

4. Confirm the auto-populated details and document any additional information needed.
5. Click the Save to Patient Record button.
6. In the Date Selection box, select today's date. Click the OK button.
7. Click on the Find Patient icon.

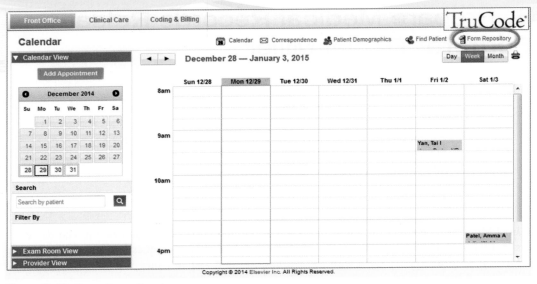

Figure 2-16 Form Repository icon.

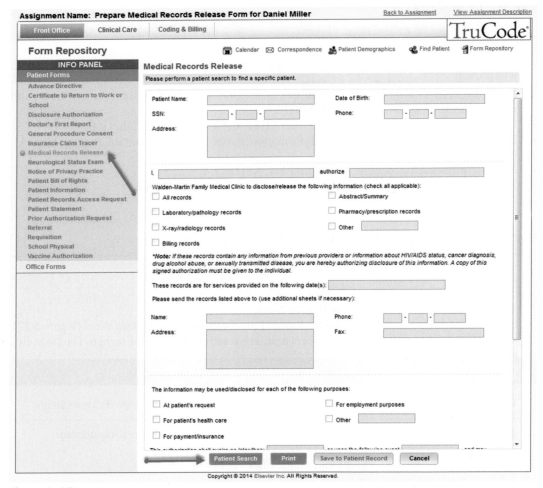

Figure 2-17 Medical Records Release from the Patient Forms section of the Info Panel.

8. Using the Patient Search fields, search for Daniel's patient record. Once you locate Daniel in the List of Patients, confirm his date of birth.

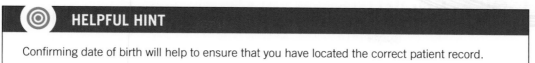

HELPFUL HINT

Confirming date of birth will help to ensure that you have located the correct patient record.

9. Select the radio button for Daniel Miller and click the Select button. Confirm the auto-populated details.
10. Scroll down to view the Forms section of the Patient Dashboard (Figure 2-18).

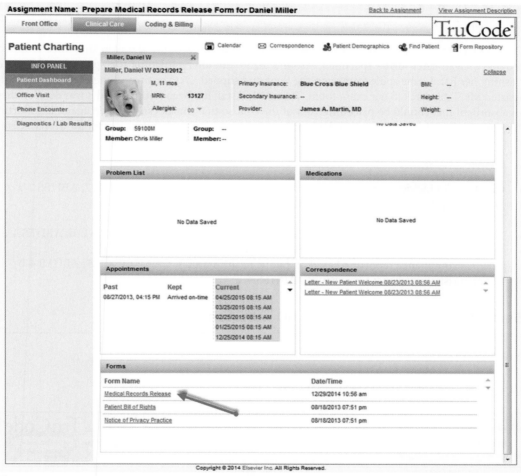

Figure 2-18 The Forms section of the Patient Dashboard.

11. Select the form you prepared. The form will open in a new window, allowing you to obtain the signature of Daniel's guardian on the printed form.

> Now use the Back to Assignment link to complete the Post-Case Quiz found on the Info Panel for this assignment!

7. Complete Incident Report for Celia Tapia

■ **Objectives**

- Search for a patient record.
- Access office forms.
- Complete an Incident Report for a patient-related incident.
- Access a saved Incident Report.

■ **Overview**

Celia Tapia experiences issues with repeated urinary tract infections. She is in the office today to provide a clean catch urine specimen. Around 10:30 am, after providing the specimen and while washing her hands, she spilled water on the floor and slipped. Dr. Martin and the Medical Assistant assisted Ms. Tapia back to her exam room. The medical staff has been notified, and it was decided that an absorbent mat should be placed in front of the sink so that this doesn't happen again. Dr. Martin determined that Ms. Tapia developed minor bruising. Complete an Incident Report for this accident.

■ **Competencies**

- Complete an incident report related to an error in patient care, CAAHEP X.P-7, ABHES 7-a
- Define the principles of standard precautions, CAAHEP III.C-5, ABHES 8-a
- Demonstrate the principles of self-boundaries, CAAHEP V.A-2, ABHES 10-b
- Describe the process in compliance reporting incident reports, CAAHEP X.C-11d, ABHES 4-e
- Identify safety signs, symbols, and labels, CAAHEP XII.C-1, ABHES 4-e
- Perform compliance reporting based on public health statutes, CAAHEP X.P-5, ABHES 4-b
- Perform risk management procedures, ABHES 4-e

Estimated completion time: 40 minutes

Measurable Steps

1. Click on the Form Repository icon (Figure 2-19).

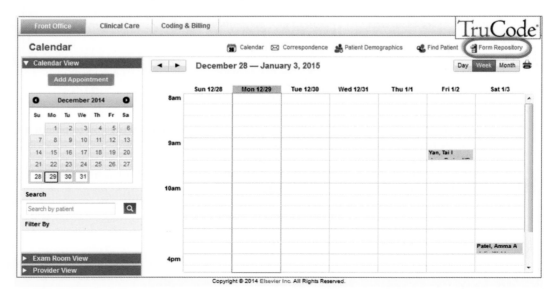

Figure 2-19 Form Repository icon.

2. Select Incident Report from the Office Forms section of the left Info Panel (Figure 2-20).

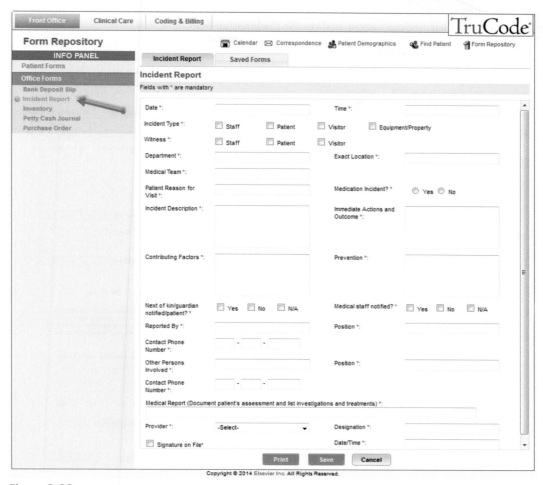

Figure 2-20 Incident Report form.

3. Document the date and time in the date and time fields.
4. Select the Patient checkbox for the Incident Type.
5. Select the Patient checkbox for the Witness.
6. Document "Urology" as the Department.
7. Document "Bathroom" as the Exact Location.
8. Document "physician, medical assistant" as the Medical Team.
9. Document "collection of the specimen" as the Patient Reason for Visit.
10. Select the No radio button to indicate that the incident is not a Medication Incident.
11. Document "Patient slipped and fell because of water spilled on the floor after washing her hands." in the Incident Description field.
12. Document "Physician and medical assistant assisted patient to exam room. Physician determined that there was minor bruising from the fall." in the Immediate Actions and Outcome field.
13. Document "Spilled water on the floor." in the Contributing Factors field.
14. Document "Place absorbent mat in front of the sink." in the Prevention field.
15. Select the No checkbox to indicate that the next of kin/guardian has not been notified.
16. Select the Yes checkbox to indicate that the medical staff has been notified.
17. Document your name in the Reported By field.
18. Document "medical assistant" in the Position field.
19. Document "123-123-1234" in the Contact Phone Number field.
20. Document "Dr. Martin" in the Other Persons Involved.
21. Document "physician" in the Position field.

22. Document "123-123-1234" in the Contact Phone Number field.
23. Document "Minor bruising, no treatment" in the Medical Report field.
24. Select James A. Martin, MD from the Provider dropdown.
25. Document "Self-inflicted, accidental" in the Designation field.
26. Select the Signature on File checkbox and document the date and time in the Date/Time field.
27. Click the Save button.
28. Within the Saved Forms tab, select the Incident Report from the dropdown menu (Figure 2-21).

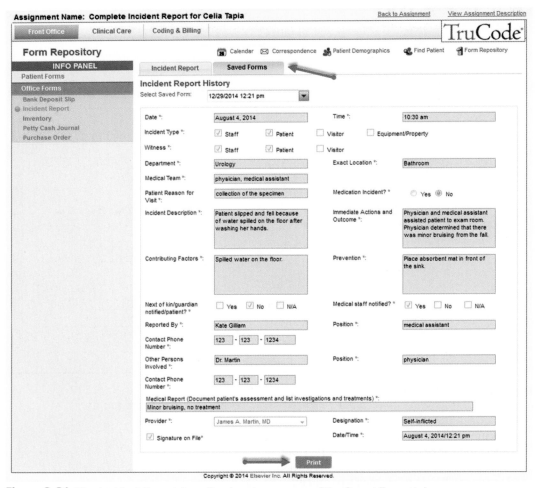

Figure 2-21 The Incident Report from the dropdown menu of the Saved Forms tab.

29. Click the Print button to print the saved Incident Report.

> ⭐ Now use the Back to Assignment link to complete the Post-Case Quiz found on the Info Panel for this assignment!

8. Complete Incident Report for Employee

■ **Objectives**

- Access office forms.
- Complete an incident report for an employee-related incident.
- Access a saved incident report.

■ **Overview**

Around 9:30 am, an employee dropped a bottle of bleach in the laboratory while preparing a 1:10 bleach solution used as a disinfectant, causing it to splash in their face and eyes. After a 15-minute eyewash and basic first aid, Dr. Walden assessed the employee and determined that no additional treatments were needed. The medical staff has been notified. Additional training on the best way to handle chemical bottles will be reviewed with the staff. Complete an incident report for this accident.

■ **Competencies**

- Complete an incident report related to an error in patient care, CAAHEP X.P-7, ABHES 4-a
- Demonstrate the proper use of eyewash equipment, CAAHEP XII.P-2a, ABHES 8-g
- Describe basic principles of first aid as they pertain to the ambulatory healthcare setting, CAAHEP I.C-14, ABHES 8-g
- Describe the process in compliance reporting incident reports, CAAHEP X.C-11d, ABHES 4-e
- Perform compliance reporting based on public health statutes, CAAHEP X.P-5, ABHES 4-b
- Recognize and respond to medical office emergencies, ABHES 8-g
- Recognize the physical and emotional effects on persons involved in an emergency situation, CAAHEP XII.A-1, ABHES 10-b

Estimated completion time: 35 minutes

Measurable Steps

1. Click on the Form Repository icon (Figure 2-22).

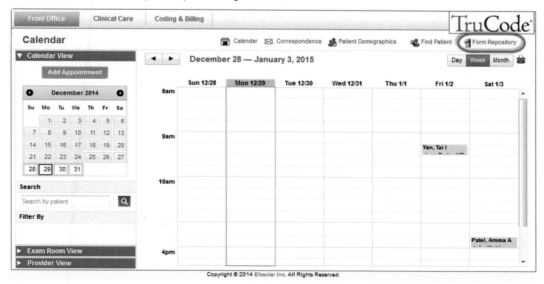

Figure 2-22 Form Repository icon.

2. Select Incident Report from the Office Forms section of the left Info Panel (Figure 2-23).

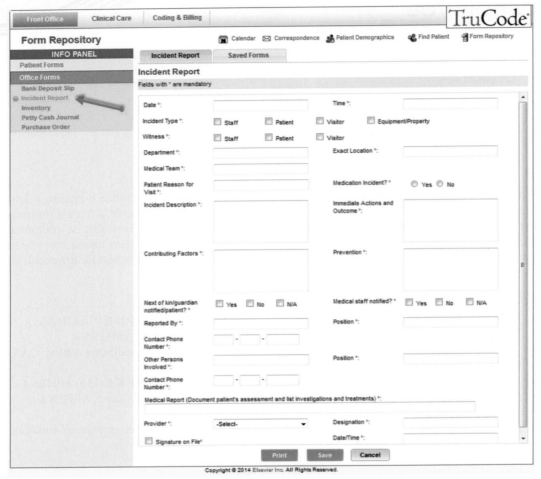

Figure 2-23 Incident Report form.

3. Document the data and time in the Date and Time fields.
4. Select Staff for the Incident Type.
5. Select Staff for the Witness.
6. Document "Laboratory" as the Department and exact location.
7. Document "physician, medical assistant" as the Medical Team.
8. Document "N/A" as the Patient Reason for Visit.
9. Select the No radio button to indicate that the incident is not a Medication Incident.
10. Document "Employee dropped bottle of bleach causing the bleach to splash into their face and eyes." in the Incident Description field.
11. Document "Employee was assisted at the eyewash station and the eyes were flushed with water for 15 minutes." in the Immediate Actions and Outcome field.
12. Document "N/A" in the Contributing Factors field.
13. Document "Employee training on the best way to handle chemical bottles." in the Prevention field.
14. Select the No checkbox to indicate that the next of kin/guardian has not been notified.
15. Select the Yes checkbox to indicate that the medical staff has been notified.
16. Document your name in the Reported By field.
17. Document "medical assistant" in the Position field.
18. Document "123-123-1234" in the Contact Phone Number field.
19. Document "none" in the Other Persons Involved field.
20. Document "N/A" in the Position field.

21. Document "000-000-0000" in the Contact Phone Number field.
22. Document "No additional treatment needed." in the Medical Report field.
23. Select Julie Walden, MD from the Provider dropdown.
24. Document "Self-inflicted, accidental" in the Designation field.
25. Select the Signature on File checkbox.
26. Document the date and time in the Date/Time field and click the Save button.
27. Within the Saved Forms tab, select the Incident Report from the dropdown menu (Figure 2-24).

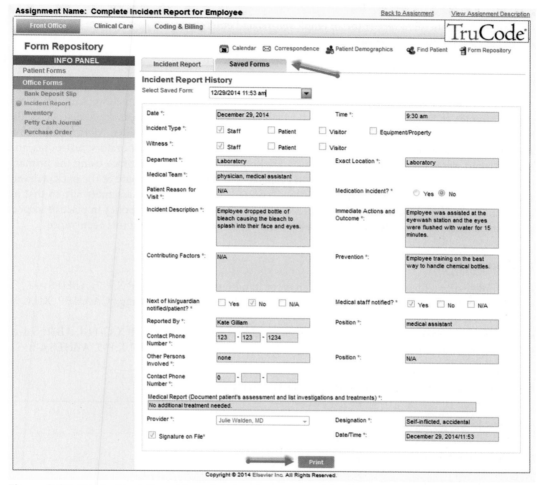

Figure 2-24 The Incident Report from the dropdown menu of the Saved Forms tab.

28. Click the Print button to print the saved Incident Report.

⭐ Now use the Back to Assignment link to complete the Post-Case Quiz found on the Info Panel for this assignment!

9. Complete Incident Report for Medical Office Evacuation

■ Objectives

- Access office forms.
- Complete an incident report for an employee-related emergency.
- Access a saved incident report.

■ Overview

A frayed cord on the coffee maker in the employee break room caused a fire, which went unnoticed for several minutes and started to spread. A medical assistant walking past the break room discovered the fire around 2:00 pm, shut the door to the room, and sounded the alarm. The Walden-Martin staff evacuated the patients following the established evacuation plan. The exam rooms, laboratory, restrooms, and waiting room were checked for patients and staff, who then left the medical office using the primary route of the front stairway and entrance when available and the secondary route of the back stairway and entrance when needed. All staff and visitors reported to the designated assembly site so that all individuals could be accounted for. Dr. Walden decided that there should be a policy in place to inspect all electrical cords on a weekly basis. Complete an incident report to document this occurrence.

■ Competencies

- Complete an incident report related to an error in patient care, CAAHEP X.P-7, ABHES 4-a
- Describe fundamental principles for evacuation of a healthcare setting, CAAHEP XII.C-4, ABHES 8-g
- Describe the process in compliance reporting incident reports, CAAHEP X.C-11d, ABHES 4-e
- Perform compliance reporting based on public health statutes, CAAHEP X.P-5, ABHES 4-b

Estimated completion time: 40 minutes

Measurable Steps

1. Click on the Form Repository icon (Figure 2-25).

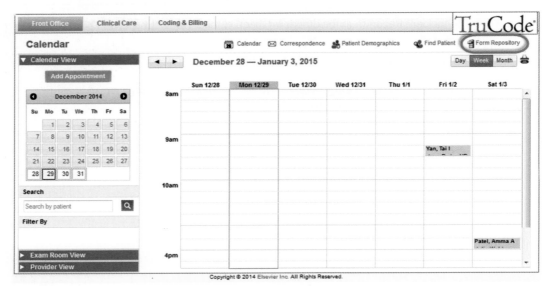

Figure 2-25 Form Repository icon.

2. Select Incident Report from the Office Forms section of the left Info Panel (Figure 2-26).

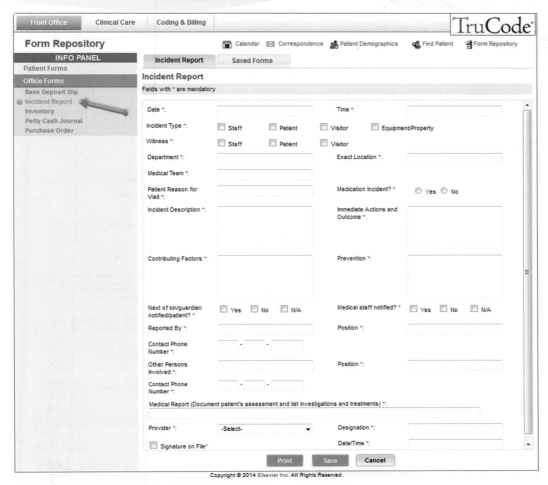

Figure 2-26 Incident Report form.

3. Document the date and time in the Date and Time fields.
4. Select Equipment/Property for the Incident Type.
5. Select Staff for the Witness.
6. Document "Break room" as the Department and Exact Location.
7. Document "Medical assistant" as the Medical Team.
8. Document "N/A" as the Patient Reason for Visit.
9. Select the No radio button to indicate that the incident is not a Medication Incident.
10. Document "Fire discovered in the empty break room." in the Incident Description field.
11. Document "Employee closed the door to the break room, sounded the alarm, and initiated evacuation of patients." in the Immediate Actions and Outcome field.
12. Document "Frayed cord on coffee maker." in the Contributing Factors field.
13. Document "Weekly inspection of all electrical cords in the medical office." in the Prevention field.
14. Select the No checkbox to indicate that the next of kin/guardian has not been notified.
15. Select the Yes checkbox to indicate that the medical staff has been notified.
16. Document your name in the Reported By field.
17. Document "Medical assistant" in the Position field.
18. Document "123-123-1234" in the Contact Phone Number field.
19. Document "None" in the Other Persons Involved field.
20. Document "N/A" in the Position field.
21. Document "000-000-0000" in the Contact Phone Number field.
22. Document "No additional treatment needed." in the Medical Report field.
23. Select Julie Walden, MD from the Provider dropdown.

24. Document "accidental" in the Designation field.
25. Select the Signature on File checkbox.
26. Document the date and time in the Date/Time field and Click the Save button.
27. Within the Saved Forms tab, select the Incident Report from the dropdown menu (Figure 2-27).

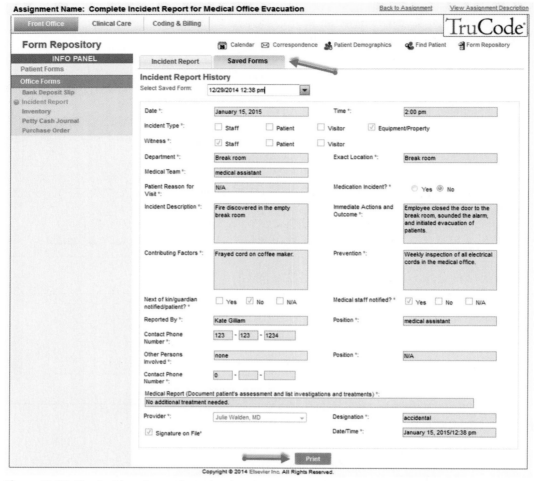

Figure 2-27 The Incident Report from the dropdown menu of the Saved Forms tab.

28. Click the Print button to print the saved Incident Report.

> ✦ Now use the Back to Assignment link to complete the Post-Case Quiz found on the Info Panel for this assignment!

10. Prepare Office Memorandum

Objectives

- Compose a Memorandum for the medical assistant staff.
- Compose professional communication.

Overview

Using today's date, compose an email Memorandum to inform the entire office staff that the refrigerator will be cleaned on Friday and that any items left in the refrigerator when the office closes will be disposed of.

Competencies

- Compose professional correspondence utilizing electronic technology, CAAHEP V.P-8, ABHES 7-g, 7-h
- Perform basic keyboarding skills by locating the keys on a keyboard, ABHES 7-h
- Utilize an EMR, CAAHEP VI.P-6, ABHES 7-b

Estimated completion time: 20 minutes

Measurable Steps

1. Click on the Correspondence icon (Figure 2-28).
2. Select the Memorandum template from the Emails section of the left Info Panel.

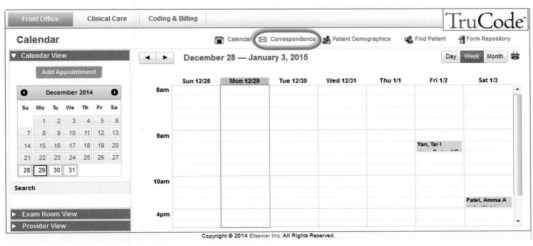

Figure 2-28 Correspondence icon.

3. In the body of the email, document "All staff" in the To field.
4. Document your name in the From field.
5. Document the current date in the Date field.
6. Document "Refrigerator Cleaning" in the Subject field.
7. Compose a professional business letter notifying the staff of the refrigerator cleaning in the message field.
8. Click the Send button. A confirmation message will appear.
9. Within the Sent Memorandums tab, select the saved memorandum (Figure 2-29).

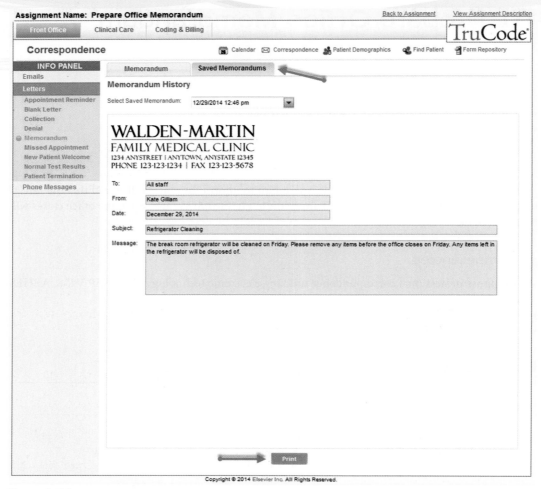

Figure 2-29 Saved Memorandums.

10. Click the Print button if instructed to print.

 Now use the Back to Assignment link to complete the Post-Case Quiz found on the Info Panel for this assignment!

11. Complete Office Inventory Form

■ **Objectives**

• Maintain an inventory supply list.

■ **Overview**

As the lead medical assistant at Walden-Martin, it is your responsibility to complete an Inventory form every week. The supplier is McKesson (123-123-4579) and the PO Number is S00425662. Use the information collected below to complete the Inventory form and determine the supplies needed based on the Quantity on Hand and the Reorder Levels. Then, use this information to complete a Purchase Order.

• Table paper, Unit – Case/12, Manufacturer – Medi-Pak, Quantity on Hand – 1, Reorder Levels – 2, Quantity to Reorder – 5, Price/Unit - $49.19
• Anti-micro soap, Unit – each, Manufacturer – Lab Guard, Quantity on Hand – 6, Reorder Levels – 5, Quantity to Reorder – 10, Price/Unit - $6.19
• Alcohol prep pads, Unit – Box/200, Manufacturer – Webcol, Quantity on Hand – 5, Reorder Levels – 10, Quantity to Reorder – 20, Price/Unit - $3.39
• Non-sterile 2x2 gauze squares, Unit – Pkg/200, Manufacturer – Curity, Quantity on Hand – 20, Reorder Levels – 15, Quantity to Reorder – 30, Price/Unit - $4.75
• Sterile 4x4 gauze squares, Unit – Box/100, Manufacturer – Curity, Quantity on Hand – 8, Reorder Levels – 10, Quantity to Reorder – 30, Price/Unit - $30.69
• 25G x ⅝" 3cc syringes, Unit – Box/100, Manufacturer – VanishPoint, Quantity on Hand – 3, Reorder Levels – 5, Quantity to Reorder – 10, Price/Unit - $73.89
• Tuberculin 27G x ½" 1cc syringes, Unit – Box/100, Manufacturer – VanishPoint, Quantity on Hand – 7, Reorder Levels – 5, Quantity to Reorder – 10, Price/Unit - $80.99
• Nitrile Powder-free exam gloves, Unit – Box/100, Manufacturer – Kimberly-Clark, Quantity on Hand – 2, Reorder Levels – 5, Quantity to Reorder – 20, Price/Unit - $12.49
• Surpass facial tissues, Unit – Case/30, Manufacturer – Kimberly-Clark, Quantity on Hand – 1, Reorder Levels – 2, Quantity to Reorder – 4, Price/Unit - $52.89

■ **Competencies**

• Input patient data utilizing a practice management system, CAAHEP VI.P-7, ABHES 7-b
• Perform an inventory with documentation, CAAHEP VI.P-9, ABHES 7-f
• List steps involved in completing an inventory, CAAHEP VI.C-10, ABHES 7-f

Estimated completion time: 20 minutes

Measurable Steps

1. Click on the Form Repository icon (Figure 2-30).
2. Select Inventory from the Office Forms section of the left Info Panel.
3. Document your name in the Submitter field.
4. Document today's date in the Date field.
5. Document "S00425662" in the PO Number field.
6. Document "McKesson" in the Supplier field.
7. Document "123-123-4579" in the Phone Number field.
8. Within the first row of the inventory grid, document "table paper" in the Product column.
9. Document "case/12" in the Units column.
10. Document "Medi-Pak" in the Manufacturer column.
11. Document "1" in the Quantity on Hand column.

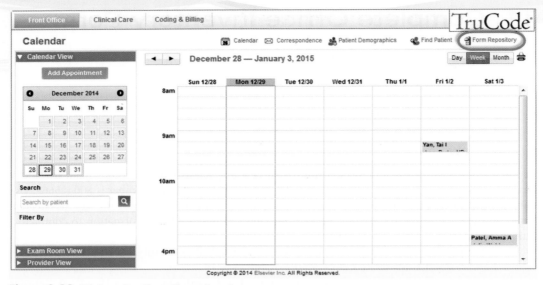

Figure 2-30 Click on the Form Repository icon.

12. Document "2" in the Reorder Levels column.
13. Document "5" in the Quantity to Reorder column.
14. Document "49.19" in the Price/Unit column.
15. Click the Add button.
16. Within the second row of the inventory grid, document "anti-micro soap" in the Product column.
17. Document "each" in the Units column.
18. Document "Lab Guard" in the Manufacturer column.
19. Document "6" in the Quantity on Hand column.
20. Document "5" in the Reorder Levels column.
21. Document "10" in the Quantity to Reorder column.
22. Document "6.19" in the Price/Unit column (Figure 2-31).
23. Document the rest of the inventory needs as directed in row two through nine. Follow the same steps as used to document the table paper.

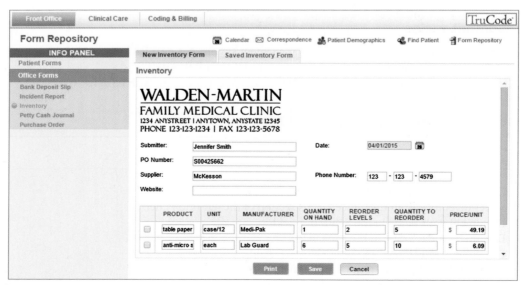

Figure 2-31 Inventory Form.

24. Click the Save button after entering the inventory (Figure 2-32).

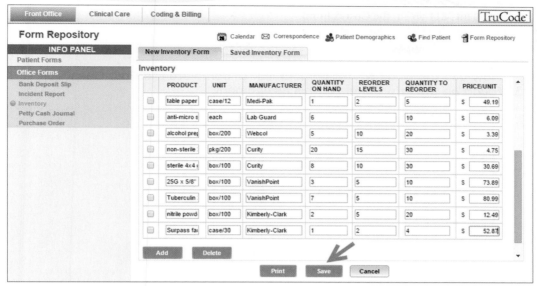

Figure 2-32 Click the Save button after entering in the inventory.

25. Determine which items to reorder and complete the Purchase Order by selecting Purchase Order from the Form Repository.
26. Document your name in the Submitter field.
27. Document "S00425662" in the PO Number field.
28. Document today's date in the Date field.
29. Document "McKesson" in the Supplier field.
30. Document "123-123-4579" in the Phone Number field.
31. Document "table paper" in the Product column.
32. Document "5" in the Quantity column.
33. Document "case" in the Unit column.
34. Document "49.19" in the Price/Unit column.
35. Document "245.95" in the Cost column.
36. In the next row, document "alcohol prep pads" in the Product column.
37. Document "20" in the Quantity column.
38. Document "box" in the Unit column.
39. Document "3.39" in the Price/Unit column.
40. Document "67.80" in the Cost column.
41. In the next row, document "sterile 4x4 gauze squares" in the Product column.
42. Document "30" in the Quantity column.
43. Document "box" in the Unit column.
44. Document "30.69" in the Price/Unit column.
45. Document "920.70" in the Cost column.
46. In the next row, document "25G x 5/8" 3cc syringes" in the Product column.
47. Document "10" in the Quantity column.
48. Document "box" in the Unit column.
49. Document "73.89" in the Price/Unit column.
50. Document "738.90" in the Cost column.
51. In the next row, document "nitrile powder-free exam gloves" in the Product column.
52. Document "20" in the Quantity column.
53. Document "box" in the Unit column.
54. Document "12.49" in the Price/Unit column.
55. Document "249.80" in the Cost column.
56. In the next row, document "surpass facial tissues" in the Product column.
57. Document "4" in the Quantity column.

58. Document "case" in the Unit column.
59. Document "52.89" in the Price/Unit column.
60. Document "211.56" in the Cost column.
61. Document "2434.71"in the Total field.
62. Click the Save button.

 Now use the Back to Assignment link to complete the Post-Case Quiz found on the Info Panel for this assignment!

12. Complete New Patient Registration for Malcolm Little

■ Objectives

1. Search for a patient record.
2. Register a patient.

■ Overview

Malcolm Little moved into the area five months ago and has been with his new employer for four months. Now that his new insurance plan is effective, he would like to see Dr. Martin. He faxed his completed Patient Information form to the Walden-Martin office this morning. Complete the new patient registration process for Malcolm Little using the Patient Information form and insurance card provided. Refer to Malcolm Little's insurance card and Patient Information Form at the end of the Measurable Steps to complete this assignment.

■ Competencies

- Apply the Patient's Bill of Rights as it relates to choice of treatment, consent for treatment, and refusal of treatment, CAAHEP X.P-4, ABHES 4-b, 4-g
- Obtain accurate patient billing information, CAAHEP VII.P-3, ABHES 5-h, 7-a, 7-c
- Utilize an EMR, CAAHEP VI.P-6, ABHES 7-b

Estimated completion time: 25 minutes

Measurable Steps

1. Click on the Patient Demographics icon (Figure 2-33).

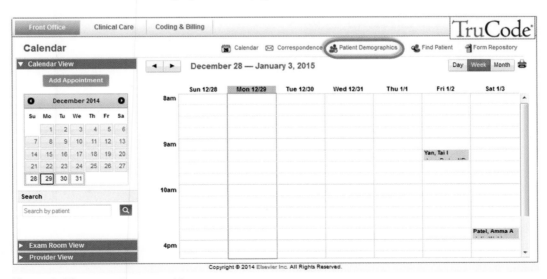

Figure 2-33 Patient Demographics.

2. Perform a patient search to confirm that Malcolm Little is not an existing patient.
3. Click the Add Patient button (Figure 2-34).
4. Using the insurance card (Figure A) and completed Patient Information Form (Figure B) provided at the end of this assignment as a reference, complete the required fields within the Patient, Guarantor, and Insurance tabs to add Malcolm Little as a new patient. Once the information

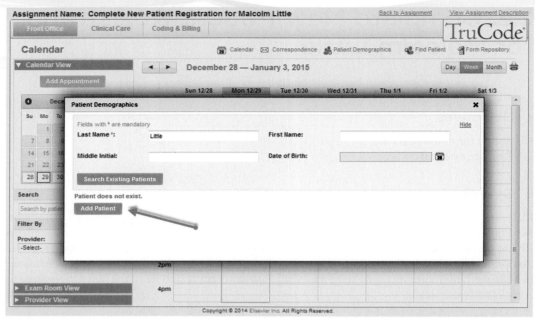

Figure 2-34 Add patient.

in all of the three tabs has been provided, click the Save Patient button to save Malcolm Little's demographic information (Figure 2-35).

5. Click the X to close out of the Patient Demographics.

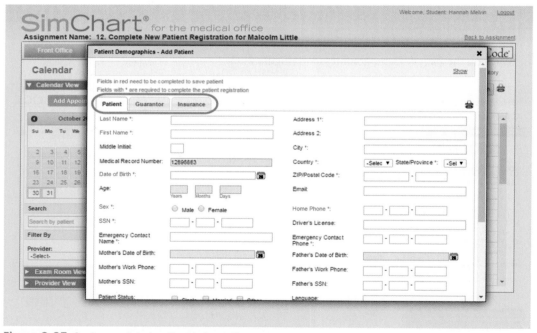

Figure 2-35 Saving updated patient information.

BLUE CROSS BLUE SHIELD

1234 Insurance Place

MEMBER: Little, Malcolm T

POLICY #: ML7582015

GROUP #: 66452L

EFFECTIVE DATE: 08/30/2013

CO-PAY: $25
SPECIALIST CO-PAY: $35
XRAY/LAB BENEFIT: $250

DRUG CO-PAY
GENERIC: $10
NAME BRAND: $50

CLAIMS/INQUIRIES: 1-800-123-1111

Figure A Insurance card for Malcolm Little.

WALDEN-MARTIN
FAMILY MEDICAL CLINIC
1234 ANYSTREET | ANYTOWN, ANYSTATE 12345
PHONE 123-123-1234 | FAX 123-123-5678

Instructor: Becky Swisher

PATIENT INFORMATION

PATIENT INFORMATION (Please use full legal name.)

Last Name:	Little		**Address 1:**	1814 Sister Avenue
First Name:	Malcolm		**Address 2:**	--
Middle Initial:	T		**City:**	Anytown
Medical Record Number:	10206460		**Country:**	United States **State/Province:** AL
Date of Birth:	10/12/1960		**Zip:**	12345 ---
Age:	56 10 28		**Email:**	--
Sex:	Male		**Home Phone:**	123-227-7245
SSN:	667-68-6855		**Driver's License:**	--
Emergency Contact Name:	Delores LIttle		**Emergency Contact Phone:**	123-693-8887
Mother's Date of Birth:	--		**Father's Date of Birth:**	--
Mother's Work Phone:	--------		**Father's Work Phone:**	--------
Mother's SSN:	--------		**Father's SSN:**	--------
Language:	--		**Race:**	--
Patient Status:	Married		**Ethnicity:**	--
Employer Name:	Anytown High School			
School Name:	--			

GUARANTOR INFORMATION (Please use full legal name.)

Relationship of Guarantor to Patient:	Self			
Guarantor/Account #:	Little, Malcolm T / 12179738			
Account Number:	12179738			
Last Name:	Little		**Address 1:**	1814 Sister Avenue
First Name:	Malcolm		**Address 2:**	--
Middle Initial:	T		**City:**	Anytown
Date of Birth:	10/12/1960		**Country:**	United States **State/Province:** AL
Age:	56 10 28		**Zip:**	12345 ---
Sex:	Male		**Email:**	--
SSN:	667-68-6855		**Home Phone:**	123-227-7245
Employer Name:	Anytown High School		**Cell Phone:**	--------
School Name:	--		**Work Phone:**	--------

Figure B Patient information form for Malcolm Little.

Front Office

OTHER EMPLOYMENT INFORMATION

Father's Employer:	--	**Mother's Employer:**	--
Employer's Address 1:	--	**Employer's Address 1:**	--
Employer's Address 2:	--	**Employer's Address 2:**	--
City:	--	**City:**	--
Country:	-- **State/Province:** --	**Country:**	-- **State/Province:** --
ZIP:	-- ---	**ZIP:**	-- ---

PROVIDER INFORMATION

Primary Provider:	James A. Martin, MD	**Provider's Address 1:**	1234 Anystreet
Referring Provider:	--	**Provider's Address 2:**	--
Date of Last Visit:	--	**City:**	Anytown
Phone:	123-123-1234	**Country:**	United States **State/Province:** AL
		Zip:	12345 ---

INSURANCE INFORMATION (If the patient is not the Insured party, please include date of birth for claims.)

PRIMARY INSURANCE

Insurance:	Blue Cross Blue Shield	**Claims Address 1:**	1234 Insurance Place
Name of Policy Holder:	Malcolm T LIttle	**Claims Address 2:**	--
SSN:	667-68-6855	**City:**	Anytown
Policy/ID Number:	ML7582015	**Country:**	United States **State/Province:** AL
Group Number:	66452L	**ZIP:**	12345 - 1234
		Claims Phone:	800-123-1111

SECONDARY INSURANCE

Insurance:	--	**Claims Address 1:**	--
Name of Policy Holder:	--	**Claims Address 2:**	--
SSN:	--------	**City:**	--
Policy/ID Number:	--	**Country:**	-- **State/Province:** --
Group Number:	--	**ZIP:**	-- ---
		Claims Phone:	--------

DENTAL INSURANCE

Dental Insurance:	--	**Claims Address 1:**	--
Name of Policy Holder:	--	**Claims Address 2:**	--
SSN:	--------	**City:**	--
Policy/ID Number:	--	**Country:**	-- **State/Province:** --
Group Number:	--	**ZIP:**	-- ---
		Claims Phone:	--------

WORKERS' COMPENSATION

Insurance:	--	**Claims Address 1:**	--
Employer:	--	**Claims Address 2:**	--
Contact:	--	**City:**	--
Policy / ID Number:	--	**Country:**	-- **State/Province:** --
Claims Phone Number:	--------	**ZIP:**	-- ---

"I hereby authorize direct payment of all insurance benefits otherwise payable to me for services rendered. I understand that I am financially responsible for all charges not covered by insurance for services rendered on my behalf to my dependents. I authorize the above providers to release any information required to secure payment of benefits.I authorize the use of this signature on all insurance submissions."

Signature: **Date:** --

Figure B, cont'd Patient information form for Malcolm Little.

⭐ Now use the Back to Assignment link to complete the Post-Case Quiz found on the Info Panel for this assignment!

13. Update Demographics and Complete Advance Directive Form for Amma Patel

■ Objectives

- Search for a patient record.
- Update patient demographics.
- Access patient forms.
- Update patient information using the correct form.

■ Overview

Amma Patel was hospitalized one week ago and is in the office for a follow-up visit. She does not have an Advance Directive on file. She would like to complete the form and name her brother, Robert Patel, as her primary representative and her mother, Indira Patel, as her alternate power of attorney. She would also like to update her phone number because she no longer has a landline telephone. Her cell phone number is 123-315-1572. Complete an Advance Directive form for Amma Patel and update her demographic information.

■ Competencies

- Define living wills/advanced directives, CAAHEP X.C-7f, ABHES 3-a, 4-f
- Define medical durable power of attorney, CAAHEP X.C-7g, ABHES 3-a, 4-f
- Input patient data utilizing a practice management system, CAAHEP VI.P-7, ABHES 7-b

Estimated completion time: 20 minutes

Measurable Steps

1. Click on the Form Repository icon (Figure 2-36).
2. Select Advance Directive from the Patient Forms section of the left Info Panel.

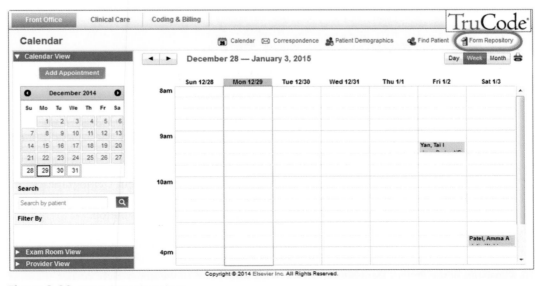

Figure 2-36 Form Repository icon.

3. Print the form to obtain Amma Patel's signature. After obtaining the signature, scan and save the signed form to your desktop.
4. Click the Patient Search button to perform a patient search and assign the form to Amma Patel (Figure 2-37).

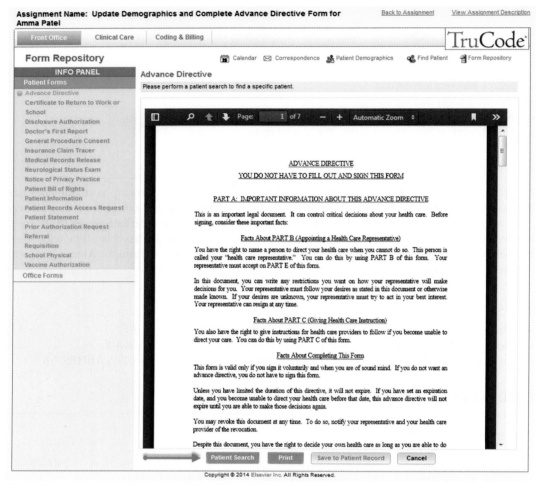

Figure 2-37 Using the Patient Search fields to find Amma Patel.

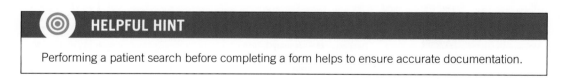

HELPFUL HINT

Performing a patient search before completing a form helps to ensure accurate documentation.

5. Click the Upload Complete Form link and then click the Browse button to select Amma Patel's signed Advance Directive and save the form to her patient record. Click the Upload Button. (Figure 2-38).
6. Click Ok.
7. In order to update Amma Patel's patient demographics, click the Patient Demographics link (Figure 2-39).
8. Enter Patel in the Last Name field and select the Search Existing Patients button.
9. Once you locate Amma Patel in the List of Patients, confirm her date of birth and select her first name (Figure 2-40). Within the Patient tab, change Amma Patel's phone number to 123-315-1572. Click the Save Patient button.
10. Close out of the Patient Demographics box by clicking the X in the upper-right corner.

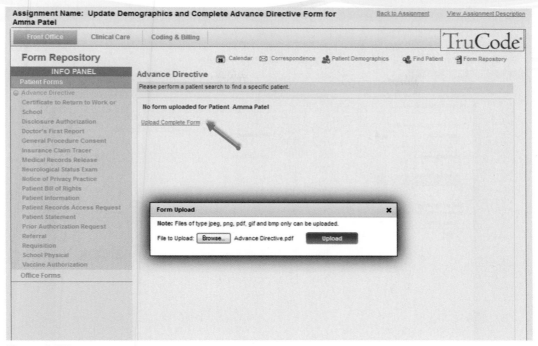

Figure 2-38 Uploading Amma Patel's Advance Directive to her patient record.

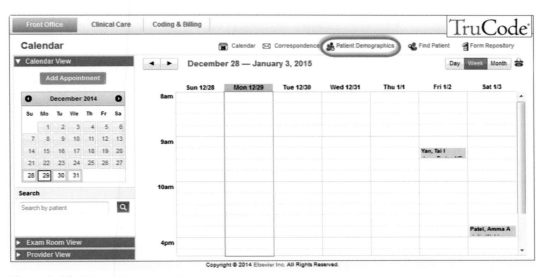

Figure 2-39 Patient Demographics.

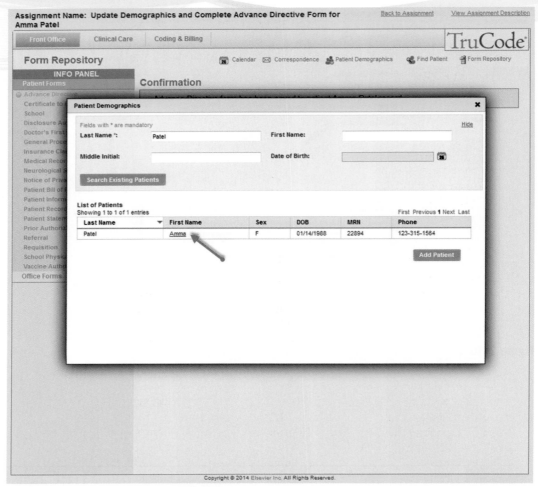

Figure 2-40 Confirming Amma Patel's information.

Now use the Back to Assignment link to complete the Post-Case Quiz found on the Info Panel for this assignment!

14. Schedule Appointment and Prepare New Patient Forms for Al Neviaser

■ Objectives

- Search for a patient record.
- Schedule an appointment.
- Access patient forms.
- Prepare patient paperwork.

■ Overview

Al Neviaser moved into the area five months ago and has been with his new employer for four months. Now that his new insurance plan is effective, he would like to schedule an appointment with Dr. Martin. New patient appointments are 30 minutes and there is an available time at 11:15 am next Thursday. Prepare for the appointment by printing one copy each of the Notice of Privacy Practice and Patient Bill of Rights forms for Al Neviaser to review once he arrives.

■ Competencies

- Apply the Patient's Bill of Rights as it relates to choice of treatment, consent for treatment, and refusal of treatment, CAAHEP X.P-4, ABHES 4-b, 4-g
- Describe components of the Health Information Portability & Accountability Act (HIPAA), CAAHEP X.C-3, ABHES 4-h
- Display sensitivity when managing appointments, CAAHEP VI.A-1, ABHES 5-h, 7-e
- Identify different types of appointment scheduling methods, CAAHEP VI.C-1, ABHES 7-e
- Manage appointment schedule, using established priorities, CAAHEP VI.P-1, ABHES 7-e
- Perform basic keyboarding skills by locating the keys on a keyboard, ABHES 7-h
- Utilize an EMR, CAAHEP VI.P-6, ABHES 7-b

Estimated completion time: 30 minutes

Measurable Steps

1. Within the Calendar of the Front Office module, click the Add Appointment button or anywhere within the calendar to open the New Appointment window (Figure 2-41).
2. Select the Patient Visit radio button as the Appointment Type.
3. Select New Patient Visit from the Visit Type dropdown.
4. Document "New patient visit" in the Chief Complaint text box.
5. Select the Search Existing Patients radio button.
6. Using the Patient Search fields, search for Al Neviaser's patient record. Once you locate him in the List of Patients, confirm his date of birth and select the radio button for Al Neviaser.

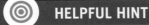 **HELPFUL HINT**

Confirming date of birth will help to ensure that you have located the correct patient record.

7. Select James A. Martin, MD from the Provider dropdown.
8. Use the calendar picker to confirm or select the appointment day.
9. Select a start and end time for the appointment using the Start Time and End Time dropdowns.
10. Click the Save button.

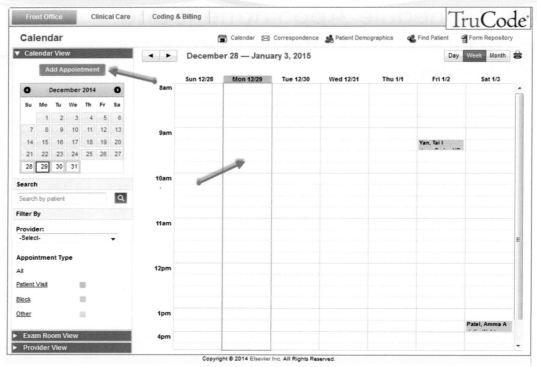

Figure 2-41 Add Appointment.

11. Al Neviaser's appointment will be displayed on the calendar.
12. Click on the Form Repository icon (Figure 2-42).

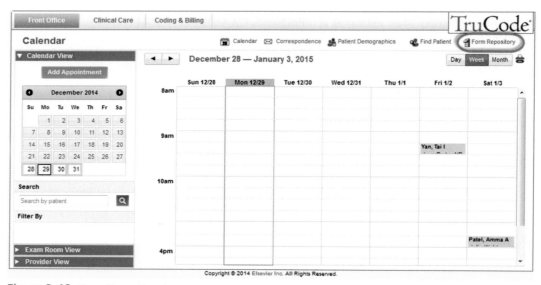

Figure 2-42 Form Repository icon.

13. Select the Notice of Privacy Practice form from the left Info Panel.
14. Click the Patient Search button.
15. Using the Patient Search fields, search for Al Neviaser's patient record. Once you locate him in the List of Patients, confirm his date of birth.
16. Select the radio button for Al Neviaser and click the Select button.
17. Click the Save to Patient Record button and select the date. Click OK.
18. Select the Patient Bill of Rights from the left Info Panel.

19. Click the Patient Search button.
20. Using the Patient Search fields, search for Al Neviaser's patient record. Once you locate him in the List of Patients, confirm his date of birth.
21. Select the radio button for Al Neviaser and click the Select button.
22. Click the Save to Patient Record button and select the date. Click OK.
23. Click on the Find Patient icon (Figure 2-43).
24. Using the Patient Search fields, search for Al Neviaser's patient record. Once you locate him in the List of Patients, confirm his date of birth.
25. Select the radio button for Al Neviaser and click the Select button. Confirm the auto-populated details.

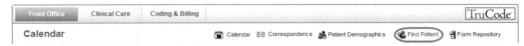

Figure 2-43 Find Patient icon.

26. Scroll down to view the Forms section of the Patient Dashboard (Figure 2-44).
27. Select the forms you prepared. The forms will open in a new window, allowing you to print.

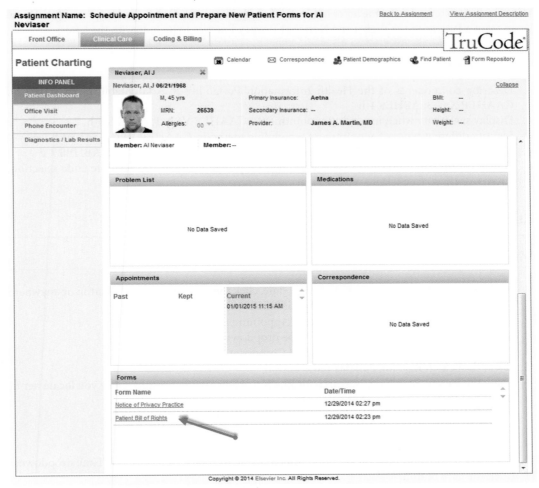

Figure 2-44 The Forms section of the Patient Dashboard.

Now use the Back to Assignment link to complete the Post-Case Quiz found on the Info Panel for this assignment!

15. Schedule Appointment and Prepare New Patient Forms for Ella Rainwater

■ **Objectives**

- Search for a patient record.
- Schedule an appointment.
- Compose professional communication.
- Access patient forms.
- Prepare patient paperwork.

■ **Overview**

New patient Ella Rainwater is fully registered and would like an appointment with Dr. Martin next Monday. She is available at 9:00 am and new patient appointments are 30 minutes. It is Walden-Martin policy to send a welcome letter before the first appointment. Create the New Patient Welcome letter. Print a Patient Bill of Rights and Notice of Privacy Practice to include with the letter.

■ **Competencies**

- Describe components of the Health Information Portability & Accountability Act (HIPAA), CAAHEP X.C-3, ABHES 4-h
- Display sensitivity when managing appointments, CAAHEP VI.A-1, ABHES 5-h, 7-e
- Identify different types of appointment scheduling methods, CAAHEP VI.C-1, ABHES 7-e
- Manage appointment schedule, using established priorities, CAAHEP VI.P-1, ABHES 7-e
- Utilize tactful communication skills with medical providers to ensure accurate code selection, CAAHEP IX. A-1, ABHES 5-h, 7-d

Estimated completion time: 25 minutes

Measurable Steps

1. Within the Calendar of the Front Office module, click the Add Appointment button or anywhere within the calendar to open the New Appointment window (Figure 2-45).
2. Select the Patient Visit radio button as the Appointment Type.
3. Select New Patient Visit from the Visit Type dropdown.
4. Document "New patient visit" in the Chief Complaint text box.
5. Select the Search Existing Patients radio button.
6. Using the Patient Search fields, search for Ella Rainwater's patient record. Once you locate her in the List of Patients, confirm her date of birth.
7. Select the radio button for Ella Rainwater and click the Select button.
8. Select James A. Martin, MD from the Provider dropdown.
9. Use the calendar picker to confirm or select the appointment day.
10. Select a start and end time for the appointment using the Start Time and End Time dropdowns.
11. Click the Save button.
12. Ms. Rainwater's appointment will be displayed on the calendar.

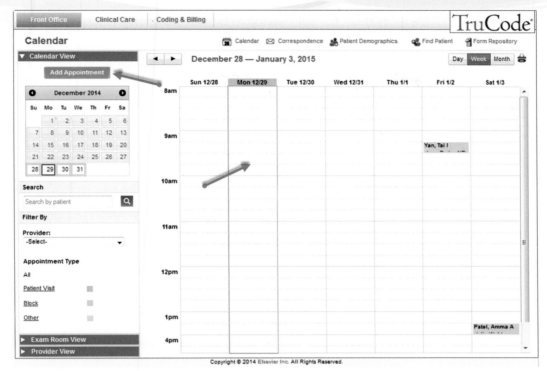

Figure 2-45 Add Appointment.

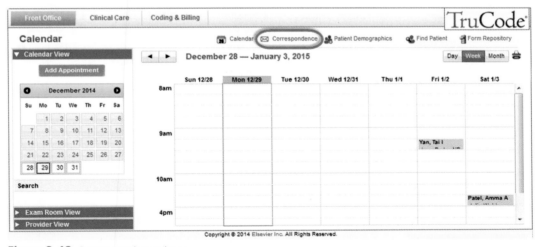

Figure 2-46 Correspondence icon.

13. Click on the Correspondence icon (Figure 2-46).
14. Select the New Patient Welcome template from the Letters section of the left Info Panel.
15. Click the Patient Search button at the bottom to assign the letter to Ms. Rainwater. The patient demographics are auto-populated (Figure 2-47).
16. Confirm the auto-populated details and click the Save to Patient Record button. Select the date and click OK.
17. Click on the Form Repository icon and select the Notice of Privacy Practice from the left Info Panel (Figure 2-48).
18. Click the Patient Search button.

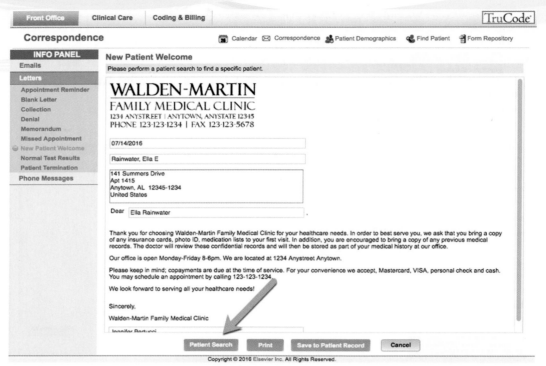

Figure 2-47 The New Patient Welcome template.

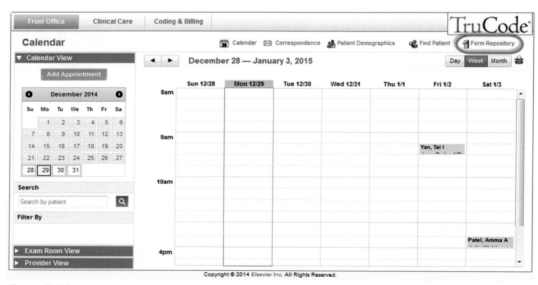

Figure 2-48 Form Repository icon.

19. Using the Patient Search fields, search for Ella Rainwater's patient record. Once you locate her in the List of Patients, confirm her date of birth.
20. Select the radio button for Ella Rainwater and click the Select button.
21. Click the Save to Patient Record button. Select the date and click OK.
22. Select the Patient Bill of Rights from the left Info Panel.
23. Click the Patient Search button.
24. Using the Patient Search fields, search for Ella Rainwater's patient record. Once you locate her in the List of Patients, confirm her date of birth.
25. Select the radio button for Ella Rainwater and click the Select button.

26. Click the Save to Patient Record button. Select the date and click OK.
27. Click on the Find Patient icon.
28. Using the Patient Search fields, search for Ella Rainwater's patient record. Once you locate her in the List of Patients, confirm her date of birth.
29. Select the radio button for Ella Rainwater and click the Select button. Confirm the auto-populated details.
30. Scroll down to view the Forms section of the Patient Dashboard.
31. Select the forms you prepared. The forms will open in a new window, allowing you to print.

 Now use the Back to Assignment link to complete the Post-Case Quiz found on the Info Panel for this assignment!

16. Schedule Appointment and Prepare Appointment Reminder Letter for Anna Richardson

■ Objectives

- Search for a patient record.
- Schedule an appointment.
- Create Appointment Reminder letter.
- Compose professional communication.

■ Overview

Anna Richardson was released from the hospital two days ago following a vaginal delivery with postpartum hemorrhage complications. She is calling to request a follow-up appointment with Dr. Martin within the next two weeks and states that Monday afternoons are best for her. She states that she is feeling great and is not currently experiencing any complications. Schedule the appointment for 30 minutes and prepare an Appointment Reminder letter.

■ Competencies

- Display sensitivity when managing appointments, CAAHEP VI.A-1, ABHES 5-h, 7-e
- Identify different types of appointment scheduling methods, CAAHEP VI.C-1, ABHES 7-e
- Manage appointment schedule, using established priorities, CAAHEP VI.P-1, ABHES 7-e
- Utilize an EMR, CAAHEP VI.P-6, ABHES 7-b
- Explain the importance of data backup, CAAHEP VI.C-11

Estimated completion time: 25 minutes

Measurable Steps

1. Within the Calendar of the Front Office module, click the Add Appointment button or anywhere within the calendar to open the New Appointment window (Figure 2-49).
2. Select the Patient Visit radio button as the Appointment Type.
3. Select Follow-Up/Established Visit from the Visit Type dropdown.
4. Document "Postpartum hemorrhage follow-up" in the Chief Complaint text box.
5. Select the Search Existing Patients radio button.
6. Using the Patient Search fields, search for Anna Richardson's patient record. Once you locate her in the List of Patients, confirm her date of birth.

> ◎ **HELPFUL HINT**
>
> Confirming date of birth will help to ensure that you have located the correct patient record.

7. Select the radio button for Anna Richardson and click the Select button. Confirm the auto-populated details.
8. Select James A. Martin, MD from the Provider dropdown.
9. Use the calendar picker to confirm or select the appointment day.
10. Select a start and end time for the appointment using the Start Time and End Time dropdowns.
11. Click the Save button.
12. Anna Richardson's appointment will be displayed on the calendar.

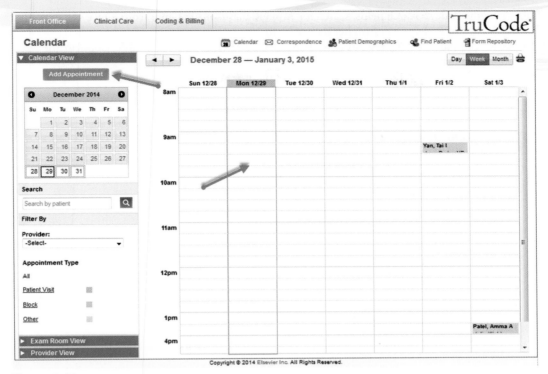

Figure 2-49 Add Appointment.

13. Click on the Correspondence icon (Figure 2-50).

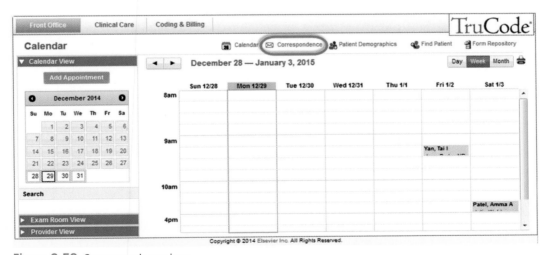

Figure 2-50 Correspondence icon.

14. Select the Appointment Reminder template from the Letters section of the left Info Panel.
15. Click the Patient Search button to assign the letter to Anna Richardson. The patient demographics are auto-populated.
16. Confirm the auto-populated details. Select the upcoming appointment from the left-hand side. Click the Save to Patient Record button. Select the date and click OK.
17. Click on the Find Patient icon (Figure 2-51).

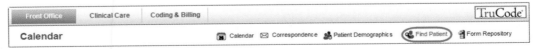

Figure 2-51 Find Patient icon.

18. Using the Patient Search fields, search for Anna Richardson's patient record. Once you locate her in the List of Patients, confirm her date of birth.
19. Select the radio button for Anna Richardson and click the Select button. Confirm the auto-populated details.
20. Scroll down to view the Correspondence section of the Patient Dashboard.
21. Select the letter you prepared.
22. The letter will open in a new window, allowing you to print.

 Now use the Back to Assignment link to complete the Post-Case Quiz found on the Info Panel for this assignment!

17. Send Missed Appointment Email to Ella Rainwater

■ Objectives

- Search for a patient record.
- Create an email for a patient.
- Compose professional communication.

■ Overview

Ella Rainwater missed her 11:00 am appointment yesterday to discuss hypertension with Dr. Martin. It is Walden-Martin policy to notify patients when they miss an appointment and her preferred method of communication is email. Prepare a Missed Appointment email for Ella Rainwater.

■ Competencies

- Coach patients regarding office policies, CAAHEP V.P-4a, ABHES 5-c, 5-h
- Discuss applications of electronic technology in professional communication, CAAHEP V.C-8, ABHES 7-g, 7-h
- Perform basic keyboarding skills by locating the keys on a keyboard, ABHES 7-h
- Manage appointment schedule, using established priorities, CAAHEP VI.P-1, ABHES 7-e
- Utilize an EMR, CAAHEP VI.P-6, ABHES 7-b
- Display sensitivity when managing appointments, CAAHEP VI.A-1

Estimated completion time: 15 minutes

Measurable Steps

1. Click on the Correspondence icon (Figure 2-52).

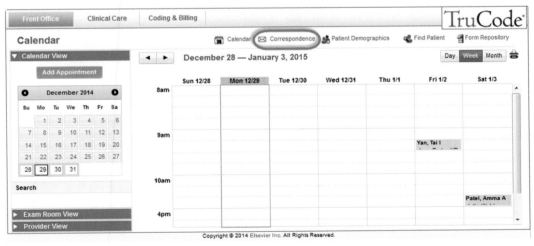

Figure 2-52 Correspondence icon.

2. Select the Missed Appointment template from the Emails section of the left Info Panel (Figure 2-53).
3. Click the Patient Search button to perform a patient search and assign the email to Ella Rainwater.
4. Confirm the auto-populated details and document any additional information needed.
5. Click the Send button to send the Missed Appointment email to Ella Rainwater (Figure 2-54). Select the date and click OK.

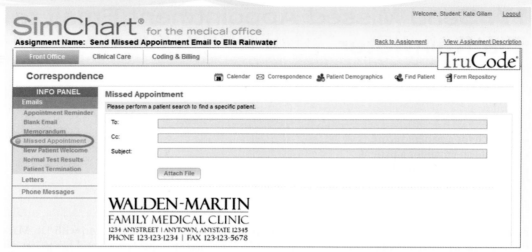

Figure 2-53 Missed Appointment template.

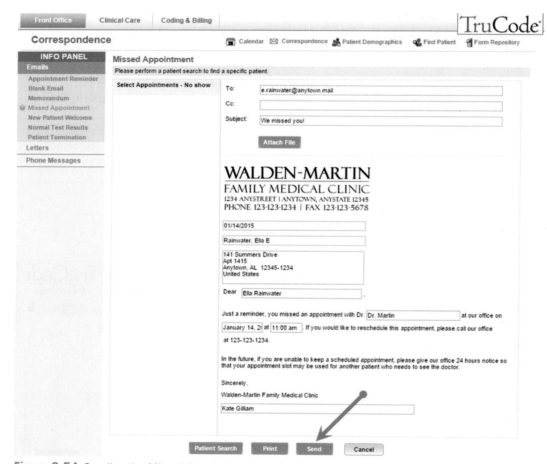

Figure 2-54 Sending the Missed Appointment email to Ella Rainwater.

Now use the Back to Assignment link to complete the Post-Case Quiz found on the Info Panel for this assignment!

18. Complete New Patient Registration and Schedule Appointment for Lisa Rae

■ Objectives

- Search for a patient record.
- Register a patient.
- Schedule an appointment.

■ Overview

Lisa Rae just moved to Anytown in order to live closer to her daughter and grandchildren. She would like to find a physician and her friend, Norma Washington, recommended Dr. Walden. She has completed the Patient Information form and would like to schedule an appointment for next Monday morning. Refer to Lisa Rae's insurance card and Patient Information Form at the end of the Measurable Steps to update the Patient Demographics and then schedule her appointment.

■ Competencies

- Apply the Patient's Bill of Rights as it relates to choice of treatment, consent for treatment, and refusal of treatment, CAAHEP X.P-4, ABHES 4-b, 4-g
- Differentiate between electronic medical records (EMR) and a practice management system, CAAHEP VI.C-8, ABHES 7-b
- Input patient data utilizing a practice management system, CAAHEP VI.P-7, ABHES 7-b
- Obtain accurate patient billing information, CAAHEP VII.P-3, ABHES 5-h, 7-a, 7-c
- Perform basic keyboarding skills by locating the keys on a keyboard, ABHES 7-h
- Utilize an EMR, CAAHEP VI.P-6, ABHES 7-b

Estimated completion time: 30 minutes

Measurable Steps

1. Click the Patient Demographics icon (Figure 2-55).
2. Perform a patient search to confirm that Lisa Rae is not an existing patient.

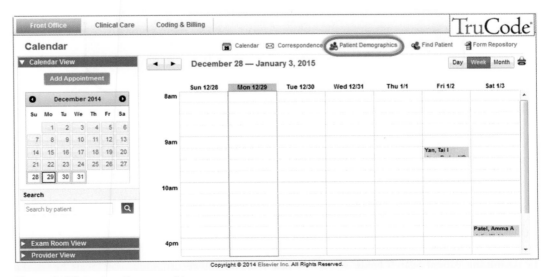

Figure 2-55 Patient Demographics.

3. Click the Add Patient button (Figure 2-56).

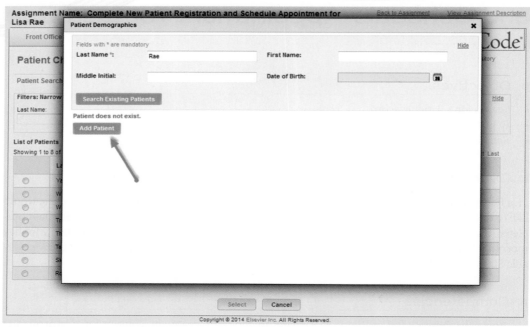

Figure 2-56 Add Patient.

4. Using the insurance card (Figure C) and completed Patient Information form (Figure D) provided at the end of this assignment as reference, complete the required fields within the Patient, Guarantor, and Insurance tabs to add Lisa Rae as a new patient. Click the Save Patient button after completing each tab.

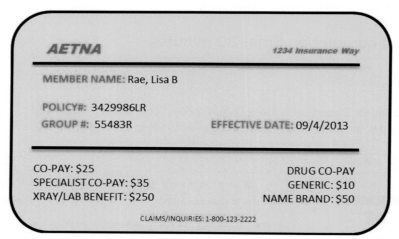

Figure C Insurance card for Lisa Rae.

5. Click the X to close out of the Patient Demographics.
6. Click the Calendar icon at the top of the screen (Figure 2-57).
7. Click the Add Appointment button or anywhere within the calendar to open the New Appointment window (Figure 2-58).
8. Select the Patient Visit radio button as the Appointment Type.
9. Select New Patient Visit from the Visit Type dropdown.
10. Document "New patient visit" in the Chief Complaint text box.
11. Select the Search Existing Patients radio button.
12. Using the Patient Search fields, search for Lisa Rae's patient record. Once you locate her in the List of Patients, confirm her date of birth.

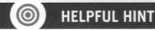

<table>
<tr><td>⊚</td><td>**HELPFUL HINT**</td></tr>
</table>

Confirming date of birth will help to ensure that you have located the correct patient record.

13. Select the radio button for Lisa Rae and click the Select button. Confirm the auto-populated details.

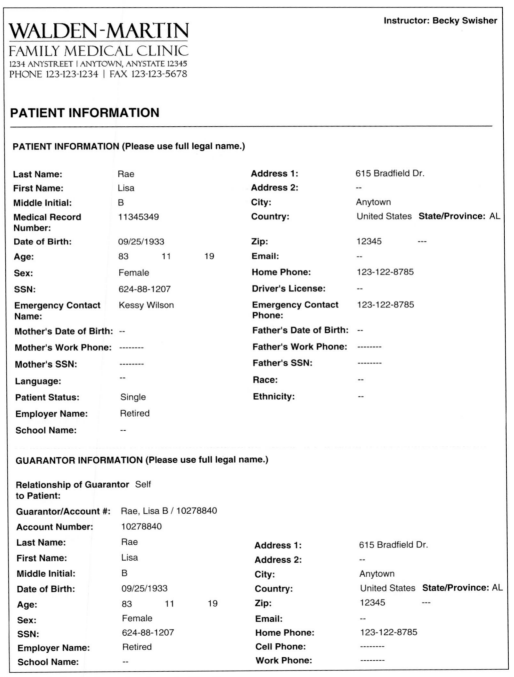

Figure D Patient information form for Lisa Rae.

Continued

OTHER EMPLOYMENT INFORMATION

Father's Employer:	--	Mother's Employer:	--
Employer's Address 1:	--	Employer's Address 1:	--
Employer's Address 2:	--	Employer's Address 2:	--
City:	--	City:	--
Country: --	State/Province: --	Country: --	State/Province: --
ZIP: --	---	ZIP: --	---

PROVIDER INFORMATION

Primary Provider:	Julie Walden, MD	Provider' s Address 1:	1234 ANYSTREET
Referring Provider:	--	Provider' s Address 2:	--
Date of Last Visit:	--	City:	ANYTOWN
Phone:	123-123-1234	Country:	United States State/Province: AL
		Zip:	12345 - 0000

INSURANCE INFORMATION (If the patient is not the Insured party, please include date of birth for claims.)

PRIMARY INSURANCE

Insurance:	Aetna	Claims Address 1:	1234 Insurance Way
Name of Policy Holder:	Lisa Rae	Claims Address 2:	--
SSN:	624-88-1207	City:	Anytown
Policy/ID Number:	3429986LR	Country:	United States State/Province: AL
Group Number:	55483R	ZIP:	12345 - 1234
		Claims Phone:	800-123-2222

SECONDARY INSURANCE

Insurance:	Aetna	Claims Address 1:	1234 Insurance Way
Name of Policy Holder:	Lisa Rae	Claims Address 2:	--
SSN:	624-88-1207	City:	Anytown
Policy/ID Number:	3429986LR	Country:	United States State/Province: AL
Group Number	55483R	ZIP:	12345 - 1234
		Claims Phone:	800-123-2222

DENTAL INSURANCE

Dental Insurance:	--	Claims Address 1:	--
Name of Policy Holder:	--	Claims Address 2:	--
SSN:	--------	City:	--
Policy/ID Number:	--	Country: --	State/Province: --
Group Number:	--	ZIP: --	---
		Claims Phone:	--------

WORKERS' COMPENSATION

Insurance:	--	Claims Address 1:	--
Employer:	--	Claims Address 2:	--
Contact:	--	City:	--
Policy / ID Number:	--	Country: --	State/Province: --
Claims Phone Number:	--------	ZIP: --	---

"I hereby authorize direct payment of all insurance benefits otherwise payable to me for services rendered. I understand that I am financially responsible for all charges not covered by insurance for services rendered on my behalf to my dependents. I authorize the above providers to release any information required to secure payment of benefits. I authorize the use of this signature on all insurance submissions."

Signature: Date: --

Figure D, cont'd Patient information form for Lisa Rae.

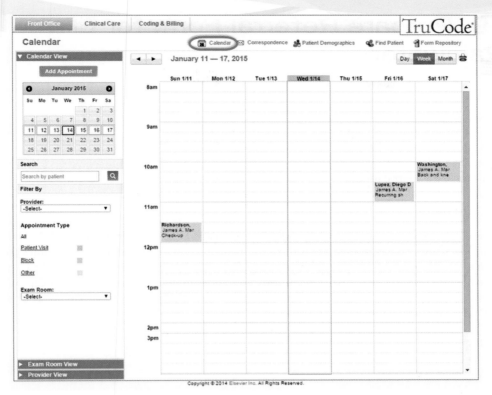

Figure 2-57 Calendar icon.

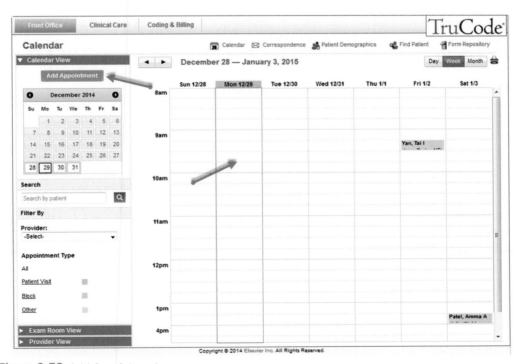

Figure 2-58 Add Appointment.

14. Select Julie Walden, MD from the Provider dropdown.
15. Use the calendar picker to confirm or select the appointment day.
16. Select a start and end time for the appointment using the Start Time and End Time dropdowns.
17. Click the Save button.
18. Lisa Rae's appointment will appear on the calendar.

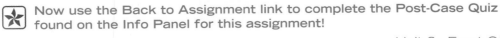
Now use the Back to Assignment link to complete the Post-Case Quiz found on the Info Panel for this assignment!

19. Prepare Referral Form for Ella Rainwater

■ Objectives

- Search for a patient record.
- Access patient forms.
- Complete a referral form.

■ Overview

Ella Rainwater continues to have trouble with bronchitis (ICD-10 J40). Dr. Martin (NPI 234216738) would like her to have a consultation with Dr. Bronchi, the pulmonologist. Dr. Martin notes the following information for the referral: "Significant Clinical Symptoms: Chest x-ray shows infiltrate of the left lung. Previous Clinical Treatments: Two courses of antibiotics (Augmentin and Cipro)." Ella Rainwater's insurance company has authorized three visits to the pulmonologist. Complete a referral form for Ella's consultation with Dr. Bronchi.

> Dr. Bronchi
> Respiratory Care Associates
> 333 Lobar Lane
> Anytown, AL 12345

■ Competencies

- Report relevant information concisely and accurately, CAAHEP V.P-11, ABHES 7-a, 7-g
- Utilize an EMR, CAAHEP VI.P-6, ABHES 7-b
- Facilitate referrals to community resources in the role of a patient navigator, CAAHEP V.P-10

Estimated completion time: 20 minutes

Measurable Steps

1. Click on the Form Repository icon (Figure 2-59).
2. Select Referral from the Patient Forms section of the left Info Panel.
3. Click the Patient Search button to perform a patient search and assign the form to Ella Rainwater.

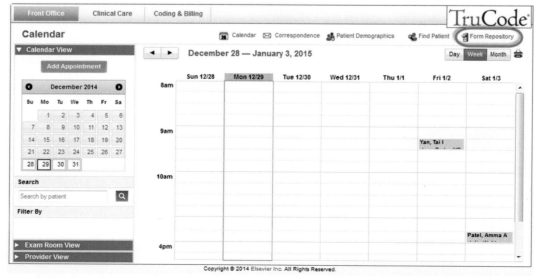

Figure 2-59 Form Repository icon.

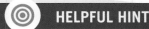

HELPFUL HINT

Performing a patient search before completing a form helps to ensure accurate documentation.

4. Confirm the auto-populated details and document any additional information needed.
5. Document Bronchitis J40 in the Diagnosis/Code field.
6. Document "Chest x-ray shows infiltrate of the left lung" in the Significant Clinical Information/ Symptoms field.
7. Document "Two courses of antibiotics (Augmentin and Cipro)" in the Previous Clinical Treatments field.
8. Document "Respiratory Care Associates, Dr. Bronchi" in the Place of Service field.
9. Document "333 Lobar Lane, Anytown, AL 12345" in the Address field.
10. Document "3" in the Number of Visits field.
11. Document "James A. Martin, MD" in the Referring Provider field.
12. Document "123-123-1234" in the Phone field.
13. Document "234216738" in the NPI Number field.
14. Select the Same as Referring Physician checkbox.
15. Click the Save to Patient Record button. Select the date and click OK.
16. Click on the Find Patient icon (Figure 2-60).

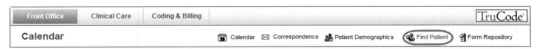

Figure 2-60 Find Patient icon.

17. Using the Patient Search fields, search for Ella Rainwater's patient record. Once you locate her in the List of Patients, confirm her date of birth.
18. Select the radio button for Ella Rainwater and click the Select button. Confirm the auto-populated details.
19. Scroll down to view the Forms section of the Patient Dashboard.
20. Select the form you prepared. The form will open in a new window, allowing you to print (Figure 2-61).

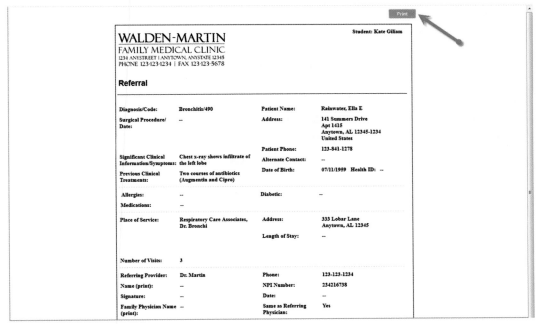

Figure 2-61 Printing the completed form.

 Now use the Back to Assignment link to complete the Post-Case Quiz found on the Info Panel for this assignment!

20. Prepare Prior Authorization Request Form for Mora Siever

▪ Objectives

- Search for a patient record.
- Access patient forms.
- Update patient information using the correct form.

▪ Overview

Mora Siever fell off her bike and injured her right knee yesterday. The physical therapist at Range of Motion Physical Therapy Group recommended a course of treatment (CPT 97110 Therapeutic exercises) including three visits over the next two weeks for the diagnosis of "right knee sprain" (ICD-10 S83.91xD). Jean Burke, NP asks you to prepare a Prior Authorization Request.

> Range of Motion
> 565 Rehab Way
> Anytown, AL 12345

▪ Competencies

- Identify types of third party claims, information required to file a third party claim, and the steps for filing a third party claim, CAAHEP VIII.C-1, ABHES 7-d
- Interact professionally with third party representatives, CAAHEP VIII.A-1, ABHES 5-h, 7-d
- Obtain precertification or preauthorization including documentation, CAAHEP VIII.P-3, ABHES 7-a, 7-d
- Organize a patient's medical record, CAAHEP VI.P-4, ABHES 7-a, 7-b
- Describe processes for verification of eligibility for services, precertification, and preauthorization, CAAHEP VIII.C-3

Estimated completion time: 20 minutes

Measurable Steps

1. Click on the Form Repository icon (Figure 2-62).

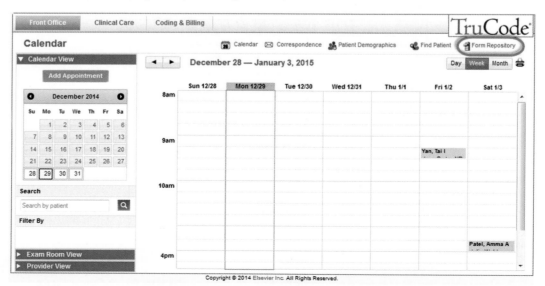

Figure 2-62 Form Repository icon.

2. Select Prior Authorization Request from the Patient Forms section of the left Info Panel.
3. Click the Patient Search button to perform a patient search and assign the form to Mora Siever.

◎ **HELPFUL HINT**

Performing a patient search before completing a form helps to ensure accurate documentation.

---

4. Confirm the auto-populated details.
5. Document "Jean Burke, NP" in the Ordering Physician Field.
6. Document your name in the Provider Contact Name field.
7. Document "Range of Motion, 565 Rehab Way, Anytown, AL 12345" in the Place of Service/Treatment and Address field.
8. Document "Therapeutic exercises" in the Service Requested field.
9. Document the current date as the Starting Service Date field.
10. Document the date two weeks from the current date as the Ending Service Date field.
11. Document "Three visits" in the Service Frequency field.
12. Document "S83.91xD Sprain of unspecified site of right knee" in the Diagnosis/ICD Code field.
13. Document "97110" in the Procedure/CPT Code(s) field.
14. Select the Yes radio button to indicate that this treatment is injury related.
15. Select the No radio button to indicate that this injury is not Worker's Compensation related (Figure 2-63).

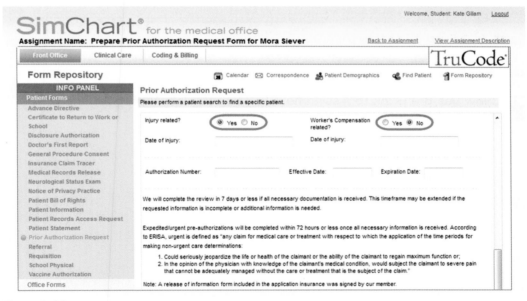

Figure 2-63 Injury and Worker's Compensation radio buttons.

16. Document yesterday's date as the Date of Injury.
17. Click the Save to Patient Record button. Select the date and click OK.
18. Click on the Find Patient icon.
19. Using the Patient Search fields, search for Mora Siever's patient record. Once you locate her in the List of Patients, confirm her date of birth.
20. Select the radio button for Mora Siever and click the Select button. Confirm the auto-populated details.

21. Scroll down to view the Forms section of the Patient Dashboard (Figure 2-64).

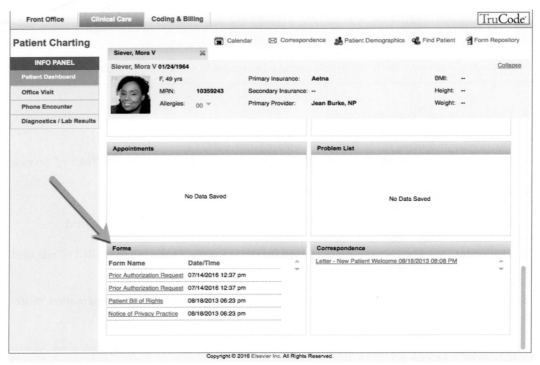

Figure 2-64 Select the form you prepared.

22. Select the form you prepared. The form will open in a new window, allowing you to print.

⊡ Now use the Back to Assignment link to complete the Post-Case Quiz found on the Info Panel for this assignment!

Unit 3 | Clinical Care

Objectives

- Search for a patient record.
- Schedule an appointment.
- Compose professional communication.
- Document patient information and education in the patient record.
- Order a procedure and document orders in the patient record.
- Create a lab requisition.
- Upload and document lab and test results.
- Document and update the problem list.
- Document diagnostic codes.
- Prepare a prescription refill.

Module Overview

The Clinical Care module features all of the clinical charting for a patient record. Students can update administered vaccines in Immunizations, in addition to documenting a comprehensive medical history in Health History. The Vital Signs record section is presented in the same order that a medical assistant would obtain this information in an exam room. Progress Notes are displayed using the SOAP format in order to help differentiate between subjective and objective information.

To enter this module, click the Clinical Care tab or the Find Patient icon at the top of the screen.

 HELPFUL HINT

Selecting a patient directs you to the Patient Dashboard, which displays patient demographics, a summary of charted information, and encounters. You must create a patient encounter before documenting in order to tie documentation to a specific date and time. Encounter types are Annual Exam, Comprehensive Visit, Follow-Up/Established Visit, New Patient Visit, Urgent Visit, Wellness Exam, 6 Month Visit, and Phone Encounter. You can also document test results by selecting the Diagnostic/Lab Results tab in the Info Panel.

When you create a patient encounter, the Record dropdown menu is automatically expanded to display the record sections available for documentation.

See the following pages for assignments related to the Clinical Care module.

Clinical Care

21. Schedule Appointment and Order X-Ray for Mora Siever

■ Objectives

- Search for a patient record.
- Schedule an appointment.
- Order a procedure.

■ Overview

Jean Burke, NP is treating Mora Siever for depression. At their last visit, Jean suggested she spend some time with her friends. Mora Siever took her advice and went cycling with friends last Monday. During the trip, she fell off her bike and injured her left knee. Schedule an appointment, order a left knee x-ray (ICD-10 code of M25.562) to be done prior to the appointment, and complete the Requisition form located in the Form Repository. She can come in any time today.

■ Competencies

- Create a patient's medical record, CAAHEP VI.P-3, ABHES 7-b
- Display sensitivity when managing appointments, CAAHEP VI.A-1, ABHES, 5-h, 7-e, 10-b
- Identify critical information required for scheduling patient procedures, CAAHEP VI.C-3, ABHES 7-a, 7-e
- Identify different types of appointment scheduling methods, CAAHEP VI.C-1, ABHES 7-e
- Manage appointment schedule, using established priorities, CAAHEP VI.P-1, ABHES 7-e
- Use medical terminology correctly and pronounced accurately to communicate information to providers and patients, CAAHEP V.P-3, ABHES 3-a, 7-g
- Utilize medical necessity guideline, CAAHEP IX.P-3, ABHES 7-d

Estimated completion time: 30 minutes

Measurable Steps

1. Click on the Add Appointment button or anywhere within the calendar to open the New Appointment window (Figure 3-1).
2. Select the Patient Visit radio button as the Appointment Type.
3. Select Urgent Visit from the Visit Type dropdown.
4. Document "left knee injury" in the Chief Complaint text box.
5. Select the Search Existing Patients radio button.
6. Using the Patient Search fields, search for Mora Siever's patient record. Once you locate her in the List of Patients, confirm her date of birth.

> ◎ **HELPFUL HINT**
>
> Confirming date of birth will help to ensure that you have located the correct patient record.

7. Select the radio button for Mora Siever and click the Select button. Confirm the auto-populated details.
8. Select Jean Burke, NP from the Provider dropdown.
9. Use the calendar picker to confirm or select the appointment day.
10. Select a start and end time for the appointment using the Start Time and End Time dropdowns.
11. Click the Save button.
12. Mora Siever's appointment will appear on the calendar.
13. Click on the Find Patient icon (Figure 3-2).

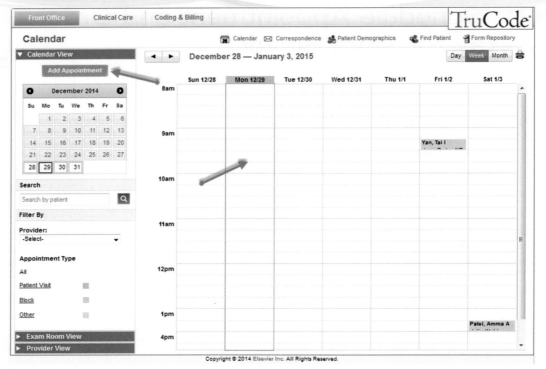

Figure 3-1 Add Appointment.

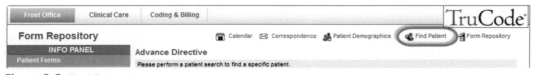

Figure 3-2 Find Patient icon.

14. Using the Patient Search fields, search for Mora Siever's patient record.
15. Select the radio button for Mora Siever and click the Select button.
16. Confirm the auto-populated details such as date of birth.
17. Create a new encounter by clicking Office Visit in the left Info Panel (Figure 3-3).

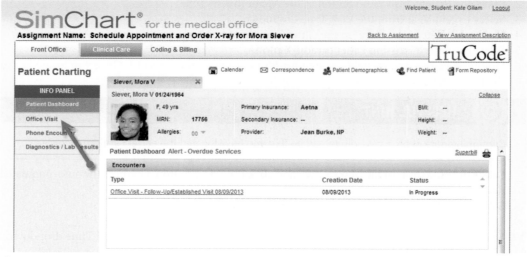

Figure 3-3 Office Visit in the left Info Panel.

18. Select Add New to create the encounter.
19. In the Create New Encounter window, select Urgent Visit from the Visit Type dropdown.
20. Select Jean Burke, NP in the Provider dropdown.
21. Click the Save button.
22. Select Order Entry from the Record dropdown menu that is already open. The menu will close once you navigate away from this screen.
23. Click the Add button below the Out-of-Office grid to add an order.
24. In the Add Order window, select Requisitions from the Order dropdown menu.
25. Select Radiology from the Requisition Type dropdown menu.
26. Document "left knee x-ray" in the Notes field.
27. Document any additional information provided and click the Save button. The grid will display the new order.

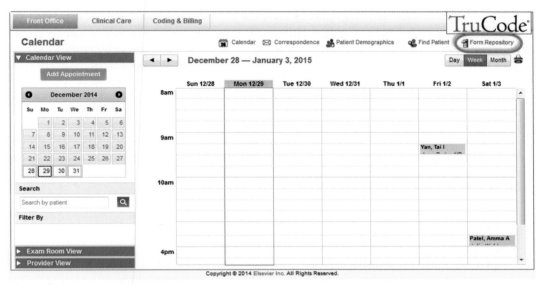

Figure 3-4 Form Repository.

28. Click the Form Repository icon (Figure 3-4).
29. Select the Requisition form from the left Info Panel.
30. Select Radiology from the Requisition Type dropdown menu.
31. Click the Patient Search button to assign the form to Mora Siever. Patient demographics will auto-populate.
32. Confirm the auto-populated details.
33. In the Diagnosis field, document "left knee pain."
34. In the Diagnosis Code field, document the ICD-10 code of M25.562.
35. In the X-ray field, select the 'L' checkbox for Knee.
36. Complete any additional necessary fields and click the Save to Patient Record button. Select the date and click OK.
37. Click on the Find Patient icon.
38. Using the Patient Search fields, search for Mora Siever's patient record. Once you locate her in the List of Patients, confirm her date of birth.
39. Select the radio button for Mora Siever and click the Select button. Confirm the auto-populated details.
40. Scroll down to view the Forms section of the Patient Dashboard.
41. Select the form you prepared.
42. The form will open in a new window, allowing you to print.

 Now use the Back to Assignment link to complete the Post-Case Quiz found on the Info Panel for this assignment.

22. Schedule Appointment and Order Procedures for Aaron Jackson

■ **Objectives**

- Search for a patient record.
- Document an order.
- Schedule an appointment.

■ **Overview**

Patricia Jackson has brought her son Aaron in to see Dr. Walden due to an increased ostomy output and decreased appetite. Aaron was born at 38 weeks gestation by cesarean section due to Patricia Jackson's worsening hypertension. He was diagnosed with Hirschsprung's disease (ICD-10 code of Q43.1) at two months of age and a colostomy was placed at that time. He was hospitalized at Anytown Hospital six weeks ago for the same issue. Aaron is on breast milk that is supplemented with formula and is up to date with vaccinations. He is sleeping throughout the night. Some activities are slightly delayed for his age. His stool is usually green and foul smelling from colostomy. Dr. Walden orders an outpatient abdominal x-ray from Anytown Radiology, a CBC, and a stool culture from Anytown Lab. Schedule a follow-up appointment four days from today's date, enter the orders in Order Entry, and create requisitions (in the Form Repository) for the orders. The appointment should be for 15 minutes at 9:30 am.

■ **Competencies**

- Create a patient's medical record, CAAHEP VI.P-3, ABHES 7-b
- Display sensitivity when managing appointments, CAAHEP VI.A-1, ABHES, 5-h, 7-e, 10-b
- Identify critical information required for scheduling patient procedures, CAAHEP VI.C-3, ABHES 7-e
- Manage appointment schedule, using established priorities, CAAHEP VI.P-1, ABHES 7-e
- Recognize and understand various treatment protocols, ABHES 7-d
- Identify the anatomical location of major organs in each body system, CAAHEP I.C-5
- Instruct and prepare a patient for a procedure or a treatment, CAAHEP I.P-8
- Describe dietary nutrients including carbohydrates, fat, protein, minerals, electrolytes, vitamins, fiber, and water, CAAHEP IV.C-1
- Instruct a patient according to patient's special dietary needs, CAAHEP IV.P-1
- Show awareness of patient's concerns regarding a dietary change, CAAHEP IV.A-1

Estimated completion time: 40 minutes

Measurable Steps

1. Click on the Add Appointment button or anywhere within the calendar to open the New Appointment window.
2. Select the Patient Visit radio button as the Appointment Type.
3. Select Follow-Up/Established Visit from the Visit Type dropdown.
4. Document "increased ostomy output and decreased appetite" in the Chief Complaint text box.
5. Select the Search Existing Patients radio button.
6. Using the Patient Search fields, search for Aaron's patient record. Once you locate Aaron in the List of Patients, confirm his date of birth.
7. Select the radio button for Aaron Jackson and click the Select button. Confirm the auto-populated details.

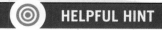 **HELPFUL HINT**

Confirming date of birth will help to ensure that you have located the correct patient record.

8. Select Julie Walden, MD from the Provider dropdown.
9. Use the calendar picker to confirm or select the appointment day.
10. Select a start and end time for the appointment using the Start Time and End Time dropdowns.
11. Click the Save button.
12. Aaron's appointment will appear on the calendar.
13. Click on the Find Patient icon.
14. Using the Patient Search fields, search for Aaron's patient record.
15. Select the radio button for Aaron Jackson and click the Select button.
16. Confirm the auto-populated details such as date of birth.
17. Create a new encounter by clicking Office Visit in the left Info Panel (Figure 3-5).

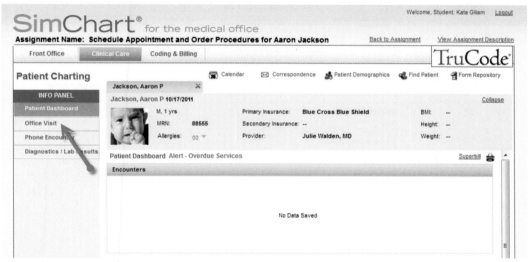

Figure 3-5 Office Visit in the left Info Panel.

18. In the Create New Encounter window, select Follow-Up/Established from the Visit Type dropdown.
19. Select Julie Walden, MD in the Provider dropdown.
20. Click the Save button.
21. Select Order Entry from the Record dropdown menu that is already open.
22. Click the Add button below the Out-of-Office grid to add an order.
23. In the Add Order window, select Requisitions from the Order dropdown menu.
24. Select Radiology from the Requisition Type dropdown menu.
25. Document "Anytown Radiology" in the Facility field.
26. Document "abdominal x-ray" in the Notes field.
27. Click the Save button.
28. Click the Add button below the Out-of-Office grid to add an order.
29. In the Add Order window, select Requisitions from the Order dropdown menu.
30. Select Laboratory from the Requisition Type dropdown menu.
31. Document "Anytown Lab" in the Facility field.
32. Document "CBC and stool culture" in the Notes field.
33. Document any additional information provided and click the Save button. The Out-of-Office grid will display the new order.
34. Click the Form Repository icon (Figure 3-6).

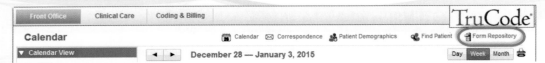

Figure 3-6 Form Repository.

35. Select the Requisition form from the left Info Panel.
36. Select Radiology from the Requisition Type dropdown menu.

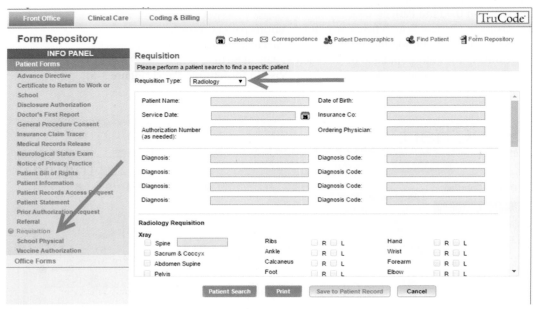

Figure 3-7 Select the Requisition Type and do a patient search.

37. Click the Patient Search button to assign the form to Aaron. Patient demographics will auto-populate. Confirm the auto-populated details before documenting in the form.
38. Document "Hirschsprung's disease" in the Diagnosis field.
39. In the Diagnosis Code field, document the ICD-10 code of Q43.1 (Figure 3-8).
40. In the X-ray field, select the Abdomen Supine checkbox.
41. Complete any additional necessary fields and click the Save to Patient Record button. Confirm the date and click OK.
42. Select the Requisition form from the left Info Panel.
43. Select Laboratory from the Requisition Type dropdown menu.
44. Click the Patient Search button to assign the form to Aaron. Patient demographics will auto-populate.
45. Document "Hirschsprung's disease" in the Diagnosis field.
46. In the Diagnosis Code field, document the ICD-10 code of Q43.1.
47. In the Microbiology field, select the Occult Blood Stool checkbox.
48. In the Laboratory Tests field, select the CBC checkbox.
49. Complete any additional necessary fields and click the Save to Patient Record button. Confirm the date and click OK.
50. Click on the Find Patient icon.

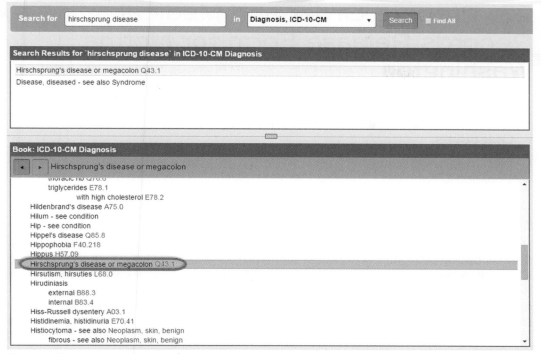

Search for [hirschsprung disease] in [Diagnosis, ICD-10-CM ▼] [Search] ☰ Find All

Search Results for "hirschsprung disease" in ICD-10-CM Diagnosis

Hirschsprung's disease or megacolon Q43.1
Disease, diseased - see also Syndrome

Book: ICD-10-CM Diagnosis

◀ ▶ | Hirschsprung's disease or megacolon

thoracic rib Q76.6
   triglycerides E78.1
       with high cholesterol E78.2
Hildenbrand's disease A75.0
Hilum - see condition
Hip - see condition
Hippel's disease Q85.8
Hippophobia F40.218
Hippus H57.09
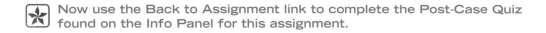
Hirschsprung's disease or megacolon Q43.1
Hirsutism, hirsuties L68.0
Hirudiniasis
       external B88.3
       internal B83.4
Hiss-Russell dysentery A03.1
Histidinemia, histidinuria E70.41
Histiocytoma - see also Neoplasm, skin, benign
       fibrous - see also Neoplasm, skin, benign

Figure 3-8 Expand the Q43.1 code.

51. Using the Patient Search fields, search for Aaron's patient record. Once you locate Aaron in the List of Patients, confirm his date of birth.
52. Select the radio button for Aaron Jackson and click the Select button. Confirm the auto-populated details.
53. Within the Patient Dashboard, scroll down to view saved forms in the Forms section.
54. Select the form you prepared. The form will open in a new window, allowing you to print.

✦ Now use the Back to Assignment link to complete the Post-Case Quiz found on the Info Panel for this assignment.

23. Prepare Order and Medical Records Release Form for Norma Washington

■ Objectives

- Search for a patient record.
- Document an order.
- Access patient forms.

■ Overview

Norma Washington is calling the medical office because her right knee pain (Right Knee Degenerative Joint Disease-unilateral primary osteoarthritis) makes it difficult for her to get around in public. She would like to have a standard wheelchair to help her ambulate and decrease her risk of falling. Norma Washington is eligible for a grant to cover the wheelchair cost and must prove medical necessity in order to qualify. The committee offering the grant, Happy Helpers, requests copies of her most recent progress note. Happy Helpers also requires a signed doctor's order from Dr. Martin for the wheelchair. Document the phone message, input an order for the wheelchair via Order Entry, and complete the Medical Records Release form.

> Happy Helpers
> 107 Hope Drive
> Anytown, AL 12345
> 123-123-8956

■ Competencies

- Apply HIPAA rules in regard to privacy and the release of information, CAAHEP X.P-2, ABHES 4-h
- Define medical necessity as it applies to procedural and diagnostic coding, CAAHEP IX.C-5, ABHES 7-d
- Protect the integrity of the medical record, CAAHEP X.A-2, ABHES 4-a
- Use medical terminology correctly and pronounced accurately to communicate information to providers and patients, CAAHEP V.P-3, ABHES 3-a, 7-g

Estimated completion time: 40 minutes

Measurable Steps

1. Click on the Find Patient icon.
2. Using the Patient Search fields, search for Ms. Washington's patient record. Once you locate her in the List of Patients, confirm her date of birth.

 HELPFUL HINT

Confirming date of birth will help to ensure that you have located the correct patient record.

3. Select the radio button for Norma Washington and click the Select button.
4. Create a new encounter by clicking Phone Encounter in the left Info Panel.
5. In the Create New Encounter window, document "Norma Washington" in the Caller field.
6. Select James A. Martin, MD from the Provider dropdown.
7. Document "Patient requesting documentation to get wheelchair for ambulation and to decrease risk of falls. Needs progress note and order sent to Happy Helpers." in the Message field.

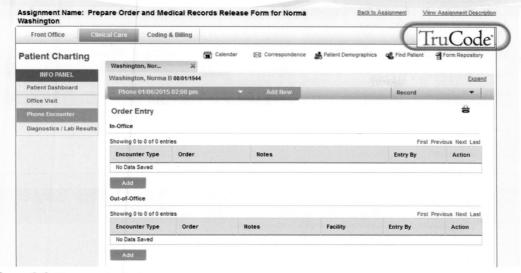

Figure 3-9 The encoder tool.

8. Click the Save button.
9. Select Order Entry from the Record dropdown menu that is already open.
10. Select the TruCode encoder link in the top right corner. The encoder tool will open in a new tab (Figure 3-9).
11. Enter "Right Knee DJD" in the Search field and select Diagnosis ICD-10-CM from the corresponding dropdown menu.
12. Click the Search button.
13. Click the code M17.9 that appears in red to expand this code and confirm that it is the most specific code available (Figure 3-10).

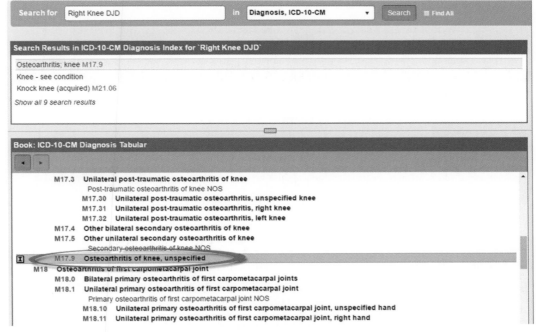

Figure 3-10 Expand the M17.9 code.

Clinical Care

14. Copy the code M17.11 for "Unilateral primary osteoarthritis, right knee" that populates in the search results (Figure 3-11).

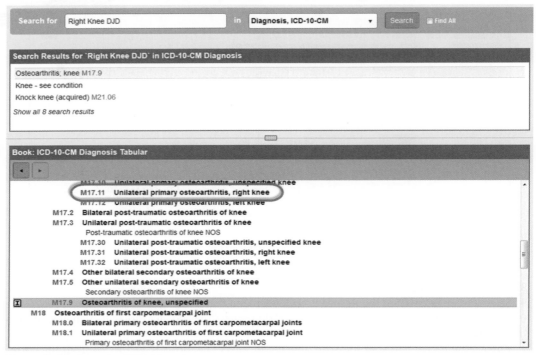

Figure 3-11 Copy the M17.11 code.

15. Click the Add button below the Out-of-Office grid to add an order.
16. In the Add Order window, select Blank Prescription from the Order dropdown menu.
17. Paste the diagnosis code retrieved from TruCode into the Blank Prescription.
18. Return to the TruCode tab and enter "Standard Wheelchair" in the Search field and select HCPCS Tabular from the corresponding dropdown menu. Click Search.
19. Click Show all 25 search results (Figure 3-12).

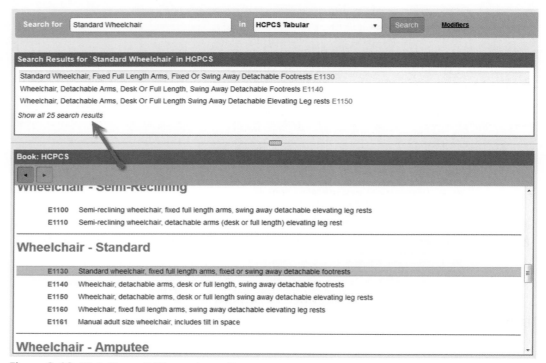

Figure 3-12 Click Show all 25 search results.

20. Click on the code Standard Wheelchair K0001 to confirm that this is the correct code.
21. Copy the code for Standard Wheelchair K0001 that populates in the search results (Figure 3-13).

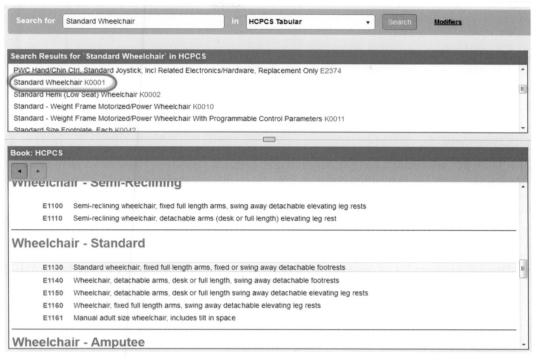

Figure 3-13 K0001 code for Standard Wheelchair.

22. Paste the HCPCS code retrieved from the encoder into the Blank Prescription.
23. Compose the text for the order of the standard wheelchair to be used due to Rt knee DJD.
24. Document "Wheelchair" in the Notes field.
25. Fill out remaining fields as appropriate.
26. Click the Save button. The Out-of-Office grid will display the new order.
27. Select the Edit icon for the order you prepared and hit the Print button.
28. Click the Form Repository icon.
29. Select the Medical Records Release form from the left Info Panel.
30. Click the Patient Search button to assign the record to Norma Washington. Patient demographics will auto-populate.
31. Confirm the auto-populated details, document any additional information needed, and click the Save to Patient Record button. Confirm the date and click OK.
32. Click on the Find Patient icon.
33. Using the Patient Search fields, search for Norma Washington's patient record. Once you locate her in the List of Patients, confirm her date of birth.
34. Select the radio button for Norma Washington and click the Select button. Confirm the auto-populated details.
35. Select the form you prepared. The form will open in a new window, allowing you to print.

> Now use the Back to Assignment link to complete the Post-Case Quiz found on the Info Panel for this assignment.

Clinical Care

24. Schedule Appointment and Update Problem List for Ella Rainwater

■ Objectives

- Search for a patient record.
- Schedule an appointment.
- Update the problem list.

■ Overview

Ella Rainwater has decided that she needs to quit smoking cigarettes. She would like to make an appointment with Dr. Martin for Friday at 4:00 pm to discuss available resources for her tobacco dependence. Schedule an appointment for 15 minutes, document the phone encounter, and add tobacco dependence to Ella Rainwater's problem list using ICD-10 coding.

■ Competencies

- Develop a current list of community resources related to patients' healthcare needs, CAAHEP V.P-9, ABHES 8-i
- Display sensitivity when managing appointments, CAAHEP VI.A-1, ABHES, 5-h, 7-e, 10-b
- Document patient care accurately in the medical record, CAAHEP X.P-3, ABHES 4-a
- Identify different types of appointment scheduling methods, CAAHEP VI.C-1, ABHES 7-e
- Manage the appointment schedule, using established priorities, CAAHEP VI.P-1, ABHES 7-e
- Report relevant information concisely and accurately, CAAHEP V.P-11, ABHES 7-d
- Utilize an EMR, CAAHEP VI.P-6, ABHES 7-b

Estimated completion time: 25 minutes

Measurable Steps

1. Click on the Add Appointment button or anywhere within the calendar to open the New Appointment window (Figure 3-14).
2. Select the Patient Visit radio button as the Appointment Type.
3. Select Follow-Up /Established Visit from the Visit Type dropdown.
4. Document "tobacco dependence" in the Chief Complaint text box.
5. Select the Search Existing Patients radio button.
6. Using the Patient Search fields, search for Ella Rainwater's patient record. Once you locate her in the List of Patients, confirm her date of birth.

 HELPFUL HINT

Confirming date of birth will help to ensure that you have located the correct patient record.

7. Select the radio button for Ella Rainwater and click the Select button. Confirm the auto-populated details.
8. Select James A. Martin, MD from the Provider dropdown.
9. Use the calendar picker to select Friday for the appointment day.
10. Select a start time of 4:00 pm and end time of 4:15 pm for the appointment using the Start Time and End Time dropdowns.

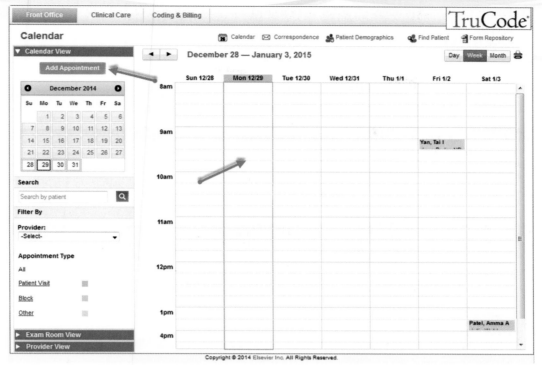

Figure 3-14 Add Appointment.

11. Click the Save button.
12. Ella Rainwater's appointment will be displayed on the calendar.
13. Click on the Find Patient icon (Figure 3-15).

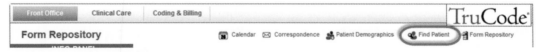

Figure 3-15 Find Patient icon.

14. Using the Patient Search fields, search for Ella Rainwater's patient record. Once you locate her patient record in the List of Patients, confirm her date of birth.
15. Select the radio button for Ella Rainwater and click the Select button.
16. Create a new encounter by clicking Phone Encounter in the left Info Panel.
17. Document "Ella Rainwater" in the Caller field.
18. Document "Ella Rainwater wants to quit smoking and would like to discuss available resources." Click the Save button.
19. Select Problem List from the Record dropdown menu.
20. Click the Add Problem button to add a problem.
21. In the Add Problem window, document "Tobacco dependence" in the Diagnosis field.
22. Select the ICD-10 Code radio button and place the cursor in the text box to access the TruCode encoder.

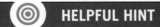 **HELPFUL HINT**

Accessing the encoder tool this way will auto-populate any selected codes where the cursor is placed.

23. Enter "tobacco dependency" in the Search field and select Diagnosis, ICD-10-CM from the dropdown menu.
24. Click the Search button.
25. Click "Dependence, drug, nicotine (Figure 3-16).

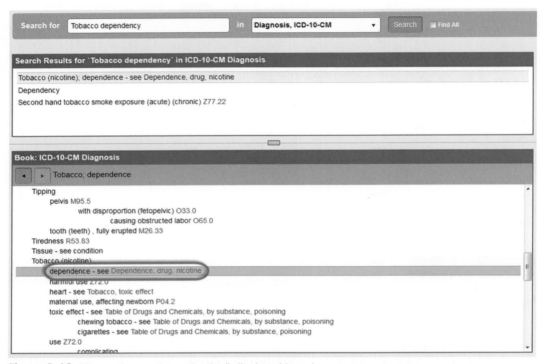

Figure 3-16 "Dependence, drug, nicotine" displayed in red.

26. Click the code F17.200 to expand this code and confirm that it is the most specific code available (Figure 3-17).

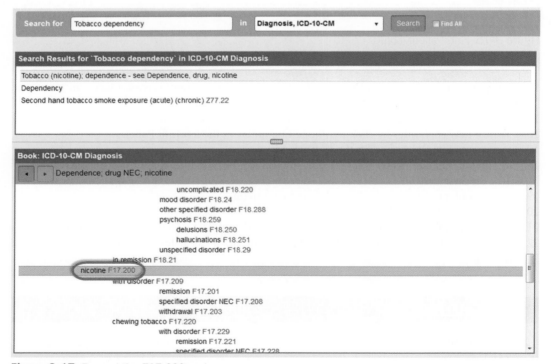

Figure 3-17 Expand the F17.200 code.

27. Click the code F17.200 for "Nicotine dependence, unspecified, uncomplicated" that appears in the tree. This code will auto-populate in the ICD-10 field of the Add Problem window (Figure 3-18).

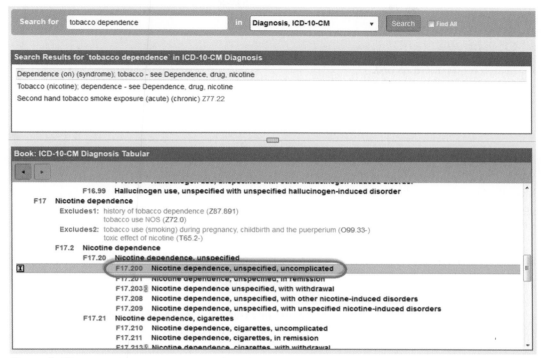

Figure 3-18 Populating the code in the ICD-10 field of the Add Problem window.

28. Document the current date in the Date Identified field.
29. Select the Active radio button in the Status field.
30. Click the Save button. The Problem List table will display the new problem.

 Now use the Back to Assignment link to complete the Post-Case Quiz found on the Info Panel for this assignment.

25. Upload Test Results and Prepare Lab Results Letter for Julia Berkley

■ Objectives

- Search for a patient record.
- Upload test results.
- Create a patient letter.
- Compose professional communication.

■ Overview

Walden-Martin just received the report for Julia Berkley's mammogram and the results are normal. It is office policy to notify patients of normal lab results via mail. Upload the results (the results are posted on the assignment description page in SimChart) to Julia Berkley's patient record and prepare a normal lab results letter.

■ Competencies

- Describe filing indexing rules, CAAHEP VI.C-7, ABHES 7-a
- Utilize an EMR, CAAHEP VI.P-6, ABHES 7-b
- Instruct and prepare a patient for a procedure or a treatment, CAAHEP I.P-8
- Reassure a patient of the accuracy of the test results, CAAHEP II.A-1

Estimated completion time: 30 minutes

Measurable Steps

1. On the assignment description page, locate Julia Berkley's test results in the Assignment Attachments section. Save the results to your computer. You will need to upload the results to Julia's patient record.
1. Click on the Find Patient icon.
2. Using the Patient Search fields, search for Julia Berkley's patient record. Once you locate her in the List of Patients, confirm her date of birth.

 HELPFUL HINT

Confirming date of birth will help to ensure that you have located the correct patient record.

3. Select the radio button for Julia Berkley and click the Select button.
4. Select Diagnostics/Lab Results in the left Info Panel (Figure 3-19).
5. Click the Add button.
6. Document the date in the Date field.
7. Select Radiology from the Type dropdown menu.
8. Document "Mammogram results" in the Notes field.
9. Click the Browse button to upload the results. Select the file to upload.
10. Click the Save button. The Diagnostic/Lab Results grid will display the new order.
11. Click on the Correspondence icon (Figure 3-20).
12. Select the Normal Test Results template from the Letters section of the left Info Panel.
13. Click the Patient Search button to perform a patient search and assign the letter to Julia Berkley.

Clinical Care

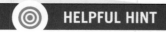
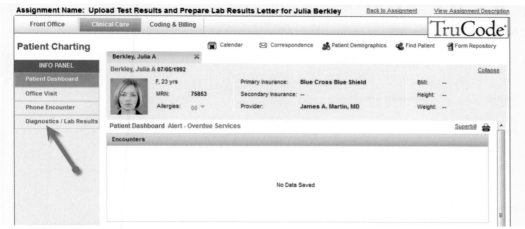

Figure 3-19 Diagnostic/Lab Results in the left Info Panel.

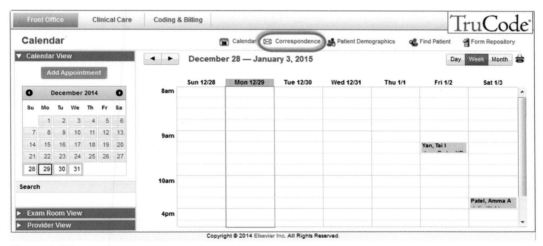

Figure 3-20 Correspondence icon.

14. Confirm the auto-populated details and document any additional information needed.
15. Click the Save to Patient Record button. Confirm the date and click OK.
16. Click on the Find Patient icon.
17. Using the Patient Search fields, search for Julia Berkley's patient record. Once you locate her in the List of Patients, confirm her date of birth.
18. Select the radio button for Julia Berkley and click the Select button. Confirm the auto-populated details.
19. Scroll down to view the Correspondence section of the Patient Dashboard.
20. Select the letter you prepared. The letter will open in a new window, allowing you to print (Figure 3-21).

WALDEN-MARTIN
FAMILY MEDICAL CLINIC
1234 ANYSTREET | ANYTOWN, ANYSTATE 12345
PHONE 123-123-1234 | FAX 123-123-5678

Normal Test Results

To:	j.berkley@anytown.mail
Cc:	--
Subject:	Mammogram results

Date:	04/02/2015
Addressee Name:	Berkley, Julia A
Address:	11 Mermaid Avenue Anytown, AL 12345-1234 United States

Dear Julia Berkley,

This letter is to inform you of recent test results. Your procedure, mammogram performed on January 23, 20XX was within normal limits.

If you have any additional questions or are still experiencing problems related to this test, please call our office at 123-123-1234 as soon as possible to speak with the Medical Assistant.

Thank you for choosing Walden-Martin Family Medical Clinic for your healthcare needs.
Our office is open Monday-Friday 8-6pm.

Sincerely,

Walden-Martin Family Medical Clinic

Jennifer Bertucci

Figure 3-21 The letter will open in a new window.

 Now use the Back to Assignment link to complete the Post-Case Quiz found on the Info Panel for this assignment.

Clinical Care

26. Update Problem List and Document Vital Signs for Aaron Jackson

■ Objectives

- Search for a patient record.
- Document in the problem list.
- Document diagnostic codes.
- Document vital signs.

■ Overview

Aaron Jackson is in the office today for an urgent visit with Dr. Walden. He was born at 38 weeks gestation by cesarean section due to Patricia Jackson's worsening hypertension. He was diagnosed with Hirschsprung's disease at two months of age and a colostomy was placed at that time. The medical assistant obtains Aaron's vital signs as HT: 24 in, WT: 16 lbs, HC: 18 in, T: 99.6°F (TA), P: 124 (Apical). Document the vital signs and update the problem list for Aaron Jackson using ICD-10 coding.

■ Competencies

- Document on a growth chart, CAAHEP II.P-4, ABHES 4-a
- Perform diagnostic coding, CAAHEP IX.P-2, ABHES 7-d
- Identify quality assurance practices in healthcare, CAAHEP I.C-12

Estimated completion time: 30 minutes

Measurable Steps

1. Click on the Find Patient icon.
2. Using the Patient Search fields, search for Aaron's patient record. Once you locate Aaron in the List of Patients, confirm his date of birth.

> **HELPFUL HINT**
>
> Confirming date of birth will help to ensure that you have located the correct patient record.

3. Select the radio button for Aaron Jackson and click the Select button.
4. Create a new encounter by clicking Office Visit in the left Info Panel.
5. In the Create New Encounter window, select Urgent Visit from the Visit Type dropdown.
6. Select Julie Walden, MD in the Provider dropdown.
7. Click the Save button.
8. Select Vital Signs from the Record dropdown menu that is already open.
9. In the Vital Signs tab, click the Add button (Figure 3-22).
10. Document "99.6" in the Temperature field and select Forehead from the Site dropdown menu.
11. Document "124" in the Pulse field and select Apical from the Site dropdown.
12. Click Save.
13. In the Height/Weight tab, click the Add button (Figure 3-23).
14. Document "24" in the Inches field for Height.
15. Document "16" in the lb field for Weight.
16. Click Save.

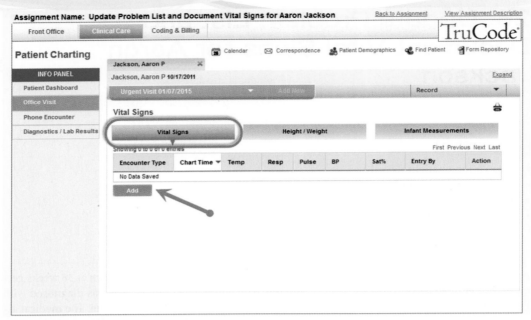

Figure 3-22 Add button in Vital Signs tab.

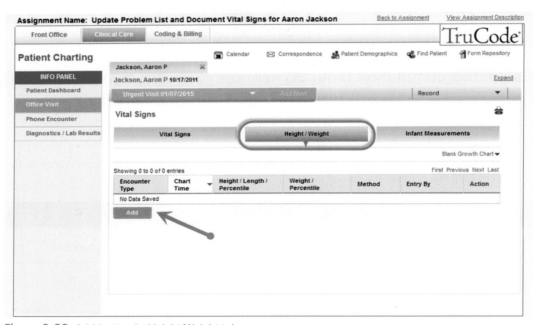

Figure 3-23 Add button in Height/Weight tab.

17. In the Infant Measurements tab, click the Add button.
18. Document "18" in the Inches field for Head Circumference.
19. Click the Save button. The Height/Weight grid will display the height and weight.
20. Select Problem List from the Record dropdown menu.
21. Click the Add Problem button to add a problem.
22. In the Add Problem window, document "Hirschsprung's disease" in the Diagnosis field.
23. Select the ICD-10 radio button and place the cursor in the text box to access the TruCode encoder (Figure 3-24).

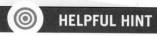

HELPFUL HINT

Accessing the encoder tool this way will auto-populate any selected codes where the cursor is placed.

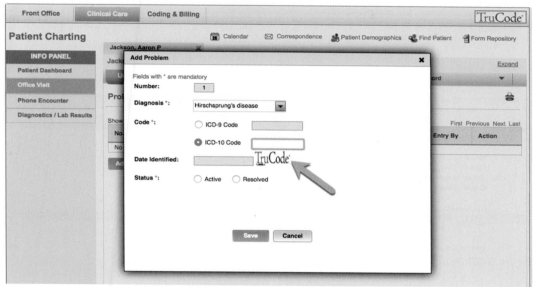

Figure 3-24 ICD-10 radio button to access TruCode encoder.

24. Enter "Hirschsprung's disease" in the Search field and select Diagnosis, ICD-10-CM from the dropdown menu.
25. Click the Search button.
26. Click the code Q43.1 to expand this code and confirm that it is the most specific code available (Figure 3-25).

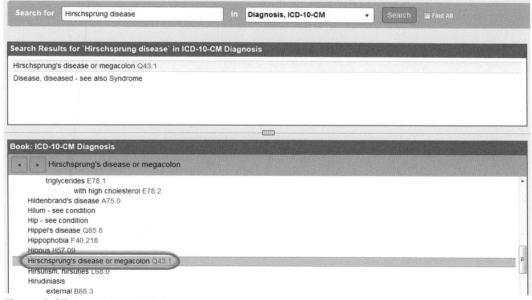

Figure 3-25 Expand the Q43.1 code.

Clinical Care

27. Click the code Q43.1 for "Hirschsprung's disease" that appears in the tree. This code will auto-populate in the ICD-10 field of the Add Problem window (Figure 3-26).

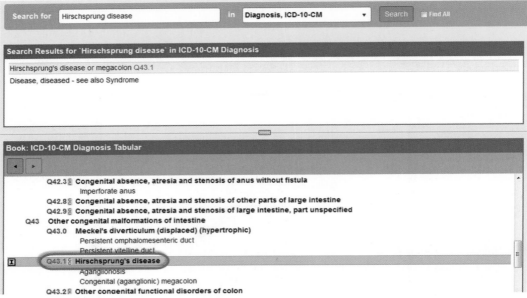

Figure 3-26 Populating the code in the ICD-10 field of the Add Problem window.

28. Document the current date in the Date Identified field.
29. Select the Active radio button in the Status field.
30. Click the Save button. The Problem List grid will display the new problem.

> Now use the Back to Assignment link to complete the Post-Case Quiz found on the Info Panel for this assignment.

27. Update Problem List for Johnny Parker

■ **Objectives**

- Search for a patient record.
- Document in the problem list.
- Document diagnostic codes.

■ **Overview**

Johnny Parker's mother, Lisa, brought him to the Walden-Martin office to see Jean Burke, NP because he presumably ingested 3900 mg of acetaminophen this morning while she was in the shower. Update the problem list for the acetaminophen poisoning using the ICD-10 CM code of T39.8x1.

■ **Competencies**

- Document patient care accurately in the medical record, CAAHEP X.P-3, ABHES 4-a
- File patient medical records, CAAHEP VI.P-5, ABHES 7-a
- Perform diagnostic coding, ABHES 8-c.3, CAAHEP IX.P-2, ABHES 7-d
- Describe compliance with public health statutes including communicable diseases, abuse, neglect, exploitation, and wounds of violence, CAAHEP X.C-12

Estimated completion time: 20 minutes

Measurable Steps

1. Click on the Find Patient icon.
2. Using the Patient Search fields, search for Johnny's patient record. Once you locate Johnny's patient record in the List of Patients, confirm his date of birth.

 HELPFUL HINT

Confirming date of birth will help to ensure that you have located the correct patient record.

3. Select the radio button for Johnny Parker and click the Select button.
4. Create a new encounter by clicking Office Visit in the left Info Panel.
5. In the Create New Encounter window, select Urgent Visit from the Visit Type dropdown.
6. Select Jean Burke, NP in the Provider dropdown.
7. Click the Save button.
8. Select Problem List from the Record dropdown menu that is already open.
9. Click the Add Problem button to add a problem.
10. In the Add Problem window, document "acetaminophen poisoning" in the Diagnosis field.
11. Select the ICD-10 radio button and place the cursor in the text box to access the TruCode encoder (Figure 3-27).

 HELPFUL HINT

Accessing the encoder tool this way will auto-populate any selected codes where the cursor is placed.

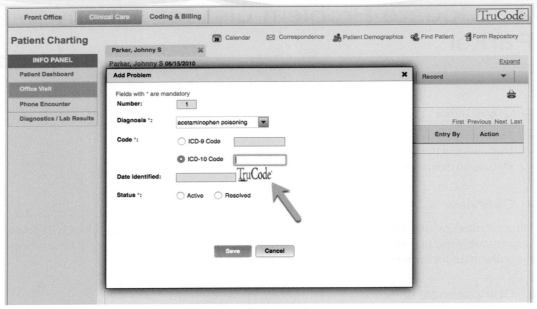

Figure 3-27 ICD-10 radio button to access TruCode encoder.

12. Enter "acetaminophen poisoning" in the Search field and select Diagnosis, ICD-10-CM from the dropdown menu.
13. Click the Search button.
14. Click the Table of Drugs and Chemicals link (Figure 3-28).

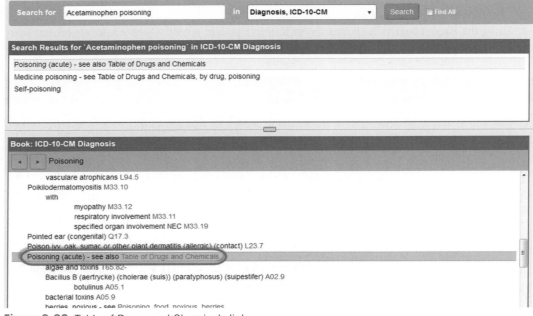

Figure 3-28 Table of Drugs and Chemicals link.

15. Scroll down to reach the row for acetaminophen and click anywhere within the row to expand the details (Figure 3-29).

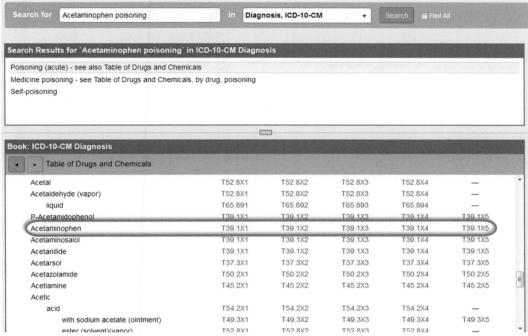

Figure 3-29 Click anywhere within the row to expand the details.

16. Click the code T39.1x1 to expand this code and confirm that it is the most specific code available (Figure 3-30).

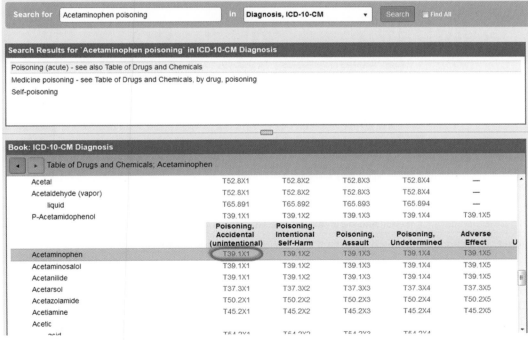

Figure 3-30 Find the most specific code available.

17. Click the black triangle to the left of the code T39.8X for "Poisoning by, adverse effect of and underdosing of other nonopioid analgesics and antipyretics, not elsewhere classified" (Figure 3-31).

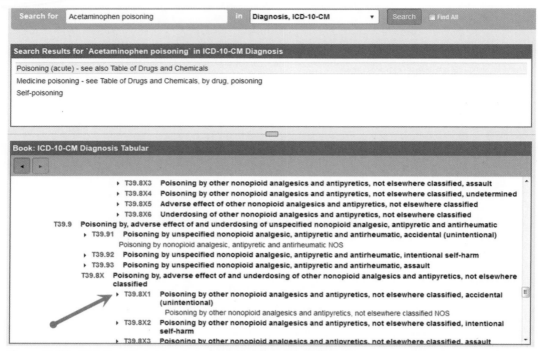

Figure 3-31 Click the black triangle to the left of the code T39.8x1A.

18. Click T38.8X1 that appears in the tree. This code will auto-populate in the ICD-10 field of the Add Problem window (or you can copy and paste this code into the field). (Figure 3-32).

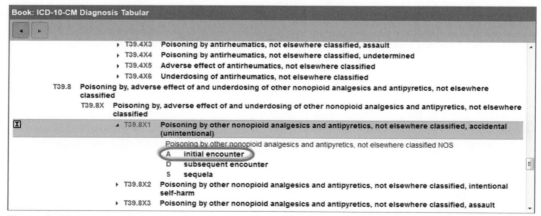

Figure 3-32 Populating the code in the ICD-10 field of the Add Problem window.

19. Document the current date in the Date Identified field.
20. Select the Active radio button in the Status field.
21. Click the Save button. The Problem List grid will display the new problem.

> ✶ Now use the Back to Assignment link to complete the Post-Case Quiz found on the Info Panel for this assignment.

28. Update Problem List for Anna Richardson

■ Objectives

- Search for a patient record.
- Document in the problem list.
- Document diagnostic codes.

■ Overview

Anna Richardson was released from the hospital two days ago following a normal vaginal delivery with postpartum hemorrhage complications. She states that she is feeling great and is not currently experiencing any pain. Document Anna Richardson's postpartum maternal care, normal vaginal delivery, and postpartum hemorrhage in the problem list using ICD-10.

■ Competencies

- Document patient care accurately in the medical record, CAAHEP X.P-3, ABHES 4-a
- Perform diagnostic coding, ABHES 8-c.3, CAAHEP IX.P-2, ABHES 7-d
- Define medical necessity as it applies to procedural and diagnostic coding, CAAHEP IX.C-5

Estimated completion time: 15 minutes

Measurable Steps

1. Click on the Find Patient icon.
2. Using the Patient Search fields, search for Anna Richardson's patient record. Once you locate her patient record in the List of Patients, confirm her date of birth.

 HELPFUL HINT

Confirming date of birth will help to ensure that you have located the correct patient record

3. Select the radio button for Anna Richardson and click the Select button.
4. Create a new encounter by clicking Office Visit in the left Info Panel. Select the Add New tab.
5. In the Create New Encounter window, select Follow-Up/Established Visit from the Visit Type dropdown.
6. Click the Save button.
7. Select Problem List from the Record dropdown menu that is already open.
8. Click the Add Problem button to add a problem.
9. In the Add Problem window, document "Postpartum maternal care" in the Diagnosis field.
10. Select the ICD-10 radio button and place the cursor in the text box to access the TruCode encoder (Figure 3-33).

 HELPFUL HINT

Accessing the encoder tool this way will auto-populate any selected codes where the cursor is placed.

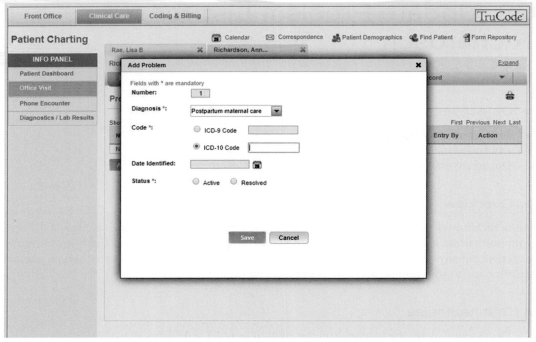

Figure 3-33 Click in text box to access TruCode encoder.

11. Enter "Postpartum maternal care" in the Search field and select Diagnosis, ICD-10-CM from the dropdown menu.
12. Click the Search button.
13. Click the code Z39.2 to expand this code and confirm that it is the most specific code available.
14. Click the code Z39.2 for "Encounter for routine postpartum follow-up" that appears in the tree. This code will auto-populate in the ICD-10 field of the Add Problem window (Figure 3-34).
15. Document the current date in the Date Identified field.
16. Select the Active radio button in the Status field.
17. Click the Save button. The Problem List grid will display the new problem.
18. Click the Add Problem button to add a problem.
19. In the Add Problem window, document "Normal vaginal delivery" in the Diagnosis field.
20. Select the ICD-10 radio button and place the cursor in the text box to access the TruCode encoder.
21. Enter "Normal vaginal delivery" in the Search field and select Diagnosis, ICD-10-CM from the dropdown menu.
22. Click the Search button.
23. Click the code O80 to expand this code and confirm that it is the most specific code available.
24. Click the code O80 for "Encounter for full-term uncomplicated delivery" that appears in the tree. This code will auto-populate in the ICD-10 field of the Add Problem window (Figure 3-35).
25. Document the current date in the Date Identified field.
26. Select the Active radio button in the Status field.
27. Click the Save button. The Problem List grid will display the new problem.
28. Click the Add Problem button to add a problem.
29. In the Add Problem window, document "Postpartum hemorrhage" in the Diagnosis field.
30. Select the ICD-10 radio button and place the cursor in the text box to access the TruCode encoder.

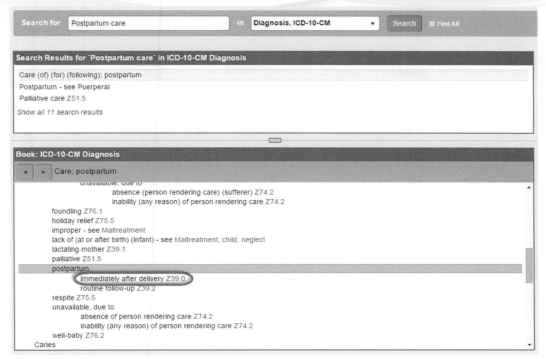

Figure 3-34 Populating the code in the ICD-10 field of the Add Problem window.

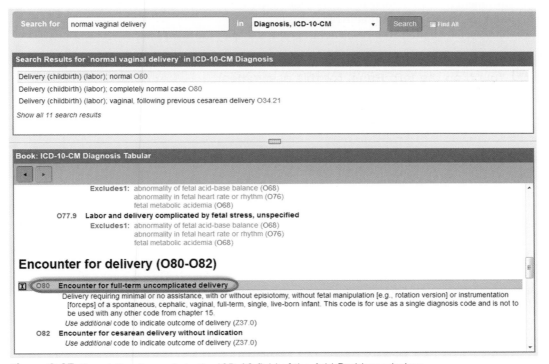

Figure 3-35 Populating the code in the ICD-10 field of the Add Problem window.

31. Enter "Postpartum hemorrhage" in the Search field and select Diagnosis, ICD-10-CM from the dropdown menu.
32. Click the Search button.
33. Click the code O72.0 to expand this code and confirm that it is the most specific code available.
34. Click the code O72.0 for "Third-stage hemorrhage" that appears in the tree. This code will auto-populate in the ICD-10 field of the Add Problem window (Figure 3-36).

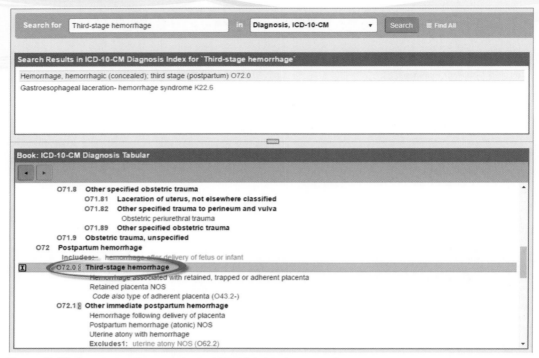

Figure 3-36 Populating the code in the ICD-10 field of the Add Problem window.

35. Document the current date in the Date Identified field.
36. Select the Active radio button in the Status field.
37. Click the Save button. The Problem List grid will display the new problem.

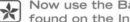 Now use the Back to Assignment link to complete the Post-Case Quiz found on the Info Panel for this assignment.

29. Update Problem List for Ella Rainwater

■ Objectives

- Search for a patient record.
- Document in the problem list.
- Document diagnostic codes.

■ Overview

Ella Rainwater has had a cold and cough for more than one week, preventing her from sleeping. After conducting an examination, Dr. Martin has determined that Ella Rainwater has bronchitis. Document her diagnosis in the problem list using ICD-10 coding.

■ Competencies

- Document patient care accurately in the medical record, CAAHEP X.P-3, ABHES 4-a
- Organize a patient's medical record, CAAHEP VI.P-4, ABHES 7-a, 7-b
- Perform diagnostic coding, CAAHEP IX.P-2, ABHES 7-d
- Define medical necessity as it applies to procedural and diagnostic coding, CAAHEP IX.C-5

Estimated completion time: 15 minutes

Measurable Steps

1. Click on the Find Patient icon.
2. Using the Patient Search fields, search for Ella Rainwater's patient record. Once you locate her in the List of Patients, confirm her date of birth.

 HELPFUL HINT

Confirming date of birth will help to ensure that you have located the correct patient record.

3. Select the radio button for Ella Rainwater and click the Select button.
4. Create a new encounter by clicking Office Visit in the left Info Panel.
5. In the Create New Encounter window, select Urgent Visit from the Visit Type dropdown.
6. Select James A. Martin, MD from the Provider dropdown.
7. Click the Save button.
8. Select Problem List from the Record dropdown menu that is already open.
9. Click the Add Problem button to add a problem.
10. In the Add Problem window, document "Bronchitis" in the Diagnosis field.
11. Select the ICD-10 radio button and place the cursor in the text box to access the TruCode encoder (Figure 3-37).

 HELPFUL HINT

Accessing the encoder tool this way will auto-populate any selected codes where the cursor is placed.

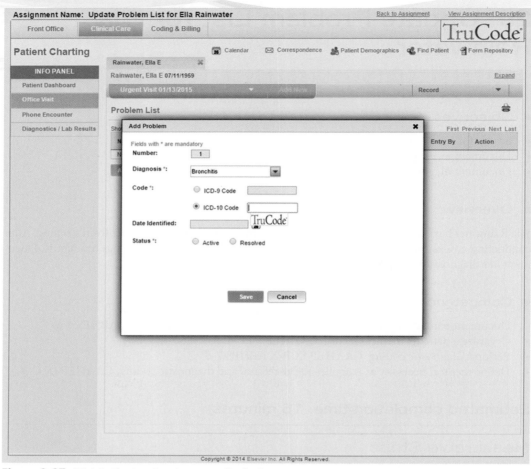

Figure 3-37 Click in the text box to access TruCode encoder.

12. Enter "Bronchitis" in the Search field and select Diagnosis, ICD-10-CM from the dropdown menu.
13. Click the Search button.
14. Click the code J40 to expand this code and confirm that it is the most specific code available (Figure 3-38).

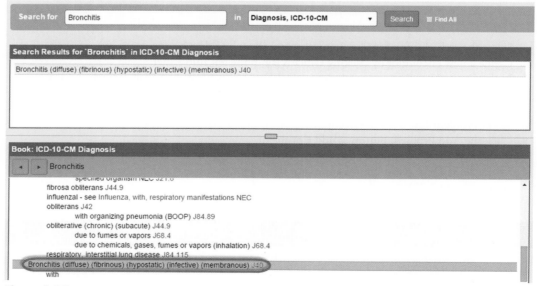

Figure 3-38 Find the most specific code available.

15. Click the code J40 for "Bronchitis, not specified as acute or chronic" that appears in the tree. This code will auto-populate in the ICD-10 field of the Add Problem window (Figure 3-39).

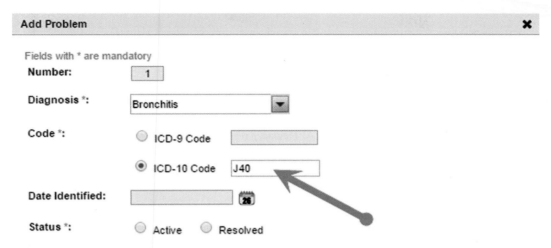

Figure 3-39 Populating the code in the ICD-10 field of the Add Problem window.

16. Document the current date in the Date Identified field.
17. Select the Active radio button in the Status field.
18. Click the Save button. The Problem List grid will display the new problem.

Now use the Back to Assignment link to complete the Post-Case Quiz found on the Info Panel for this assignment.

Clinical Care

30. Document Allergies for Al Neviaser

■ Objectives

- Search for a patient record.
- Document allergies.

■ Overview

During his appointment with Dr. Martin, Al Neviaser reported an allergy to sulfa drugs (nausea & vomiting). He also mentioned that he developed a rash from the latex gloves he wore while volunteering at the Anytown Food Pantry last week. Document Mr. Neviaser's allergies.

■ Competencies

- Document patient care accurately in the medical record, CAAHEP X.P-3, ABHES 4-a
- Explain to a patient the rationale for performance of a procedure, CAAHEP V.A-4, ABHES 5-h, 6-a
- Identify equipment and supplies needed for medical records in order to create, maintain, and store, CAAHEP VI.C-6, ABHES 7-a, 7-f
- Utilize an EMR, CAAHEP VI.P-6, ABHES 7-b

Estimated completion time: 25 minutes

Measurable Steps

1. Click on the Find Patient icon.
2. Using the Patient Search fields, search for Al Neviaser's patient record. Once you locate his patient record in the List of Patients, confirm his date of birth.

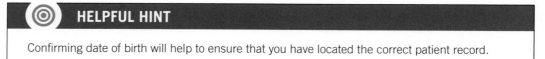

HELPFUL HINT

Confirming date of birth will help to ensure that you have located the correct patient record.

3. Select the radio button for Al Neviaser and click the Select button.
4. Create a new encounter by clicking Office Visit in the left Info Panel (Figure 3-40).

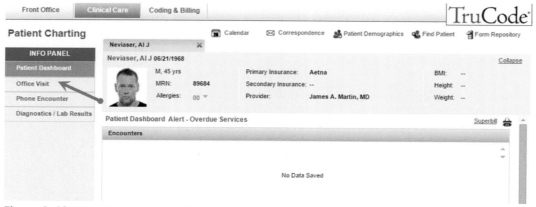

Figure 3-40 Office Visit in the Info Panel.

5. In the Create New Encounter window, select Follow-Up/Established Visit from the Visit Type dropdown.
6. Select James A. Martin, MD from the Provider dropdown.
7. Click the Save button.
8. Allergies is the first option available within the Record dropdown menu, automatically landing the user in that section of the patient chart.
9. Click the Add Allergy button to add sulfa as an allergy for Al Neviaser (Figure 3-41).

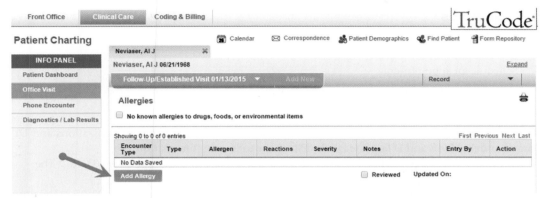

Figure 3-41 Add Allergy button.

10. Within the Add Allergy window, select the Medication radio button in the Allergy Type field.
11. Document "sulfa" in the Select Allergen field.
12. Check Nausea and Vomiting in the Reactions field.
13. Select Self in the Informant field. Select Very Reliable in the Confidence Level field.
14. Click the Save button in the Add Allergy window. The allergy you added will display in the Allergies grid (Figure 3-42).

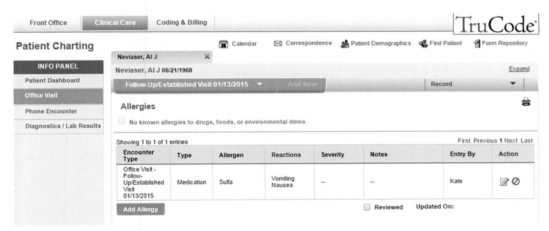

Figure 3-42 Allergies grid with added allergy.

15. Click the Add Allergy button to add latex as an allergy for Al Neviaser.
16. Select the Environmental radio button in the Allergy Type field.
17. Select Latex from the Select Allergen dropdown menu.
18. Check Itching in the Reactions field.
19. Select Self in the Informant field. Select Very Reliable in the Confidence Level field.
20. Click the Save button in the Add Allergy window. The Allergies grid will display the new allergy.

 Now use the Back to Assignment link to complete the Post-Case Quiz found on the Info Panel for this assignment.

31. Document Immunizations and Schedule Follow-up Appointment for Daniel Miller

■ Objectives

- Search for a patient record.
- Document immunizations.
- Schedule an appointment.

■ Overview

Daniel Miller has a well-child check-up with Dr. Martin. Daniel needs his immunizations and Dr. Martin orders MMR and DTaP. The labels display the following information:

MMR, Dosage: 0.5 mL. Manufacturer: Medical Corp. Lot#: K023L, Expiration: 03/15. * The dose is given IM in the left Vastus Lateralis.

DTaP, Dosage: 0.5 mL. Manufacturer: Medical Corp. Lot#: Y043L, Expiration: 02/05. * The dose is given IM in the right Vastus Lateralis.

Daniel had no reaction to the immunizations.

Dr. Martin tells Daniel's mom, Tracy Miller, to schedule another check-up in two months. Ms. Miller states Monday mornings work best for her, and well-child check-ups usually last 30 minutes.

* The year of expiration displayed on the labels should reflect an expiration date of 3 years from the current year.

■ Competencies

- Differentiate between scope of practice and standards of care for medical assistants, CAAHEP X.C-1, ABHES 1-b, 4-f
- Explain to a patient the rationale for performance of a procedure, CAAHEP V.A-4, ABHES 5-h
- Identify the abbreviations and symbols used in calculating medication dosages, CAAHEP II.C-5, ABHES 3-d, 6-c
- Maintain medication and immunization records, ABHES 4-a, 4-f
- Perform procedural coding, CAAHEP IX.P-1, ABHES 7-d
- Utilize an EMR, CAAHEP VI.P-6, ABHES 7-b

Estimated completion time: 50 minutes

Measurable Steps

1. Click on the Find Patient icon.
2. Using the Patient Search fields, search for Daniel's patient record. Once you locate Daniel's patient record in the List of Patients, confirm his date of birth.

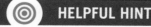

HELPFUL HINT

Confirming date of birth will help to ensure that you have located the correct patient record.

3. Select the radio button for Daniel Miller and click the Select button (Figure 3-43).
4. Confirm the auto-populated details in the Patient Header.
5. Create an encounter for Daniel by clicking Office Visit in the Info Panel to the left.

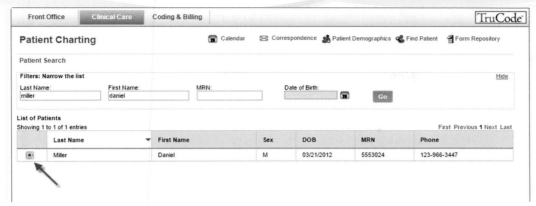

Figure 3-43 Select the radio button for Daniel Miller.

6. In the Create New Encounter window, select Follow-Up/Established Visit from the Visit Type dropdown (Figure 3-44).

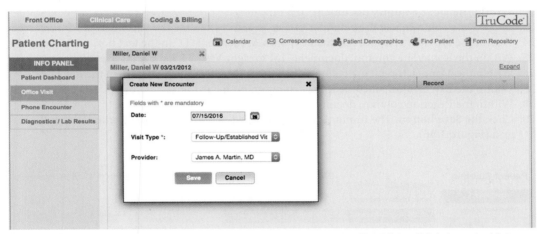

Figure 3-44 In the Create New Encounter window, select Follow-Up/Established Visit from the Visit Type dropdown, as well as a provider from the Provider dropdown.

7. Select James A. Martin, MD from the Provider dropdown (see Figure 3-44).
8. Click the Save button.
9. Select Immunizations from the Record dropdown menu that is already open.
10. Locate the row for the "MMR" vaccine and click on the green plus sign to the far right of that row. That row will become active so you can add an immunization to Daniel's record (Figure 3-45).
11. In the Type column, select MMR.
12. Within the Dose column, document "0.5 mL".
13. In the Date column, use the calendar picker to select the date the vaccine was administered.
14. Within the Provider column, document "James A. Martin, MD" in the text box.
15. Within the Route/Site column, document "left Vastus Lateralis" in the text box.
16. Within the Manufacturer/Lot# column, document "Medical Corp./K023L" in the text box.
17. Within the Exp column, document the expiration in the text box.
18. Within the Reaction column, document No Reaction in the text box.
19. Click the Save button. The immunization you added will display in the Immunization Review grid.
20. Locate the row for the "DTaP, Diptheria, Tetanus, Pertussis" vaccine and click on the green plus sign to the far right of that row. That row will become active so you can add an immunization to Daniel's record.
21. Within the Type column, select DTaP.

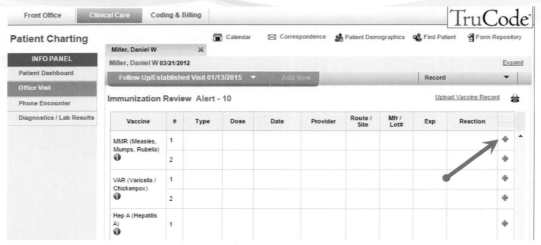

Figure 3-45 Activating a row to add an immunization.

22. Within the Dose column, document "0.5 mL".
23. In the Date column, use the calendar picker to select the date the vaccine was administered.
24. Within the Provider column, document "James A. Martin, MD" in the text box.
25. Within the Route/Site column, document "IM to right Vastus Lateralis" in the text box.
26. Within the Manufacturer/Lot# column, document "Medical Corp./Y043L" in the text box.
27. Within the Exp column, document the expiration in the text box.
28. Within the Reaction column, document No Reaction in the text box.
29. Click the Save button. The immunization you added will display in the Immunization Review grid (Figure 3-46).

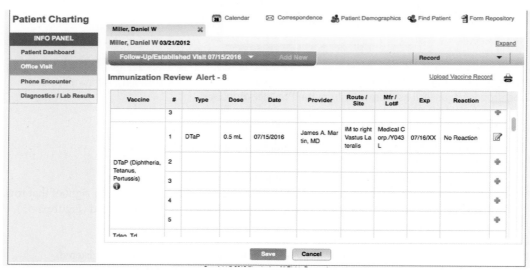

Figure 3-46 The immunization will display on the Immunization Review grid.

30. Click on the Calendar icon.
31. Within the weekly calendar, click on a time slot to open the New Appointment window.
32. Select the Patient Visit radio button as the Appointment Type.
33. Select Wellness Exam from the Visit Type dropdown.
34. Document "Well-child check-up" in the Chief Complaint text box (Figure 3-47).
35. Select the Search Existing Patients radio button.

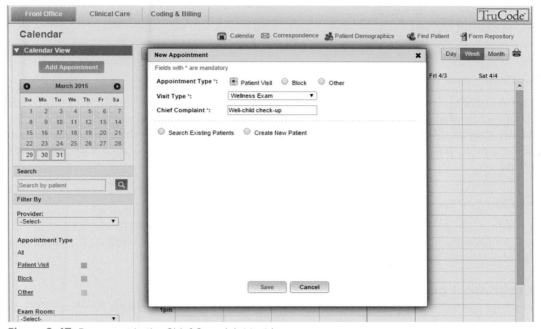

Figure 3-47 Document in the Chief Complaint text box.

36. Using the Patient Search fields, search for Daniel's patient record. Once you locate Daniel in the List of Patients, confirm his date of birth.
37. Select the radio button for Daniel Miller and click the Select button. Confirm the auto-populated details.
38. Select James A. Martin, MD from the Provider dropdown.
39. Use the calendar picker to confirm or select the appointment day.
40. Select a start and end time for the appointment using the Start Time and End Time dropdowns.
41. Click the Save button.
42. Daniel's appointment will be displayed on the calendar.

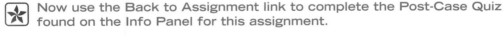

Now use the Back to Assignment link to complete the Post-Case Quiz found on the Info Panel for this assignment.

32. Document Allergies and Medications for Daniel Miller

■ Objectives

- Search for a patient record.
- Document allergies.
- Document medications.

■ Overview

Daniel Miller has a well-child check-up with Dr. Martin. Daniel's mom, Tracy Miller, says that Daniel developed hives from the amoxicillin prescribed during a previous visit. During this visit's exam, Dr. Martin diagnoses Daniel with an ear infection and prescribes cephalexin tablet for oral suspension 250 mg twice daily for seven days. Document Daniel Miller's allergy and update his medication record.

■ Competencies

- Administer parenteral (excluding IV) medications, CAAHEP I.P-7, ABHES 2-c, 8-f
- Define basic units of measurement in metric and household systems, CAAHEP II.C-3, ABHES 6-b
- Maintain medication and immunization records, ABHES 4-a, 4-f

Estimated completion time: 20 minutes

Measurable Steps

1. Click on the Find Patient icon.
2. Using the Patient Search fields, search for Daniel's patient record. Once you locate Daniel's patient record in the List of Patients, confirm his date of birth.

 HELPFUL HINT

Confirming date of birth will help to ensure that you have located the correct patient record.

3. Select the radio button for Daniel Miller and click the Select button.
4. Create a new encounter by clicking Office Visit in the left Info Panel (Figure 3-48). Click the Add New button to create a new encounter.
5. In the Create New Encounter window, select Follow-up/Established visit from the Visit Type dropdown.
6. Select James A. Martin, MD from the Provider dropdown.
7. Click the Save button.
8. Allergies is the first option available within the Record dropdown menu, automatically landing the user in that section of the patient chart.
9. Click the Add Allergy button to add amoxicillin suspension as an allergy for Daniel. An Add Allergy window will appear (Figure 3-49).
10. Select the Medication radio button in the Allergy Type field.
11. Document "amoxicillin suspension" in the Select Allergen field.

Clinical Care

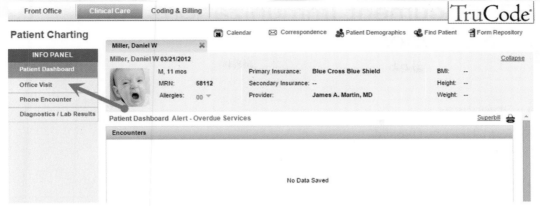

Figure 3-48 Office Visit in the Info Panel.

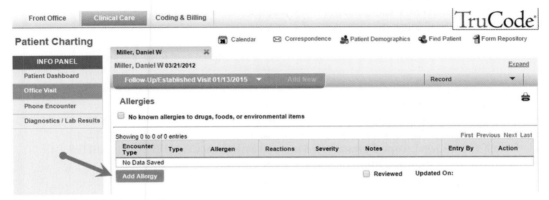

Figure 3-49 Add Allergy button.

12. Check Hives in the Reactions field.
13. Select Parent in the Informant field. Select Very Reliable in the Confidence Level field.
14. Click the Save button in the Add Allergy window. The allergy you added will display in the Allergies grid.
15. Select Medications from the Record dropdown menu.
16. Select the edit icon from the Action column for amoxicillin.
17. Select the Discontinued radio button in the Status field.
18. Document the date one week from the Start Date for the amoxicillin in the Discontinued Date field.
19. Document "Hives" in the Reason field.
20. Click the Save button. The status will be changed to Discontinued in the Medications grid.
21. Click the Add Medication button.
22. Document "cephalexin tablet for oral suspension" in the Medication field.
23. Document "250" in the Strength field.
24. Document "Suspension tablet" in the Form field.
25. Document "Oral" in the Route field.
26. Document "Every 6 hours" in the Frequency field.
27. Document today's date in the Start Date field.
28. Select the "Active" radio button in the Status field.
29. Click the Save button. The medication you added will display in the Medications grid.

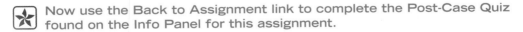

Now use the Back to Assignment link to complete the Post-Case Quiz found on the Info Panel for this assignment.

33. Document Immunizations for Al Neviaser

■ Objectives

- Search for a patient record.
- Document immunizations.

■ Overview

Dr. Martin orders a tetanus booster for Al Neviaser because he notices that it has been 10 years since his last immunization. Al Neviaser tolerates the injection well and has no reactions. Update his immunization record with the following information:

DTaP, Dosage: 0.5 mL. Manufacturer: MassBiologics, Lot#: XX923, Expiration: 06/18.* The dose is injected into the right deltoid.

* The year of expiration displayed on the labels should reflect an expiration date of three years from the current year.

■ Competencies

- Administer parenteral (excluding IV) medications, CAAHEP I.P-7, ABHES 2-c, 8-f
- Document patient care accurately in the medical record, CAAHEP X.P-3, ABHES 4-a
- Locate a state's legal scope of practice for medical assistants, CAAHEP X.P-1, ABHES 4-f
- Maintain medication and immunization records, ABHES 4-a, 4-f
- Organize a patient's medical record, CAAHEP VI.P-4, ABHES 7-a, 7-b

Estimated completion time: 20 minutes

Measurable Steps

1. Click on the Find Patient icon (Figure 3-50).
2. Using the Patient Search fields, search for Al Neviaser's patient record. Once you locate his patient record in the List of Patients, confirm his date of birth.

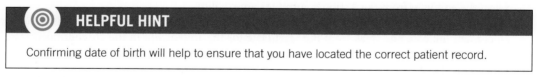

HELPFUL HINT

Confirming date of birth will help to ensure that you have located the correct patient record.

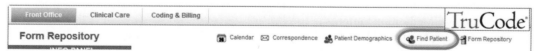

Figure 3-50 Find Patient icon.

3. Select the radio button for Al Neviaser and click the Select button.
4. Confirm the auto-populated details in the Patient Header.
5. Create an encounter for Al Neviaser by clicking Office Visit in the Info Panel to the left (Figure 3-51).
6. In the Create New Encounter window, select Follow-up/Established Visit from the Visit Type dropdown.
7. Select James A. Martin, MD in the Provider dropdown.
8. Click the Save button.

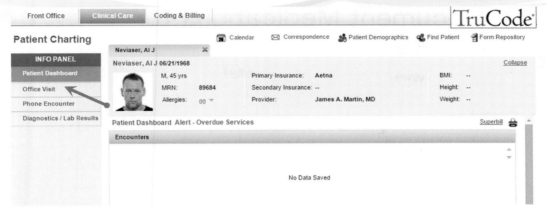

Figure 3-51 Office Visit in the left Info Panel.

9. In order to begin documenting in this encounter, select Immunizations from the Record drop-down menu that is already open.
10. Locate the row for the "DTaP (Diphtheria, Tetanus, Pertussis)" vaccine and click on the green plus sign to the far right of that row. That row will become active so you can add an immunization to Al Neviaser's record (Figure 3-52).

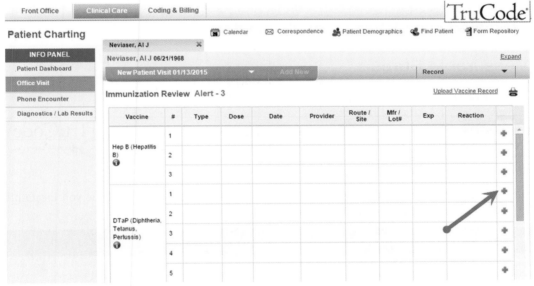

Figure 3-52 Activating a row to add an immunization.

11. Within the Type column, select DTaP.
12. Within the Dose column, document "0.5 mL".
13. Within the Date column, use the calendar picker to select the date the vaccine was administered.
14. Within the Provider column, document "James A. Martin, MD" in the text box.
15. Within the Route/Site column, document "0.5 mL to right deltoid" in the text box.
16. Within the Manufacturer/Lot# column, document "MassBiologics/XX923" in the text box.
17. Within the Exp column, document the expiration in the text box.
18. Within the Reaction column, document "Patient tolerates procedure well with no reaction" in the text box.
19. Click the Save button. The immunization you added will display in the Immunization Review grid.

 Now use the Back to Assignment link to complete the Post-Case Quiz found on the Info Panel for this assignment.

34. Document Medications for Al Neviaser

■ Objectives

- Search for a patient record.
- Document medications.

■ Overview

Al Neviaser has a history of high blood pressure and takes Diovan 160 mg daily. He also takes Nexium 20 mg daily for GERD. Document Al Neviaser's current medications.

■ Competencies

- Administer oral medications, CAAHEP I.P-6, ABHES 2-c, 8-f
- Apply mathematical computations to solve equations, CAAHEP II.C-2, ABHES 6-b
- Maintain medication and immunization records, ABHES 4-a, 4-f

Estimated completion time: 25 minutes

Measurable Steps

1. Click on the Find Patient icon (Figure 3-53).

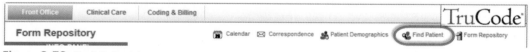

Figure 3-53 Find Patient icon.

2. Using the Patient Search fields, search for Al Neviaser's patient record. Once you locate his patient record in the List of Patients, confirm his date of birth.

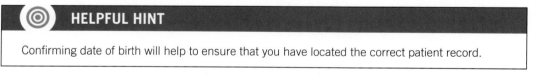

> **HELPFUL HINT**
>
> Confirming date of birth will help to ensure that you have located the correct patient record.

3. Select the radio button for Al Neviaser and click the Select button.
4. Confirm the auto-populated details in the Patient Header.
5. Create an encounter for Al Neviaser by clicking Office Visit in the Info Panel to the left (Figure 3-54).

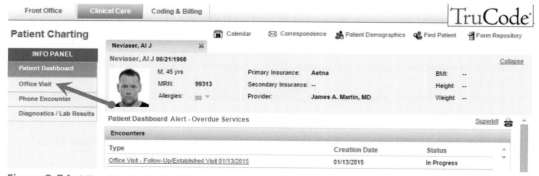

Figure 3-54 Office Visit in the Info Panel.

6. In the Create New Encounter window, select Follow-Up/Established Visit from the Visit Type dropdown menu.
7. Click the Save button.
8. Select Medications from the Record dropdown menu.
9. Within the Prescription Medications tab, click the Add Medication button to add Diovan (Valsartan) to Al Neviaser's medications (Figure 3-55). An Add Prescription Medication window will appear.

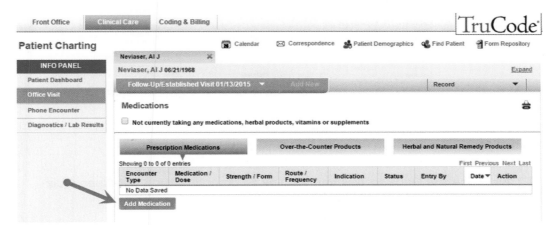

Figure 3-55 The Add Medication button in the Prescription Medications tab.

10. Select Valsartan Tablet - (Diovan) from the Medication dropdown menu.
11. Select 160 from the Strength dropdown menu.
12. Select Tablet from the Form dropdown menu.
13. Select Oral from the Route dropdown menu.
14. Select Daily from the Frequency dropdown menu.
15. Document any additional information and select the Active radio button in the Status field.
16. Click the Save button in the Add Prescription Medication window. The medication you added will display in the Prescription Medications grid.
17. Within the Prescription Medications tab, click the Add Medication button again to add Nexium. An Add Prescription Medication window will appear.
18. Select Esomeprazole Delayed Release Capsule from the Medication dropdown menu.
19. Select 20 mg from the Strength dropdown menu.
20. Select Capsule DR from the Form dropdown menu.
21. Select Oral from the Route dropdown menu.
22. Select Daily from the Frequency dropdown menu.
23. Document any additional information and select the Active radio button in the Status field.
24. Click the Save button in the Add Prescription Medication window. The medication you added will display in the Prescription Medications grid (Figure 3-56).

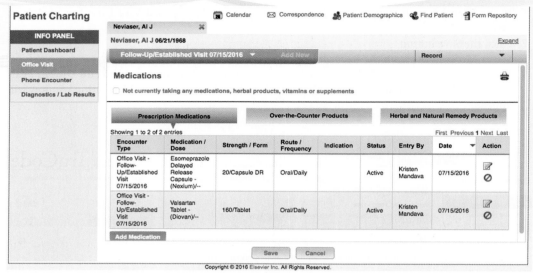

Figure 3-56 The medication will display in the Prescription Medications grid.

Now use the Back to Assignment link to complete the Post-Case Quiz found on the Info Panel for this assignment.

Clinical Care

35. Document Immunizations and Medications for Diego Lupez

■ Objectives

- Search for a patient record.
- Document medications.

■ Overview

Diego Lupez stepped on a nail that went through his shoe and punctured the bottom of his foot while he was at work. His supervisor told him to see his primary care physician for treatment. Dr. Martin orders a tetanus booster and Diego Lupez has no reactions. He also has GERD which is treated with Prilosec capsules 40 mg daily. Document Diego Lupez's medications and immunizations:

DTaP, 0.5 mL. Manufacturer: CareMed, Lot#: 89FG, Exp: 05/18.* The dose was injected into the left deltoid.

*The year of expiration displayed on the labels should reflect an expiration date of three years past the current date.

■ Competencies

- Administer oral medications, CAAHEP I.P-6, ABHES 2-c, 8-f
- Administer parenteral (excluding IV) medications, CAAHEP I.P-7, ABHES 2-c, 8-f
- Identify the abbreviations and symbols used in calculating medication dosages, CAAHEP II.C-5 ABHES 3-d, 6-c
- Maintain medication and immunization records, ABHES 4-a, 4-f
- Recognize and understand various treatment protocols, ABHES 2-c
- Perform dressing change, CAAHEP III.P-9

Estimated completion time: 20 minutes

Measurable Steps

1. Click on the Find Patient icon.
2. Using the Patient Search fields, search for Diego Lupez's patient record. Once you locate his patient record in the List of Patients, confirm his date of birth.

 HELPFUL HINT

Confirming date of birth will help to ensure that you have located the correct patient record.

3. Select the radio button for Diego Lupez and click the Select button.
4. Create a new encounter by clicking Office Visit in the left Info Panel (Figure 3-57).
5. In the Create New Encounter window, select Urgent Visit from the Visit Type dropdown.
6. Select James A. Martin, MD from the Provider dropdown.
7. Click the Save button.
8. Select Immunizations from the Record dropdown menu.

Clinical Care

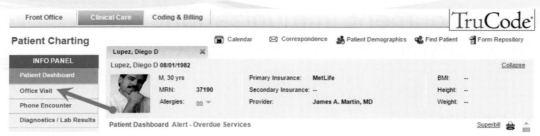

Figure 3-57 Office Visit in the left Info Panel.

9. Locate the row for the "DTaP (Diphtheria, Tetanus, Pertussis)" vaccine and click on the green plus sign to the far right of that row. That row will become active so you can add an immunization to Diego Lupez's record (Figure 3-58).
10. Within the Type column, select DTaP.
11. Within the Dose column, document "0.5 mL."

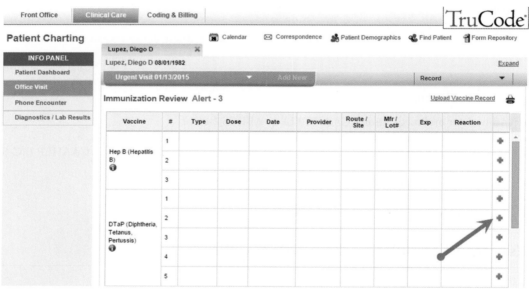

Figure 3-58 Activating a row to add an immunization.

12. Within the Date column, use the calendar picker to select the date administered.
13. Within the Provider column, document "James A. Martin, MD" in the text box.
14. Within the Route/Site column, document "injection to left deltoid" in the text box.
15. Within the Manufacturer/Lot# column, document "CareMed/89FG" in the text box.
16. Within the Exp column, document the expiration in the text box.
17. Within the Reaction column, document "No reaction".
18. Click the Save button. The Immunizations table will display the new immunization.
19. Select Medications from the Record dropdown menu.
20. Within the Prescription Medications tab, click the Add Medication button to add Prilosec (Omeprazole DR) to Diego Lupez's medications. An Add Prescription Medication window will appear (Figure 3-59).
21. Document Omeprazole Delayed Release Capsule in the Medication field.
22. Select 40 in the Strength dropdown menu.
23. Select Capsule DR in the Form dropdown menu.
24. Select Oral in the Route field.
25. Document "Daily" in the Frequency field.
26. Document any additional information and select the Active radio button in the Status field.

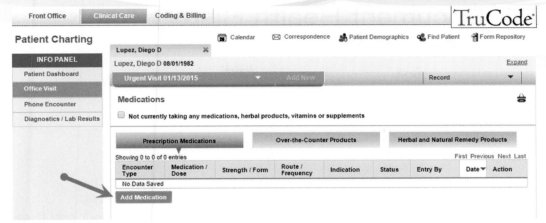

Figure 3-59 Add Prescription Medication window.

27. Click the Save button in the Add Prescription Medication window. The medication you added will display in the Prescription Medications grid.

Now use the Back to Assignment link to complete the Post-Case Quiz found on the Info Panel for this assignment.

36. Document Health History for Ella Rainwater

■ Objectives

- Search for a patient record.
- Document health history.

■ Overview

Ella Rainwater started coming to the Walden-Martin office because she heard such great things about Dr. Martin. She had been seeing a physician at a different clinic, but didn't appreciate the tone that physician used when discussing health concerns. Ella Rainwater smokes two packs of cigarettes a day and both her mother (82 years old) and father (84 years old) have hypertension. She reports a surgical history of "hemorrhoidectomy in 2007" and "inguinal hernia repair in 1999." Document Ella Rainwater's health history.

■ Competencies

- Demonstrate active listening, CAAHEP V.A-1b, ABHES 5-h
- Demonstrate empathy, CAAHEP V.A-1a, ABHES 5-h
- Document patient care accurately in the medical record, CAAHEP X.P-3, ABHES 4-a
- Locate a state's legal scope of practice for medical assistants, CAAHEP X.P-1, ABHES 4-f

Estimated completion time: 25 minutes

Measurable Steps

1. Click on the Find Patient icon (Figure 3-60).

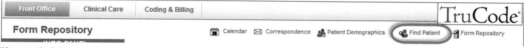

Figure 3-60 Find Patient icon.

2. Using the Patient Search fields, search for Ella Rainwater's patient record. Once you locate her patient record in the List of Patients, confirm her date of birth.

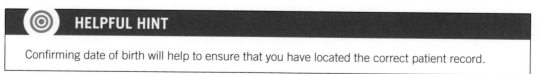

Confirming date of birth will help to ensure that you have located the correct patient record.

3. Select the radio button for Ella Rainwater and click the Select button.
4. Confirm the auto-populated details in the Patient Header.
5. Create an encounter for Ella Rainwater by clicking Office Visit in the Info Panel to the left (Figure 3-61).
6. In the Create New Encounter window, select New Patient Visit from the Visit Type dropdown.
7. Select James A. Martin, MD from the Provider dropdown.
8. Click the Save button.

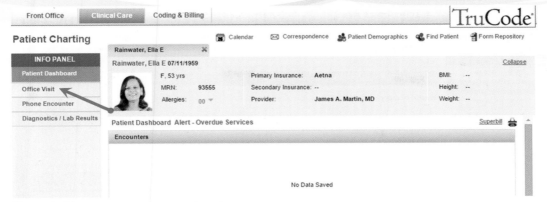

Figure 3-61 Office Visit in the Info Panel.

9. In order to begin documenting in this encounter, select Health History from the Record drop-down menu that is already open.
10. Within the Medical History tab, click the Add New button beneath the Past Surgeries section.
11. In the Add Past Surgery window, document "2007" in the Date field (Figure 3-62).

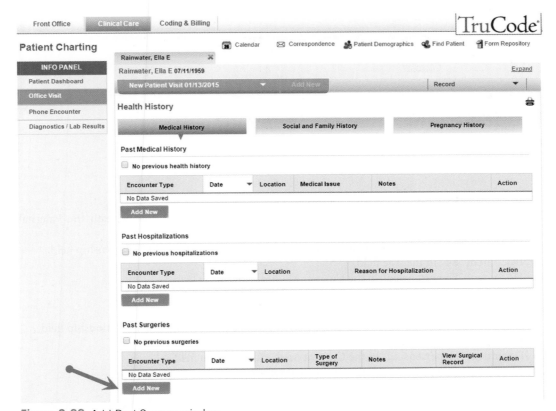

Figure 3-62 Add Past Surgery window.

12. Document "Hemorrhoidectomy" in the Type of Surgery field, along with any additional information needed.
13. Click the Save button. The Past Surgeries grid will refresh.
14. Click the Add New button beneath the Past Surgeries section (Figure 3-63).
15. In the Add Past Surgery window, document "1999" in the Date field.
16. Document "Inguinal hernia repair" in the Type of Surgery field, along with any additional information needed.

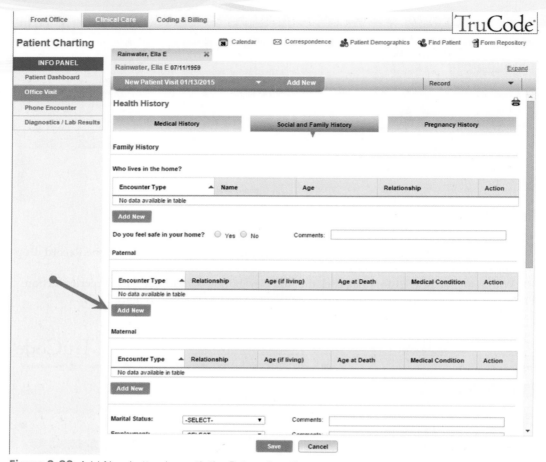

Figure 3-63 Add New button beneath the Paternal section.

17. Click the Save button. The Past Surgeries grid will refresh.
18. Within the Social and Family History tab, click the Add New button beneath the Paternal section.
19. In the Add Paternal Family Member window, document "Father" in the Relationship field.
20. Document "84" in the Age field.
21. Document "Hypertension" in the Current Medical Condition field.
22. Click the Save button. The Paternal grid will refresh.
23. Click the Add New button beneath the Maternal section.
24. In the Add Maternal Family Member window, document "Mother" in the Relationship field.
25. Document "82" in the Age field.
26. Document "Hypertension" in the Current Medical Condition field.
27. Click the Save button. The Maternal grid will refresh.

Now use the Back to Assignment link to complete the Post-Case Quiz found on the Info Panel for this assignment.

Clinical Care

37. Document Phone Encounter and Prepare Medication Refill for Casey Hernandez

■ Objectives

- Search for a patient record.
- Document a phone encounter.
- Prepare a prescription refill.

■ Overview

Casey Hernandez's mother, Maria Hernandez, is calling to request a refill for Casey's albuterol inhaler. Maria Hernandez sometimes has difficulty understanding English without the help of gestures and visual cues. Casey takes the inhaler every four to six hours as needed for asthma. Order one inhaler for Casey to keep at home and one for the school nurse to keep at school. Ms. Hernandez uses Consumer Pharmacy. Create a phone encounter and prepare the electronic transfer refill (for Albuterol) for Jean Burke, NP's approval.

■ Competencies

- Develop a current list of community resources related to patients' healthcare needs, CAAHEP V.P-9, ABHES 8-i
- Comply with legal aspects of creating prescriptions, including federal and state laws, ABHES 6-c
- Identify techniques for overcoming communication barriers, CAAHEP V.C-4, ABHES 5-h

Estimated completion time: 40 minutes

Measurable Steps

1. Click on the Find Patient icon (Figure 3-64).

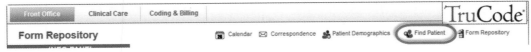

Figure 3-64 Find Patient icon.

2. Using the Patient Search fields, search for Casey's patient record. Once you locate her patient record in the List of Patients, confirm her date of birth.

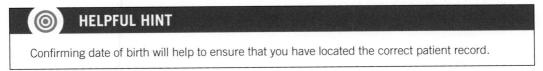

Confirming date of birth will help to ensure that you have located the correct patient record.

3. Select the radio button for Casey Hernandez and click the Select button.
4. Confirm the auto-populated details in the Patient Header.
5. Create a phone encounter for Casey by clicking Phone Encounter in the Info Panel to the left (Figure 3-65).
6. In the Create New Encounter window, document "Maria Hernandez" in the Caller field.
7. Select Jean Burke, NP from the Provider dropdown menu.

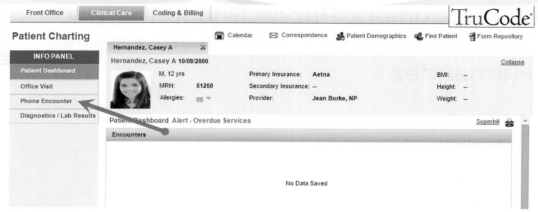

Figure 3-65 Phone Encounter in the Info Panel.

8. Document "Refill request for Casey's albuterol inhaler. Mother is requesting refill of two albuterol inhalers for Casey, one for home and one for school." in the Message field.
9. Click the Save button.
10. Select Order Entry from the Record dropdown menu that is already open.
11. Click the Add button in the Out-of-Office section (Figure 3-66).

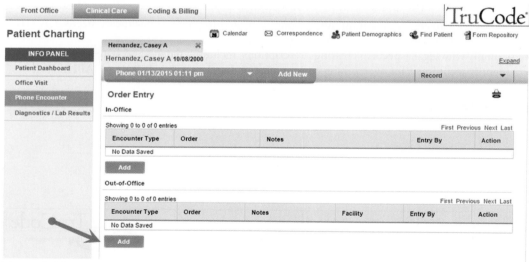

Figure 3-66 Add button in the Out-of-Office section.

12. Select Medication Prescription from the Order dropdown menu.
13. Select the checkbox for Jean Burke, NP.
14. Document "Asthma" in the Diagnosis field.
15. Document "Albuterol" in the Drug field.
16. Document "Consumer Pharmacy" in the Pharmacy field.
17. Document "Take 2 puffs every 4-6 hours as needed" in the Directions field.
18. Document "2" in the Quantity field.
19. Select the Electronic transfer radio button in the Issue Via field.
20. Provide any additional information needed and click the Save button. The order you added will display in the Out-of-Office grid.

 Now use the Back to Assignment link to complete the Post-Case Quiz found on the Info Panel for this assignment.

38. Document Patient Education for Amma Patel

■ Objectives

- Search for a patient record.
- Document patient education.

■ Overview

Amma Patel is experiencing her first urinary tract infection and seems uncomfortable while she is discussing her symptoms with Dr. Walden. She is avoiding eye contact and crossing her arms. Print the urinary tract infection patient education handout for Amma Patel so she knows what to expect.

■ Competencies

- Demonstrate empathy, CAAHEP V.A-1a, ABHES 5-h
- Demonstrate respect for individual diversity, CAAHEP V.A-3, ABHES 5-i
- Identify types of nonverbal communication, CAAHEP V.C-2, ABHES 5-h
- Instruct and prepare a patient for a procedure or a treatment, CAAHEP I.P-8, ABHES 2-c, 5-h, 7-g, 8-d, 8-h
- Use language/verbal skills that enable patients' understanding, CAAHEP V.P- 5, ABHES 5-h, 7-g

Estimated completion time: 20 minutes

Measurable Steps

1. Click on the Find Patient icon (Figure 3-67).

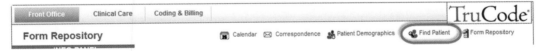

Figure 3-67 Find Patient icon.

2. Using the Patient Search fields, search for Amma Patel's patient record. Once you locate her patient record in the List of Patients, confirm her date of birth.
3. Select the radio button for Amma Patel and click the Select button.
4. Create a new encounter by clicking Office Visit in the left Info Panel (Figure 3-68). If the Create New Encounter window doesn't appear automatically, click on Add New to create a new encounter.

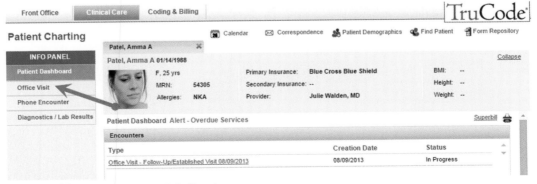

Figure 3-68 Office Visit in the Info Panel.

Clinical Care

5. In the Create New Encounter window, select Urgent Visit from the Visit Type dropdown.
6. Select Julie Walden, MD from the Provider dropdown.
7. Click the Save button.
8. Select Patient Education from the Record dropdown menu that is already open. The menu will close once you navigate away from this screen.
9. Select Diagnosis from the Category dropdown menu.
10. Select Urinary System from the Subcategory dropdown menu.
11. Select the Urinary Tract Infection (UTI) checkbox in the Teaching Topics field.
12. Fill out remaining fields as appropriate.
13. Click the Save button. This teaching topic will move from the New tab to the Saved tab (Figure 3-69).

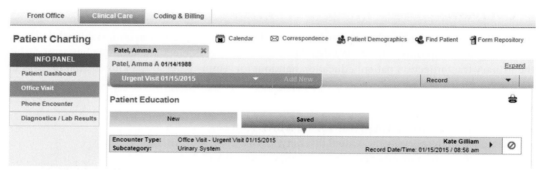

Figure 3-69 The teaching topic in the Saved tab.

14. Click the triangle on the right side of the header to expand the accordion of the saved patient education category to view and print the handout.

> ✦ Now use the Back to Assignment link to complete the Post-Case Quiz found on the Info Panel for this assignment.

39. Document Patient Education for Casey Hernandez

■ Objectives

- Search for a patient record.
- Document patient education.

■ Overview

Jean Burke, NP is discussing bike safety with Casey Hernandez and her mom. Document this patient education in the patient record and print the patient education handout.

■ Competencies

- Demonstrate empathy, CAAHEP V.A-1a, ABHES 5-h
- Demonstrate respect for individual diversity, CAAHEP V.A-3, ABHES 5-i
- Instruct and prepare a patient for a procedure or a treatment, CAAHEP I.P-8, ABHES 7-g, 8-h
- Coach patients appropriately considering cultural diversity, developmental life stage, and communication barriers, CAAHEP V.P- 5, ABHES 5-d, 5-h

Estimated completion time: 20 minutes

Measurable Steps

1. Click on the Find Patient icon (Figure 3-70).

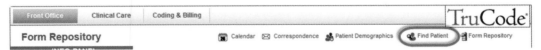

Figure 3-70 Find Patient icon.

2. Using the Patient Search fields, search for Casey Hernandez's patient record. Once you locate her patient record in the List of Patients, confirm her date of birth.

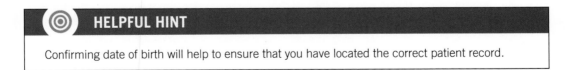

Confirming date of birth will help to ensure that you have located the correct patient record.

3. Select the radio button for Casey Hernandez and click the Select button.
4. Create a new encounter by clicking Office Visit in the left Info Panel (Figure 3-71).
5. In the Create New Encounter window, select Follow-Up/Established Visit from the Visit Type dropdown.
6. Select Jean Burke, NP from the Provider dropdown.
7. Click the Save button.
8. Select Patient Education from the Record dropdown menu.
9. Select Health Promotion from the Category dropdown menu.
10. Select Exercise or Safety from the Subcategory dropdown menu.
11. Select the Bike Safety checkbox in the Teaching Topics field.

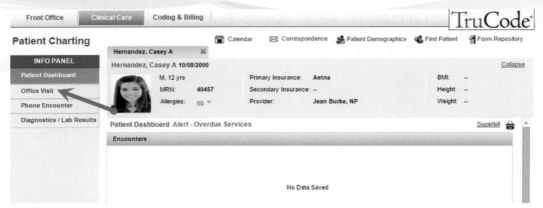

Figure 3-71 Office Visit in the Info Panel.

12. Fill out remaining fields as appropriate.
13. Click the Save button. This teaching topic will move from the New tab to the Saved tab.
14. Click the triangle on the right side of the header to expand the accordion of the saved patient education category to view and print the handout.

 Now use the Back to Assignment link to complete the Post-Case Quiz found on the Info Panel for this assignment.

40. Document Vital Signs for Amma Patel

■ Objectives

- Search for a patient record.
- Document vital signs.

■ Overview

During Amma Patel's follow-up visit with Dr. Martin, her vital signs were measured: "Ht: 5 ft 3 in, Wt: 102 pounds (standing scale), T: 98.2°F (tympanic), P: 74 regular (radial), R: 16 regular rhythm, BP: 112/72 (left arm, manual with cuff, sitting)". Document Amma Patel's vital signs.

■ Competencies

- Convert among measurement systems, CAAHEP II.C-4, ABHES 6-b
- Document patient care accurately in the medical record, CAAHEP X.P-3, ABHES 4-a
- Measure and record vital signs, CAAHEP I.P-1, ABHES 8-b

Estimated completion time: 30 minutes

Measurable Steps

1. Click on the Find Patient icon (Figure 3-72).

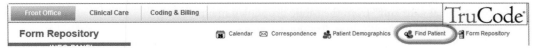

Figure 3-72 Find Patient icon.

2. Using the Patient Search fields, search for Amma Patel's patient record.
3. Select the radio button for Amma Patel and click the Select button. Once you locate her patient record in the List of Patients, confirm her date of birth.

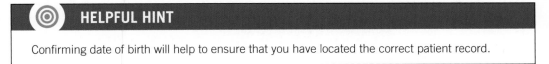

> **⊙ HELPFUL HINT**
>
> Confirming date of birth will help to ensure that you have located the correct patient record.

4. Confirm the auto-populated details such as date of birth.
5. Create a new encounter by clicking Office Visit in the left Info Panel (Figure 3-73). Click the Add New button to create a new encounter.
6. In the Create New Encounter window, select Follow-Up/Established Visit from the Visit Type dropdown.
7. Select James A. Martin, MD from the Provider dropdown.
8. Click the Save button.
9. Select Vital Signs from the Visit Type dropdown menu that is already open. The menu will close once you navigate away from this screen.
10. In the Vital Signs tab, click the Add button (Figure 3-74).
11. Document "98.2°F" in the Temperature field and select Tympanic from the Site dropdown menu.
12. Document "74 reg" in the Pulse field and select Radial from the Site dropdown.
13. Document "16 reg" in the Respiration field.

Clinical Care

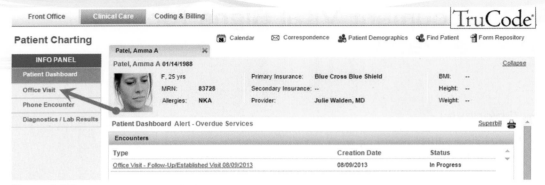

Figure 3-73 Office Visit in the Info Panel.

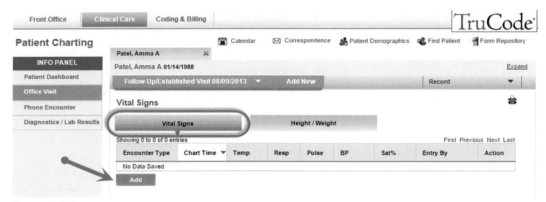

Figure 3-74 Add button in Vital Signs tab.

14. Document "112" in the Systolic field and select Left arm from the Site dropdown menu.
15. Document "72" in the Diastolic field.
16. Select "Manual with cuff" from the Mode dropdown menu.
17. Select "Sitting" from the Position dropdown menu.
18. Click the Save button. The Vital Signs grid will display the vital signs for this encounter.
19. In the Height/Weight tab, click the Add button (Figure 3-75).
20. Document "5" as the feet and "3" as the inches for the Height field.

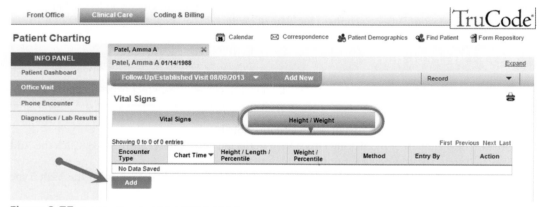

Figure 3-75 Add button in Height/Weight tab.

21. Document "102" in the Weight field.
22. Select Standing scale from the Method dropdown menu.
23. Click the Save button. The Height/Weight grid will display the height and weight for this encounter.

⭐ Now use the Back to Assignment link to complete the Post-Case Quiz found on the Info Panel for this assignment.

41. Document Vital Signs for Ella Rainwater

Objectives

- Search for a patient record.
- Document vital signs.

Overview

Ella Rainwater has been experiencing issues related to her hypertension, so Dr. Martin asked her to stop in to have her vital signs checked. Ella Rainwater thinks her high blood pressure is getting worse and appears very nervous because her neighbor recently died due to hypertensive complications. She is sifting through magazines quickly, avoiding eye contact, and tapping her foot on the floor while she waits for the medical assistant to call her name. Ella Rainwater's vital signs were measured as T: 98.7°F, Site: tympanic; P: 82 reg, bounding, Site: radial, R: 14 reg, normal, BP: 122/86, Position: sitting, Site: left arm, Mode: manual with cuff.

Competencies

- Demonstrate nonverbal communication, CAAHEP V.A-1c, ABHES 5-a, 5-h
- Identify types of nonverbal communication, CAAHEP V.C-2, ABHES 5-h, 8-j
- Measure and record vital signs, CAAHEP I.P-1, ABHES 8-b
- Organize a patient's medical record, CAAHEP VI.P-4, ABHES 7-a, 7-b

Estimated completion time: 30 minutes

Measurable Steps

1. Click on the Find Patient icon (Figure 3-76).

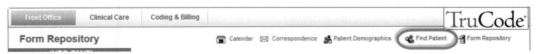

Figure 3-76 Find Patient icon.

2. Using the Patient Search fields, search for Ella Rainwater's patient record.
3. Select the radio button for Ella Rainwater and click the Select button. Once you locate her patient record in the List of Patients, confirm her date of birth.

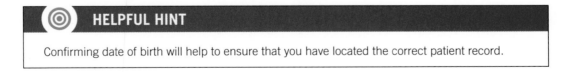

> **HELPFUL HINT**
>
> Confirming date of birth will help to ensure that you have located the correct patient record.

4. Create a new encounter by clicking Office Visit in the left Info Panel (Figure 3-77).
5. In the Create New Encounter window, select Follow-Up/Established Visit from the Visit Type dropdown.
6. Select James A. Martin, MD from the Provider dropdown.
7. Click the Save button.

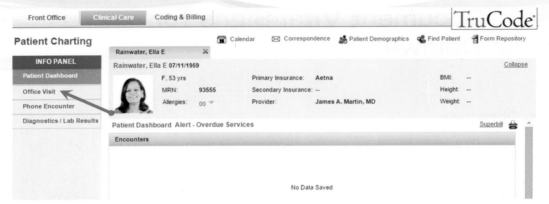

Figure 3-77 Office Visit in the Info Panel.

8. Select Vital Signs from the Record dropdown menu.
9. In the Vital Signs tab, click the Add button (Figure 3-78).

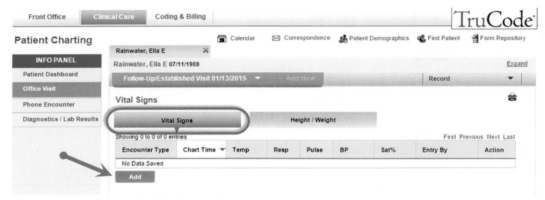

Figure 3-78 Add button in Vital Signs tab.

10. Document "98.7°F" in the Temperature field and select Tympanic from the Site dropdown menu.
11. Document "82 reg, bounding" in the Pulse field and select Radial from the Site dropdown.
12. Document "14 reg" in the Respiration field.
13. Document "122" in the Systolic field and select Left arm from the Site dropdown menu.
14. Document "86" in the Diastolic field and select Manual with cuff in the Mode dropdown menu.
15. Select Sitting from the Position dropdown menu.
16. Click the Save button. The Vital Signs grid will display the vital signs for this encounter.

> ★ Now use the Back to Assignment link to complete the Post-Case Quiz found on the Info Panel for this assignment.

Clinical Care

42. Document Preventative Services for Amma Patel

■ Objectives

- Search for a patient record.
- Document preventative services.

■ Overview

Dr. Walden asked Amma Patel to complete a stool for a fecal occult blood test to fulfill annual health maintenance recommendations. Amma Patel returned her test, which was processed in the medical office. The results of the test are three negative specimens. Document the results of this test in the patient record for Amma Patel.

■ Competencies

- Define coaching a patient, CAAHEP V.C-6, ABHES 5-c, 8-h
- Discuss applications of electronic technology in professional communication, CAAHEP V.C-8, ABHES 7-g
- Maintain laboratory test results using flow sheets, CAAHEP II.P-3, ABHES 4-a, 9-e

Estimated completion time: 20 minutes

Measurable Steps

1. Click on the Find Patient icon (Figure 3-79).

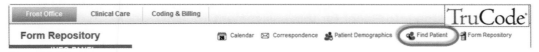

Figure 3-79 Find Patient icon.

2. Using the Patient Search fields, search for Amma Patel's patient record.
3. Select the radio button for Amma Patel and click the Select button. Once you locate her patient record in the List of Patients, confirm her date of birth.

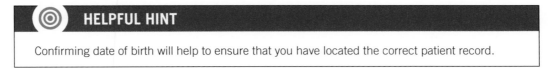

HELPFUL HINT

Confirming date of birth will help to ensure that you have located the correct patient record.

4. Create a new encounter by clicking Office Visit in the left Info Panel (Figure 3-80). Click on the Add New button to create a new encounter.
5. In the Create New Encounter window, select Follow-Up/Established Visit from the Visit Type dropdown.
6. Select Julie Walden, MD from the Provider dropdown.
7. Click the Save button.
8. Select Preventative Services from the Record dropdown menu that is already open.
9. Click the Add button below the Procedures table (Figure 3-81).
10. Select Fecal Occult Blood Test from the Health Recommendation dropdown menu.
11. Use the calendar picker to document the date in the Date Performed field.

Clinical Care

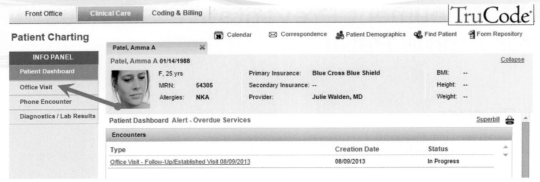

Figure 3-80 Office Visit in the Info Panel.

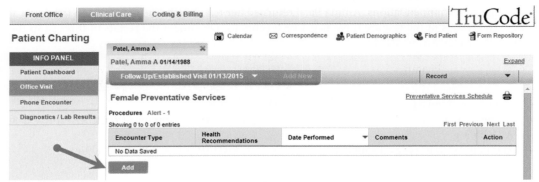

Figure 3-81 Add button below the Procedures table.

12. Document "Negative × 3" in the Comments field.
13. Click the Save button. The Preventative Services table will display the preventative services for this encounter.

> ⊞ Now use the Back to Assignment link to complete the Post-Case Quiz found on the Info Panel for this assignment.

43. Document Encounter and Schedule Appointment for Walter Biller

■ Objectives

- Search for a patient record.
- Document medications.
- Document allergies.
- Schedule an appointment.

■ Overview

It has been two years since Walter Biller's last appointment with Dr. Walden. His general health needs are met at the clinic where he works, but the nurse recommended he see his primary care physician after he failed to pass a routine eye exam and had glucose in a urine sample. Walter Biller is not currently on any medications, but he says that Darvocet gives him a headache. Dr. Walden diagnoses Walter Biller with Type II DM (without complications), uncontrolled and starts him on Metformin (extended release tablet) 500 mg PO bid. Dr. Walden would like to see Walter Biller again for 30 minutes next Friday. Document Mr. Biller's encounter and schedule a follow-up appointment.

■ Competencies

- Display sensitivity when managing appointments, CAAHEP VI.A-1, ABHES 5-h, 7-e
- Document patient care accurately in the medical record, CAAHEP X.P-3, ABHES 4-a
- Maintain medication and immunization records, ABHES 4-a, 4-f
- Manage appointment schedule, using established priorities, CAAHEP VI.P-1, ABHES 7-e
- Properly utilize PDR, drug handbook and other drug reference to identify a drug's classification, usual dosage, usual side effects, and contraindications, ABHES 6-d

Estimated completion time: 25 minutes

Measurable Steps

1. Click on the Find Patient icon (Figure 3-82).

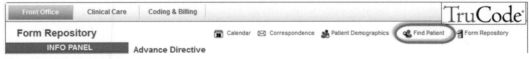

Figure 3-82 Find Patient icon.

2. Using the Patient Search fields, search for Walter Biller's patient record. Once you locate his patient record in the List of Patients, confirm his date of birth.

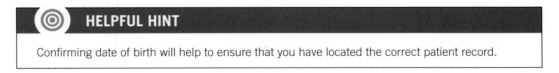

Confirming date of birth will help to ensure that you have located the correct patient record.

3. Select the radio button for Walter Biller and click the Select button. Confirm the auto-populated details in the Patient Header.

4. Create an encounter for Walter Biller by clicking Office Visit in the left Info Panel (Figure 3-83).

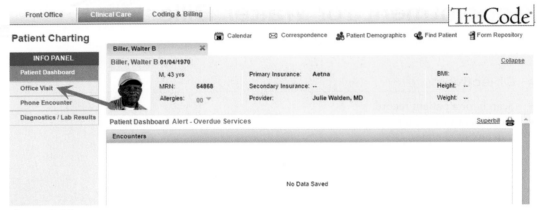

Figure 3-83 Office Visit in the Info Panel.

5. In the Create New Encounter window, select Follow-Up/Established Visit from the Visit Type dropdown.
6. Select Julie Walden, MD from the Provider dropdown.
7. Click the Save button. Allergies is the first option available within the Record dropdown menu, automatically landing the user in that section of the patient chart.

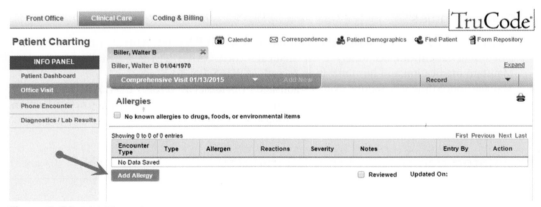

Figure 3-84 Add Allergy button.

8. Click the Add Allergy button (Figure 3-84).
9. Select the Medication radio button in the Allergy Type field.
10. Document "Darvocet" in the Allergen field. If Darvocet is not available in the list of allergies, this can be typed in manually.
11. Click the Headache checkbox in the Reactions field.
12. Document 14 reg normal.
13. Click the Save button in the Add Allergy window. The allergy you added will display in the Allergies grid.
14. Select Problem List from the Record dropdown menu.
15. Click the Add Problem button to add a problem.
16. Select "Diabetes mellitus, Type 2 without complications" from the Diagnosis dropdown menu.
17. Select the ICD-10 radio button and place the cursor in the text box to access the TruCode encoder. Accessing the encoder tool this way will auto-populate any selected codes where the cursor is placed.
18. Enter "Diabetes mellitus, Type 2 without complications" in the Search field and select Diagnosis, ICD-10-CM from the dropdown menu.
19. Click the Search button.
20. Click the code E11.9 to expand this code and confirm that it is the most specific code available.

21. Click the code E11.9 for "Diabetes mellitus, Type 2 without complications" that appears in the tree. This code will auto-populate in the ICD-10 field of the Add Problem window.
22. Document the current date in the Date Identified field.
23. Select the Active radio button in the Status field.
24. Click the Save button. The Problem List table will display the new problem.

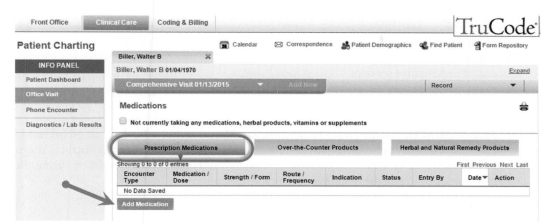

Figure 3-85 The Add Medication button in the Prescription Medications tab.

25. Select Medications from the Record dropdown menu.
26. Within the Prescription Medications tab, click the Add Medication button (Figure 3-85).
27. Document Metformin Extended Release Tablet in the Medication field.
28. Select 500 mg in the Strength dropdown.
29. Select Tablet ER in the Form dropdown.
30. Select Oral in the Route dropdown.
31. Select 2 Times/Day in the Frequency dropdown.
32. Document the indication (Diagnosis) and select the Active radio button in the Status field.
33. Click the Save button in the Add Prescription Medication window. The medication you added will display in the Prescription Medications grid.
34. Click the Calendar icon (Figure 3-86).

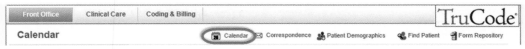

Figure 3-86 Calendar icon.

35. Within the weekly calendar, click on the instructed day to open the New Appointment window.
36. Select the Patient Visit radio button as the Appointment Type.
37. Select Follow-Up/Established Visit from the Visit Type dropdown.
38. Document "Diabetes follow-up" in the Chief Complaint text box.
39. Select the Search Existing Patients radio button.
40. Using the Patient Search fields, search for Walter Biller's patient record. Once you locate him in the List of Patients, confirm his date of birth.
41. Select the radio button for Walter Biller and click the Select button. Confirm the auto-populated details.
42. Select Julie Walden, MD from the Provider dropdown.
43. Use the calendar picker to confirm or select the appointment day.
44. Select a start and end time for the appointment using the Start Time and End Time dropdowns.
45. Click the Save button. Walter's appointment will be displayed on the calendar.

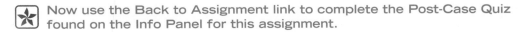

Now use the Back to Assignment link to complete the Post-Case Quiz found on the Info Panel for this assignment.

44. Document Order and Preventative Services for Diego Lupez

■ Objectives

- Search for a patient record.
- Document an order.
- Document preventative services.

■ Overview

Diego Lupez is seeing Dr. Martin today for anemia. Dr. Martin orders a fecal occult blood test to be performed during today's encounter. The test results are positive and Dr. Martin instructs Diego Lupez to complete three specimen collections. Document the Fecal Occult Blood Test (using the ICD-10 code for anemia) and preventative services for Mr. Lupez.

■ Competencies

- Define coaching a patient, CAAHEP V.C-6, ABHES 5-c, 8-h
- Differentiate between normal and abnormal test results, CAAHEP II.P-2, ABHES 2-c
- Identify body systems, CAAHEP I.C-2, ABHES 2-a
- Report relevant information concisely and accurately, CAAHEP V.P-11, ABHES 7-d, 7-g
- Define the function of dietary supplements, CAAHEP IV.C-2

Estimated completion time: 20 minutes

Measurable Steps

1. Click on the Find Patient icon (Figure 3-87).

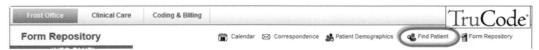

Figure 3-87 Find Patient icon.

2. Using the Patient Search fields, search for Diego Lupez's patient record. Once you locate his patient record in the List of Patients, confirm his date of birth.

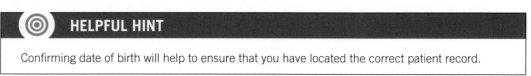

HELPFUL HINT

Confirming date of birth will help to ensure that you have located the correct patient record.

3. Select the radio button for Diego Lupez and click the Select button.
4. Create a new encounter by clicking Office Visit in the left Info Panel (Figure 3-88).
5. In the Create New Encounter window, select Follow-Up/Established Visit from the Visit Type dropdown menu.
6. Select James A. Martin, MD from the Provider dropdown.
7. Click the Save button.
8. Select Order Entry from the Record dropdown menu.
9. Select the TruCode encoder link in the top right corner. The encoder tool will open in a new tab (Figure 3-89).

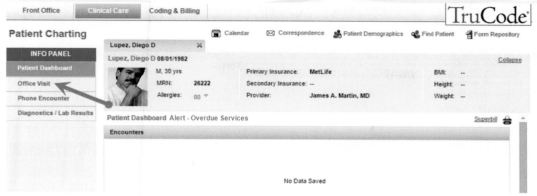

Figure 3-88 Office Visit in the Info Panel.

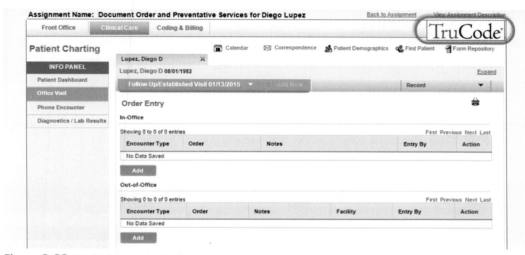

Figure 3-89 TruCode encoder tool.

10. Enter "Anemia" in the Search field and select Diagnosis, ICD-10-CM from the corresponding dropdown menu.
11. Click the Search button.
12. Click the code Anemia D64.9 that appears in red to expand this code and confirm that it is the most specific code available (Figure 3-90).
13. Copy Anemia, unspecified D64.9 that populates in the search results (Figure 3-91).
14. Within SimChart for the Medical Office, click the Add button below the In-Office grid to add an order.
15. In the Add Order window, select Fecal Occult Blood Test from the Order dropdown menu.
16. Click the Exam radio button in the Specimen Collected field.
17. Click the Positive radio button in the Results field.
18. Paste Anemia, unspecified D64.9 in the Notes field and click the Save button.
19. Select Preventative Services from the Record dropdown.
20. Click the Add button in the Procedures section.
21. Select Fecal Occult Blood Test from the Health Recommendation dropdown menu.
22. Document the date using the calendar picker.
23. Document "In office FOBT positive" in the Comments field.
24. Click the Save button. The preventative service you added will display in the Preventative Services table.

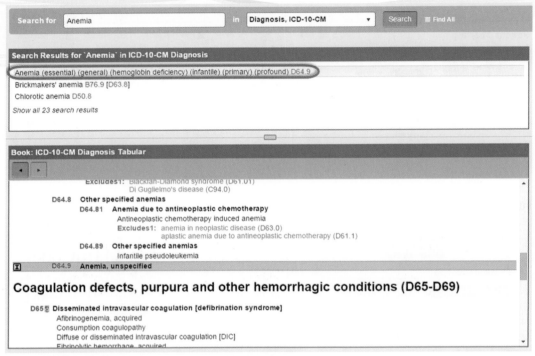

Figure 3-90 Copy appropriate code from the search results.

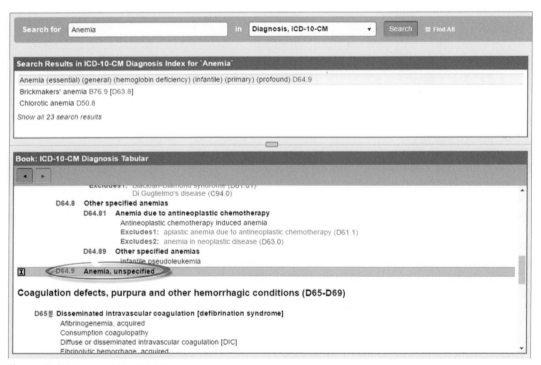

Figure 3-91 Expand the D64.9 code.

Now use the Back to Assignment link to complete the Post-Case Quiz found on the Info Panel for this assignment.

45. Document Progress Note and Order for Norma Washington

■ Objectives

- Search for a patient record.
- Document a progress note.
- Document an order.

■ Overview

Norma Washington has been experiencing lower back pain for the past two days and says the area feels tender. She was doing some spring cleaning a few days ago and slipped on her wet floor. Her vital signs are T: 99.9°F, P: 88, R: 16, BP: 130/84. Dr. Martin notices swelling and diagnoses Norma Washington with a lumbar sprain and prescribes Naprosyn 500 mg tid with food. He also orders an x-ray of the lumbar spine. Document this information in the progress note, order a spine, unenhanced x-ray (using the ICD-10 code for lumbar sprain), and complete a Requisition form for Ms. Washington.

■ Competencies

- Coach patients regarding office policies, CAAHEP V.P-4a, ABHES 5-c
- Differentiate between subjective and objective information, CAAHEP V.C-16, ABHES 5-f, 7-g
- Organize a patient's medical record, CAAHEP VI.P-4, ABHES 7-a, 7-b
- Report relevant information concisely and accurately, CAAHEP V.P-11, ABHES 2-c, 5-f, 7-d
- Perform wound care, CAAHEP III.P-8

Estimated completion time: 35 minutes

Measurable Steps

1. Click on the Find Patient icon (Figure 3-92).
2. Using the Patient Search fields, search for Norma Washington's patient record. Once you locate her patient record in the List of Patients, confirm her date of birth.

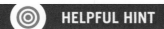

> **⊙ HELPFUL HINT**
>
> Confirming date of birth will help to ensure that you have located the correct patient record.

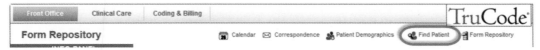

Figure 3-92 Find Patient icon.

3. Select the radio button for Norma Washington and click the Select button.
4. Create a new encounter by clicking Office Visit in the left Info Panel (Figure 3-93). Click on the Add New button to create a new encounter.
5. In the Create New Encounter window, select Urgent Visit from the Visit Type dropdown.
6. Select James A. Martin, MD from the Provider dropdown.
7. Click the Save button.
8. Select Progress Notes from the Record dropdown menu that is already open.
9. Document the date using the calendar picker.

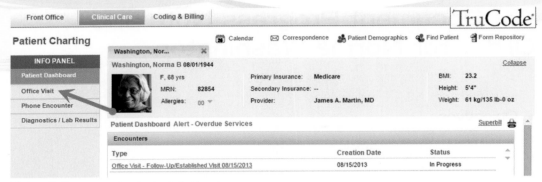

Figure 3-93 Office Visit in the Info Panel.

10. Document "CC: LBP x3-4 d. C/O swelling, and tenderness. Patient states she slipped on a wet floor while cleaning." in the Subjective field.
11. Document "VS: T: 99.9°F, P: 88, R: 16, BP 130/84" in the Objective field.
12. Document "Lumbar sprain" in the Assessment field.
13. Document "Naprosyn 500 mg TID with food, Lumbar spine x-ray" in the Plan field.
14. Click the Save button.
15. Select Medications from the Record dropdown menu.
16. Click the Add Medication button.
17. Document Naprosyn Tablet in the Medication field.
18. Select 500 from the Strength dropdown menu.
19. Select Tablet from the Form dropdown menu.
20. Select Oral from the Route dropdown menu.
21. Select Every 8 Hours from the Frequency dropdown menu.
22. Click the Active radio button in the Status field.
23. Click the Save button.
24. Select Order Entry from the Record dropdown menu.
25. Select the TruCode encoder link in the top right corner. The encoder tool will open in a new tab (Figure 3-94).

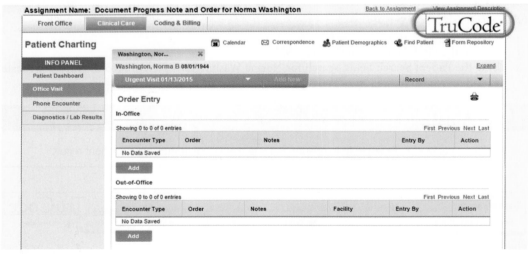

Figure 3-94 TruCode encoder tool.

26. Enter "Lumbar sprain" in the Search field and select Diagnosis, ICD-10-CM from the corresponding dropdown menu.
27. Click the Search button.
28. Click the code S33.5 that appears in red to expand this code and confirm that it is the most specific code available (Figure 3-95).
29. Copy the code Sprain of ligaments of lumbar spine S33.5 that populates in the search results (Figure 3-96).

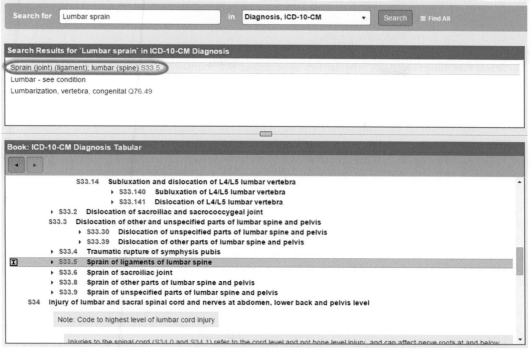

Figure 3-95 Copy appropriate code from the search results.

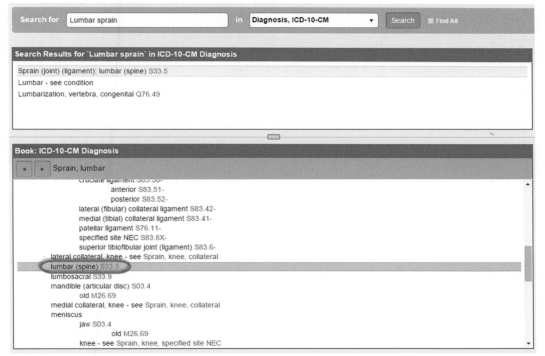

Figure 3-96 Expand the S33.5 code.

30. Within SimChart for the Medical Office, click the Add button below the Out-of-Office grid to add an order.
31. In the Add Order window, select Requisitions from the Order dropdown menu.
32. Select Radiology from the Requisition Type dropdown menu.
33. Document your name in the Entry by field.

34. Document "Spine, unenhanced" and paste the code in the Notes field so that it is available for documentation. Click the Save button.
35. Click on the Form Repository icon.
36. Select the Requisition form from the left Info Panel.
37. Select Radiology from the Requisition Type dropdown menu.
38. Click the Patient Search button to assign the requisition to Norma Washington. Confirm the auto-populated details.
39. In the Diagnosis field, document "Lumbar sprain."
40. Place the cursor in the Diagnosis Code field to access the encoder. Accessing the encoder tool this way will auto-populate any selected codes where the cursor is placed.
41. Enter "Lumbar sprain" in the Search field and select Diagnosis, ICD-10-CM from the dropdown menu.
42. Click the Search button.
43. Click the code S33.5 to expand this code and confirm that it is the most specific code available.
44. Click the code S33.5XXA for "Lumbar sprain, initial encounter" that appears in the tree. This code will auto-populate in the Diagnosis Code field.
45. In the X-ray field, select the Spine checkbox.
46. Document "Lumbar" in the Spine text box.
47. Complete any additional necessary fields and click the Save to Patient Record button. Select the date and click OK. A confirmation message will appear.
48. Click on the Find Patient icon.
49. Using the Patient Search fields, search for Norma Washington's patient record. Once you locate her in the List of Patients, confirm her date of birth.
50. Select the radio button for Norma Washington and click the Select button. Confirm the auto-populated details.
51. Within the Patient Dashboard, scroll down to view the saved forms in the Forms section.
52. Select the form you prepared. The form will open in a new window, allowing you to print.

Now use the Back to Assignment link to complete the Post-Case Quiz found on the Info Panel for this assignment.

46. Document Allergies and Medications for Ella Rainwater

■ Objectives

- Search for a patient record.
- Document medications.
- Document allergies.

■ Overview

Ella Rainwater is on lisinopril 10 mg po QD for her hypertension and is going to need a new prescription soon. Ella Rainwater also mentions that she is allergic to penicillin and broke out in hives the last time she took it. Prepare a patient refill for Dr. Martin's signature and document Ella Rainwater's allergies.

■ Competencies

- Demonstrate knowledge of basic math computations, CAAHEP II.C-1, ABHES 6-b

Estimated completion time: 35 minutes

Measurable Steps

1. Click on the Find Patient icon (Figure 3-97).

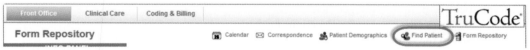

Figure 3-97 Find Patient icon.

2. Using the Patient Search fields, search for Ella Rainwater's patient record. Once you locate her patient record in the List of Patients, confirm her date of birth.

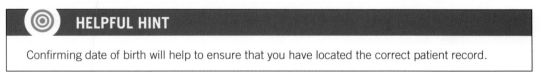

Confirming date of birth will help to ensure that you have located the correct patient record.

3. Select the radio button for Ella Rainwater and click the Select button.
4. Confirm the auto-populated details in the Patient Header.
5. Create an encounter for Ella Rainwater by clicking Office Visit in the Info Panel to the left (Figure 3-98).
6. In the Create New Encounter window, select Follow-Up/Established Visit from the Visit Type dropdown.
7. Select James A. Martin, MD from the Provider dropdown.
8. Click the Save button.
9. Allergies is the first option available within the Record dropdown menu, automatically landing the user in that section within the patient chart.
10. Click the Add Allergy button to add penicillin as an allergy for Ella Rainwater. An Add Allergy window will appear (Figure 3-99).
11. Select the Medication radio button in the Allergy Type field.

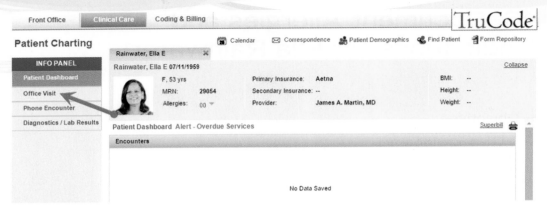

Figure 3-98 Office Visit in the Info Panel.

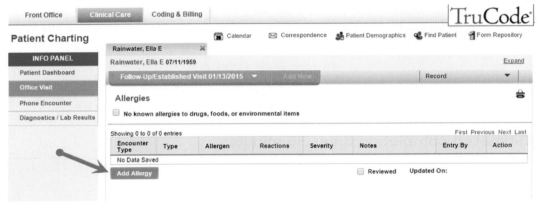

Figure 3-99 Add Allergy button.

12. Type "penicillin" in the Allergen field.
13. Click the Hives checkbox in the Reactions field.
14. Select Self in the Informant field. Select Very Reliable in the Confidence Level field.
15. Click the Save button in the Add Allergy window. The allergy you added will display in the Allergies grid (Figure 3-100).

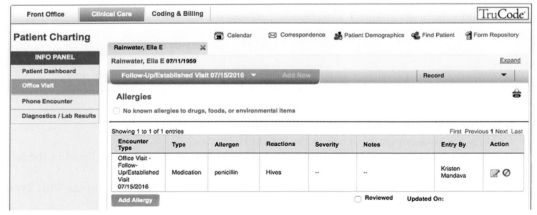

Figure 3-100 The allergy will display in the Allergies grid.

16. Select Medications from the Record dropdown menu.
17. Within the Prescription Medications tab, click the Add Medication button to add Lisinopril to Ella Rainwater's medications. An Add Prescription Medication window will appear (Figure 3-101).
18. Select Lisinopril Tablet - (Prinvil, Zestril) from the Medication dropdown menu.

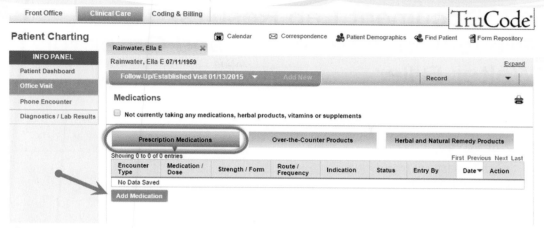

Figure 3-101 The Add Medication button in the Prescription Medications tab.

19. Select 10 mg from the Strength dropdown menu.
20. Select Tablet from the Form dropdown menu.
21. Select Oral from the Route dropdown menu.
22. Select Daily from the Frequency dropdown menu.
23. Document any additional information and select the Active radio button in the Status field.
24. Click the Save button in the Add Prescription Medication window. The medication you added will display in the Prescription Medications grid.

Now use the Back to Assignment link to complete the Post-Case Quiz found on the Info Panel for this assignment.

Clinical Care

47. Document Lab Results, Preventative Services, and Order for Walter Biller

Objectives

- Search for a patient record.
- Document lab results.
- Document preventative services.
- Create a lab requisition.

Overview

Walter Biller is a type 2, uncontrolled diabetic and the Walden-Martin office had blood work performed one week ago and just received his results. The fasting glucose was 145 mg/dL. Since these levels are elevated, Dr. Walden would like Walter Biller to have additional HbA1c and fasting blood glucose tests in one month. Document Walter Biller's lab results, preventative services, and lab order (including the requisition form).

Competencies

- Assist provider with a patient exam, CAAHEP I.P-9, ABHES 8-c, 8-d
- Create a patient's medical record, CAAHEP VI.P-3, ABHES 7-a, 7-b
- Define coaching a patient, CAAHEP V.C-6, ABHES 5-c, 8-h
- Display professionalism through written and verbal communications, ABHES 7-g
- Recognize and understand various treatment protocols, ABHES 2-c
- Instruct and prepare a patient for a procedure or a treatment, CAAHEP I.P-8
- Instruct a patient according to patient's special dietary needs, CAAHEP IV.P-1
- Show awareness of patient's concerns regarding a dietary change, CAAHEP IV.A-1
- Define common medical legal terms, CAAHEP X.C-13

Estimated completion time: 45 minutes

Measurable Steps

1. On the Assignment Description page, locate Walter Biller's lab results in the Assignment Attachments section. Save the results to your computer. You will need to upload the results to Walter's patient record.
1. Click on the Find Patient icon.
2. Using the Patient Search fields, search for Walter Biller's patient record. Once you locate his patient record in the List of Patients, confirm his date of birth.

 HELPFUL HINT

Confirming date of birth will help to ensure that you have located the correct patient record.

3. Select the radio button for Walter Biller and click the Select button.
4. Upload Walter Biller's results by clicking Diagnostics/Lab Results in the left Info Panel (Figure 3-102).
5. Click the Add button.
6. Document the date using the calendar picker.

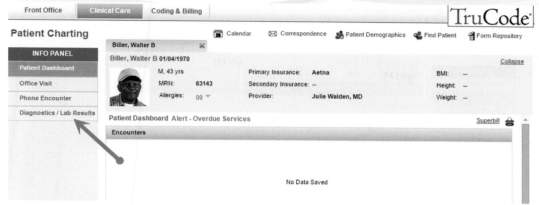

Figure 3-102 Diagnostics/Lab Results in the Info Panel.

7. Select Path/Lab from the Type dropdown menu.
8. Document test results in the Notes field.
9. Click the Browse button to upload Walter Biller's test results. Select the file to upload.
10. Click the Save button. The test results you added will display in the Diagnostic/Lab Results grid.
11. Create a new encounter by clicking Office Visit in the left Info Panel (Figure 3-103).

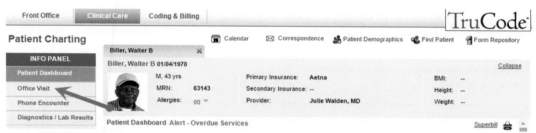

Figure 3-103 Office Visit in the Info Panel.

12. In the Create New Encounter window, select Follow-Up/Established Visit from the Visit Type dropdown.
13. Select Julie Walden, MD from the Provider dropdown.
14. Click the Save button.
15. Select Preventative Services from the Record dropdown menu that is already open.
16. Click the Add button below the Laboratory Testing grid.
17. Select Glucose from the Health Recommendation dropdown field.
18. Document the date performed using the calendar picker.
19. Document the test results in the Comments field.
20. Click the Save button. The test results you added will display in the Laboratory Testing grid.
21. Select Order Entry form the Record dropdown menu.
22. Select the TruCode encoder link in the top right corner. The encoder tool will open in a new tab (Figure 3-104).
23. Enter "Type 2 diabetes uncontrolled" in the Search field and select Diagnosis, ICD-10-CM from the corresponding dropdown menu.
24. Click the Search button.
25. Click the E11.9 code that appears in red to expand this code and confirm that it is the most specific code available (Figure 3-105).
26. Copy the E11.65 code for "Type 2 diabetes mellitus with hyperglycemia" that populates in the search results (Figure 3-106).
27. Within SimChart for the Medical Office, click the Add button below the Out-Of-Office grid to add an order.
28. Select Requisitions from the Order dropdown menu.
29. Select Laboratory from the Requisition Type menu.
30. Document your name in the Entry by field.

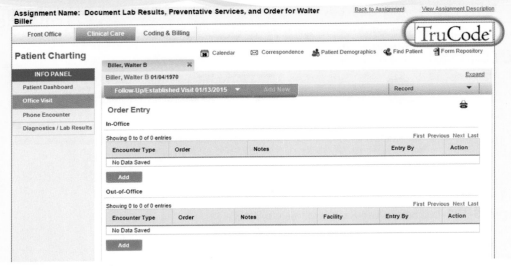

Figure 3-104 TruCode encoder tool.

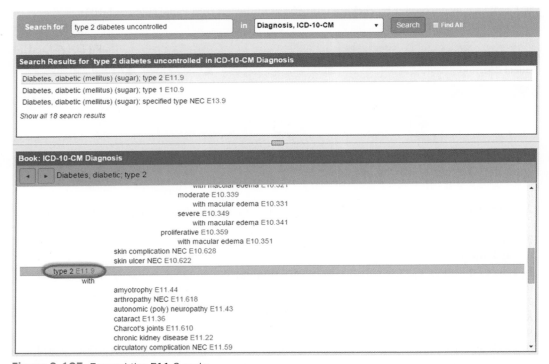

Figure 3-105 Expand the E11.9 code.

31. Document "HbA1c, fasting blood sugar" and paste the diagnosis within the Notes field so that is available for documentation.
32. Click the Save button. The order you added will display in the Out-of-Office grid.
33. Click the Form Repository icon.
34. Select the Requisition form from the left Info Panel.
35. Select Laboratory from the Requisition Type dropdown menu.
36. Click the Patient Search button to assign the form to Walter Biller. Patient demographics will auto-populate. Confirm the auto-populated details.
37. Document the Service Date as one month from the current date using the calendar picker.
38. Document "Diabetes Type 2 with hyperglycemia" in the Diagnosis field.

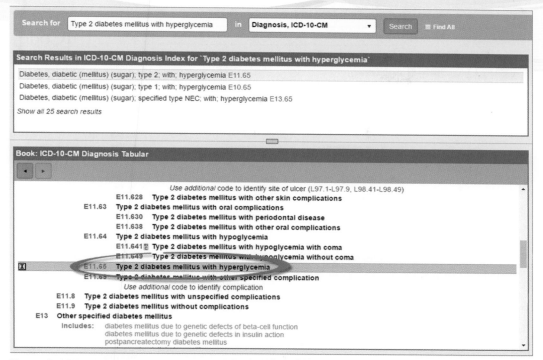

Figure 3-106 Copy appropriate code from the search results.

39. Place the cursor in the Diagnosis Code field to access the encoder. Accessing the encoder tool this way will auto-populate any selected codes where the cursor is placed.
40. Enter "Diabetes Type 2 with hyperglycemia" in the Search field and select Diagnosis, ICD-10-CM from the dropdown menu.
41. Click the Search button.
42. Click the code E11.65 to expand this code and confirm that it is the most specific code available.
43. Click the code E11.65 for "Type 2 diabetes mellitus with hyperglycemia" that appears in the tree. This code will auto-populate in the ICD-10 field of the Add Problem window.
44. In the Basic Metabolic Panel category of the Laboratory Requisition section, select the Glucose checkbox.
45. In the Laboratory Tests section, select the HbA1c (Glycohemo) checkbox.
46. Document "Due in one month, fasting" in the Patient Preparation field (Figure 3-107).
47. Complete any additional necessary fields and click the Save to Patient Record button. Select the date and click OK.
48. Click on the Find Patient icon.
49. Using the Patient Search fields, search for Walter Biller's patient record. Once you locate him in the List of Patients, confirm his date of birth.
50. Select the radio button for Walter Biller and click the Select button. Confirm the auto-populated details.
51. Within the Patient Dashboard, scroll down to view the saved forms in the Forms section.
52. Select the form you prepared. The form will open in a new window, allowing you to print.

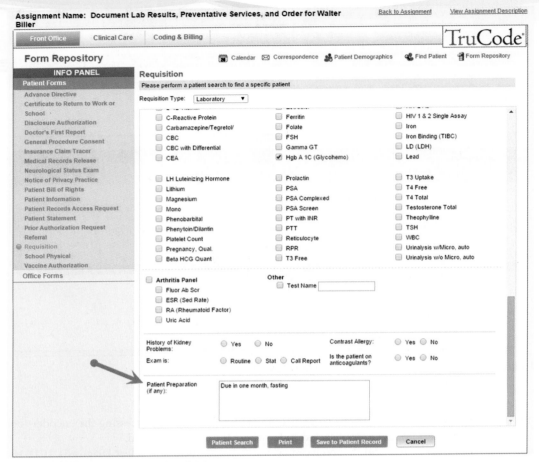

Figure 3-107 Patient Preparation field.

⭐ Now use the Back to Assignment link to complete the Post-Case Quiz found on the Info Panel for this assignment.

48. Document Preventative Services and Test Results for Diego Lupez

▪ Objectives

- Search for a patient record.
- Document preventive services.
- Document test results.

▪ Overview

During the patient interview, Diego Lupez states his last eye exam was two years ago on September 18. Dr. Martin orders a Snellen exam without corrective lenses, which yields the following results: right eye: 20/40, left eye: 20/25, both eyes: 20/25. Document Diego Lupez's preventative services and Snellen exam order with results.

▪ Competencies

- Assist physician with minor office surgical procedures, ABHES 8-e
- Define coaching a patient, CAAHEP V.C-6, ABHES 5-c, 8-h
- Demonstrate respect for individual diversity, CAAHEP V.A-3, ABHES 5-i
- Explain to a patient the rationale for performance of a procedure, CAAHEP V.A-4, ABHES 2-c, 8-h

Estimated completion time: 20 minutes

Measurable Steps

1. Click on the Find Patient icon (Figure 3-108).

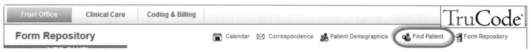

Figure 3-108 Find Patient icon.

2. Using the Patient Search fields, search for Diego Lupez's patient record. Once you locate his patient record in the List of Patients, confirm his date of birth.

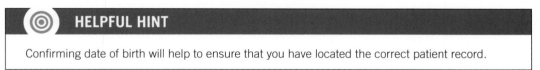

> **◎ HELPFUL HINT**
>
> Confirming date of birth will help to ensure that you have located the correct patient record.

3. Select the radio button for Diego Lupez and click the Select button.
4. Confirm the auto-populated details in the Patient Header.
5. Create a new encounter by clicking Office Visit in the left Info Panel (Figure 3-109).
6. In the Create New Encounter window, select Follow-Up/Established Visit from the Visit Type dropdown.
7. Select James A. Martin, MD from the Provider dropdown.
8. Click the Save button.
9. Select Preventative Services from the Record dropdown.
10. Click the Add button in the General Eye Exam section (Figure 3-110).
11. Document "Exam" in the Health Recommendations field.
12. Document the date as September 18 (2 years ago) using the calendar picker.

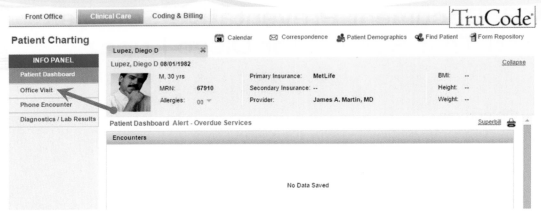

Figure 3-109 Office Visit in the Info Panel.

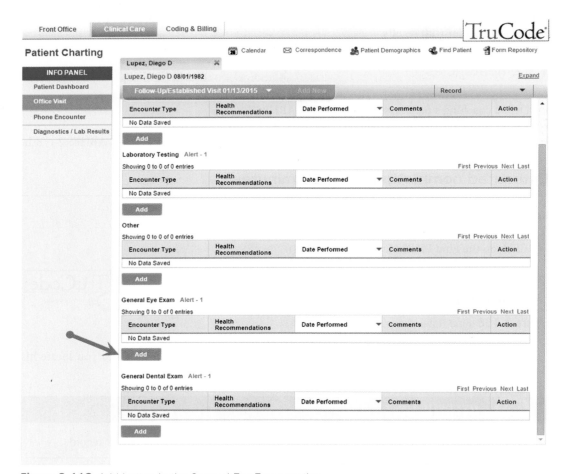

Figure 3-110 Add button in the General Eye Exam section.

13. Click the Save button. The preventative service you added will display in the General Eye Exam table.
14. Select Order Entry from the Record dropdown menu.
15. Click the Add button below the In-Office table to add an order (Figure 3-111).
16. In the Add Order window, select Snellen Exam from the Order dropdown menu.
17. Document "20/40" in the Right eye field.
18. Document "20/25" in the Left eye field.
19. Document "20/25" in the Both eyes field.

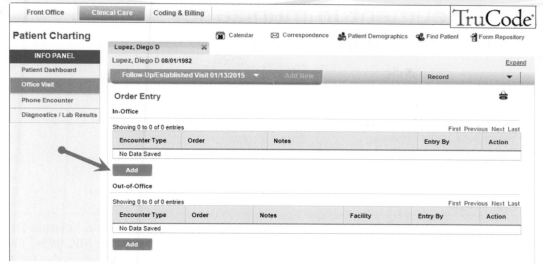

Figure 3-111 Add button below the In-Office table.

20. Document any additional information provided and click the Save button. The In-Office table will display the new order.

⊞ Now use the Back to Assignment link to complete the Post-Case Quiz found on the Info Panel for this assignment.

Clinical Care

49. Document Immunizations and Order for Celia Tapia

■ **Objectives**

- Search for a patient record.
- Document an order.
- Document immunizations.

■ **Overview**

Celia Tapia has arrived for her follow-up appointment with Dr. Martin after a bladder infection. Dr. Martin orders a clean catch urinalysis (clear, yellow) and the results are negative for RBC, WBC, nitrites, and glucose. Bilirubin 0.2, pH: 7.5, SG: 1.025, Ketones negative. Dr. Martin notices that Celia Tapia has not had a flu shot yet this year and discusses the vaccine with her. She agrees to the vaccination and has no reaction. Document the order and immunization for Celia Tapia.

Influenza (Flu), Dosage: 0.5 mL, Given IM in the left deltoid. Manufacturer: CSL Biotherapies Inc. Lot#: 105879, Expiration: 08/30.*

*The year of expiration displayed on the labels should reflect an expiration date of three years from the current year.

■ **Competencies**

- Administer parenteral (excluding IV) medications, CAAHEP I.P-7, ABHES 2-c, 8-f
- Demonstrate sensitivity to patients' rights, CAAHEP X.A-1, ABHES 4-g, 5-h
- List major types of infectious agents, CAAHEP III.C-1, ABHES 2-b
- Maintain medication and immunization records, ABHES 4-a, 4-f
- Organize a patient's medical record, CAAHEP VI.P-4, ABHES 7-a, 7-b
- Select proper sites for administering parenteral medication, CAAHEP I.P- 5, ABHES 8-f

Estimated completion time: 30 minutes

Measurable Steps

1. Click on the Find Patient icon.
2. Using the Patient Search fields, search for Celia Tapia's patient record. Once you locate her patient record in the List of Patients, confirm her date of birth.

 HELPFUL HINT

Confirming date of birth will help to ensure that you have located the correct patient record.

3. Select the radio button for Celia Tapia and click the Select button.
4. Create a new encounter by clicking Office Visit in the left Info Panel (Figure 3-112).
5. In the Create New Encounter window, select Follow-Up/Established Visit from the Visit Type dropdown.
6. Select James A. Martin, MD from the Provider dropdown.
7. Click the Save button.

Clinical Care

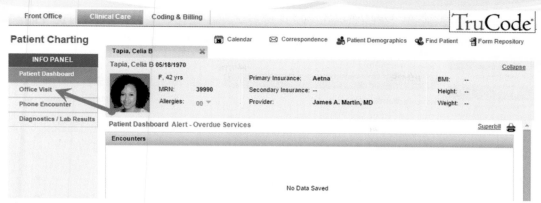

Figure 3-112 Office Visit in the Info Panel.

8. Select Order Entry from the Record dropdown menu that is already open.
9. Click the Add button below the In-Office table to add an order (Figure 3-113).

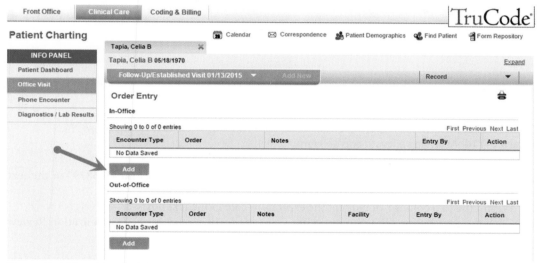

Figure 3-113 Add button below the In-Office table.

10. In the Add Order window, select Urinalysis from the Order dropdown menu.
11. Select the Clean Catch radio button in the Specimen Type field.
12. Document "Clear, yellow" in the Physical Appearance field.
13. Select the Negative radio buttons for RBCs, WBCs, Nitrites, Glucose, and Ketones.
14. Document "0.2" in the Bilirubin field.
15. Document "7.5" in the pH field.
16. Document "1.025" in the Specific Gravity field.
17. Document any additional information needed and click the Save button. The In-Office table will display the new order.
18. Select Immunizations from the Record dropdown menu that is already open.
19. Locate the row for the Influenza (Flu) vaccine and click on the green plus sign to the far right of that row. That row will become active so you can add an immunization to Ms. Tapia's record (Figure 3-114).
20. Within the Type column, select IIV.
21. Within the Dose column, document "0.5 mL".
22. Within the Date column, use the calendar picker to select the date administered.
23. Within the Provider column, document "James A. Martin, MD" in the text box.
24. Within the Route/Site column, document "IM L deltoid" in the text box.

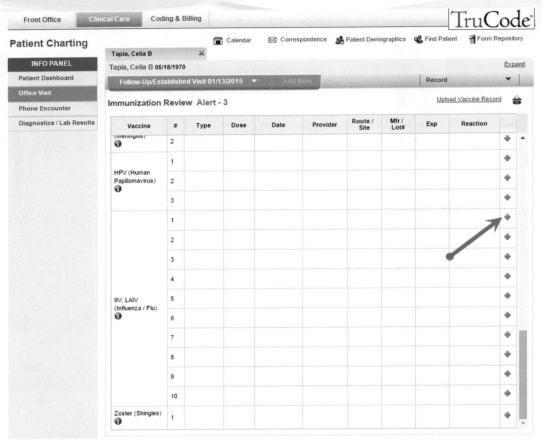

Figure 3-114 Activating a row to add an immunization.

25. Within the Manufacturer/Lot# column, document "CSL Biotherapies Inc./105879" in the text box.
26. Within the Exp column, document the expiration date in the text box.
27. Click the Save button. The immunization you added will display in the Immunization Review grid.

⊞ Now use the Back to Assignment link to complete the Post-Case Quiz found on the Info Panel for this assignment.

50. Document Preventative Services for Diego Lupez

■ Objectives

- Search for a patient record.
- Document preventative services.

■ Overview

Diego Lupez indicated that his father has a history of coronary artery disease, so Dr. Martin ordered a lipid profile. The results were total cholesterol 189, HDL: 45 and LDL: 185. Document these results in Diego Lupez's patient record. English is Diego Lupez's second language.

■ Competencies

- Coach patients regarding disease prevention, CAAHEP V.P-4c, ABHES 8-h
- Define coaching a patient, CAAHEP V.C-6, ABHES 5-c, 8-h
- Demonstrate respect for individual diversity, CAAHEP V.A-3, ABHES 5-i
- Demonstrate sensitivity to patient rights, CAAHEP X.A-1, ABHES 4-g, 5-h
- Show awareness of a patient's concerns related to the procedure being performed, CAAHEP I.A-3, ABHES 5-a, 5-h
- Verify eligibility for managed care services, CAAHEP VIII.P-2, ABHES 7-d

Estimated completion time: 25 minutes

Measurable Steps

1. Click on the Find Patient icon (Figure 3-115).

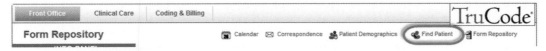

Front Office	Clinical Care	Coding & Billing					TruCode
Form Repository			📅 Calendar	✉ Correspondence	👥 Patient Demographics	🔍 Find Patient	📋 Form Repository

Figure 3-115 Find Patient icon.

2. Using the Patient Search fields, search for Diego Lupez's patient record.
3. Select the radio button for Diego Lupez and click the Select button. Once you locate his patient record in the List of Patients, confirm his date of birth.

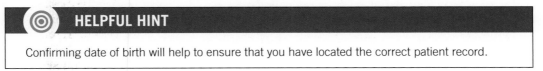

◎ HELPFUL HINT

Confirming date of birth will help to ensure that you have located the correct patient record.

4. Create a new encounter by clicking Office Visit in the left Info Panel (Figure 3-116).
5. In the Create New Encounter window, select Follow-Up/Established Visit from the Visit Type dropdown.
6. Select James A. Martin, MD from the Provider dropdown.
7. Click the Save button.
8. Select Preventative Services from the Record dropdown menu that is already open.
9. Click the Add button below the Laboratory Testing table (Figure 3-117).
10. Select Lipid Profile from the Health Recommendation dropdown menu.
11. Use the calendar picker to document the date in the Date Performed field.

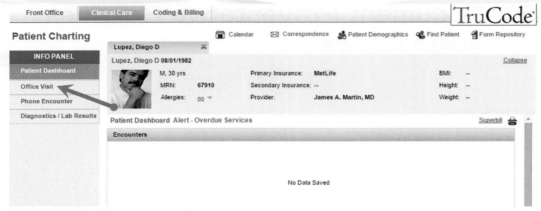

Figure 3-116 Office Visit in the Info Panel.

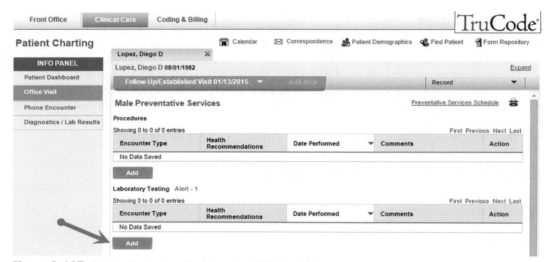

Figure 3-117 Add button below the Laboratory Testing table.

12. Document "Total Cholesterol: 189, HDL: 45, and LDL: 185" in the Comments field.
13. Click the Save button. The Preventative Services table will display the preventative services for this encounter.

> Now use the Back to Assignment link to complete the Post-Case Quiz found on the Info Panel for this assignment.

51. Document Progress Note and Order for Charles Johnson

■ **Objectives**

- Search for a patient record.
- Document in the progress note.
- Document an order.

■ **Overview**

Charles Johnson has a history of Type 2 diabetes and has an appointment with Dr. Martin to address his hyperglycemia. He states he checked his random blood glucose at home around 9:00 pm last night and it was 230. He is experiencing shakes and anxiety a few hours after meals. The vital signs are measured as T: 98.4°F (TA), P: 84 reg, strong radial, R: 14 reg, BP: 156/90 left arm, sitting. HbA1c – 7.6%. Dr. Martin orders the medical assistant to perform a glucometer test and the results are 189 mg/dL (RBS). Document a progress note, enter an order for the glucometer reading, and complete the laboratory requisition form.

■ **Competencies**

- Analyze healthcare results as reported in graphs and tables, CAAHEP II.C-6, ABHES 2-b, 2-c
- Compare and contrast physician and medical assistant roles in terms of standard of care, CAAHEP X.C-2, ABHES 1-b, 4-f
- Maintain laboratory test results using flow sheets, CAAHEP II.P-3, ABHES 4-a
- Explain meaningful use as it applies to EMR, CAAHEP VI.C-12

Estimated completion time: 30 minutes

Measurable Steps

1. Click on the Find Patient icon (Figure 3-118).

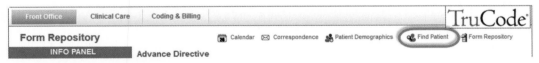

Figure 3-118 Find Patient icon.

2. Using the Patient Search fields, search for Charles Johnson's patient record. Once you locate his patient record in the List of Patients, confirm his date of birth.

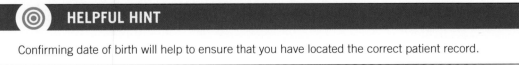

HELPFUL HINT

Confirming date of birth will help to ensure that you have located the correct patient record.

3. Select the radio button for Charles Johnson and click the Select button.
4. Create a new encounter by clicking Office Visit in the left Info Panel (Figure 3-119).
5. In the Create New Encounter window, select Follow-Up/Established Visit from the Visit Type dropdown.
6. Select James A. Martin, MD from the Provider dropdown.
7. Click the Save button.
8. Select Progress Notes from the Record dropdown menu.
9. Document the date using the calendar picker.

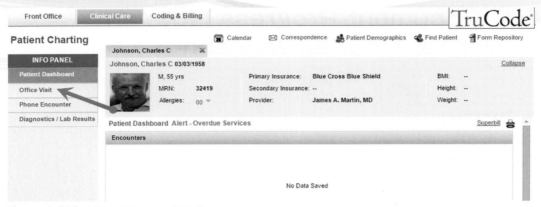

Figure 3-119 Office Visit in the Info Panel.

10. Document "CC: Elevated BS last night. 230 mg/dL at 9:00 PM. Experiencing shakes and anxiety a few hours after meals." in the Subjective field.
11. Document "T: 98.4°F (TA), P: 84 reg, strong radial, R: 14 reg, BP: 156/90 left arm, sitting, HbA1c - 7.6%. BS random 189 mg/dL." in the Objective field.
12. Click the Save button.
13. Select Order Entry from the Record dropdown menu.
14. Click the Add button below the In-Office table to add an order.
15. In the Add Order window, select Glucometer Reading from the Order dropdown menu.
16. Document "189 mg/dL" in the Results field.
17. Select the RBS radio button.
18. Document any additional information provided and click the Save button. The In-Office table will display the new order.
19. Click the Form Repository icon.
20. Select the Requisition form from the left Info Panel.
21. Select Laboratory from the Requisition Type dropdown menu.
22. Click the Patient Search button to assign the form to Charles Johnson. Confirm the auto-populated patient demographics.
23. Use the calendar picker to document the correct date in the Service Date field.
24. In the Diagnosis field, document "Type 2 diabetes with hyperglycemia."
25. Place the cursor in the Diagnosis Code field to access the encoder (Figure 3-120).

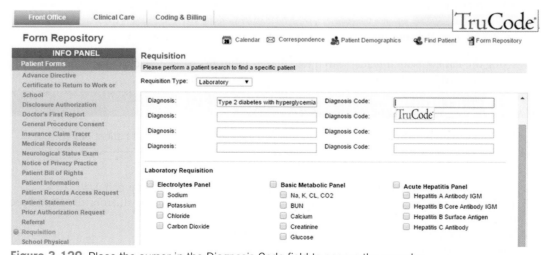

Figure 3-120 Place the cursor in the Diagnosis Code field to access the encoder.

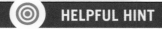

HELPFUL HINT

Accessing the encoder tool this way will auto-populate any selected codes where the cursor is placed.

26. Enter "Type 2 diabetes with hyperglycemia" in the Search field and select Diagnosis, ICD-10-CM from the dropdown menu.
27. Click the Search button.
28. Click the code E11.65 to expand this code and confirm that it is the most specific code available (Figure 3-121).

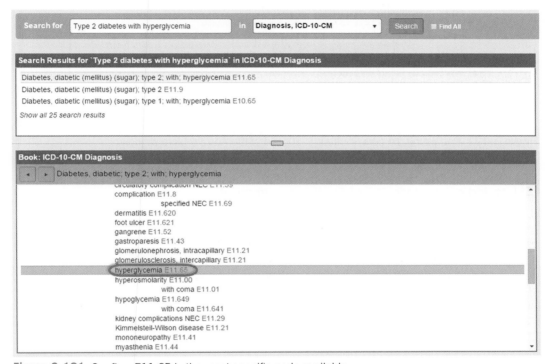

Figure 3-121 Confirm E11.65 is the most specific code available.

29. Click the code E11.65 for "Type 2 diabetes mellitus with hyperglycemia" that appears in the tree. This code will auto-populate in the ICD-10 field of the Diagnosis Code field. (Figure 3-122).
30. Select the Hgb A 1C (Glycohemo) checkbox in the Laboratory Tests section.
31. Document any additional information needed and click the Save to Patient Record button. Confirm the date and click OK.
32. Click the Clinical Care tab.
33. Using the Patient Search fields, search for Charles Johnson's patient record. Once you locate him in the List of Patients, confirm his date of birth.
34. Select the radio button for Charles Johnson and click the Select button. Confirm the auto-populated details.
35. Within the Patient Dashboard, scroll down to view the saved forms in the Forms section. Select the form you prepared. The form will open in a new window, allowing you to print.

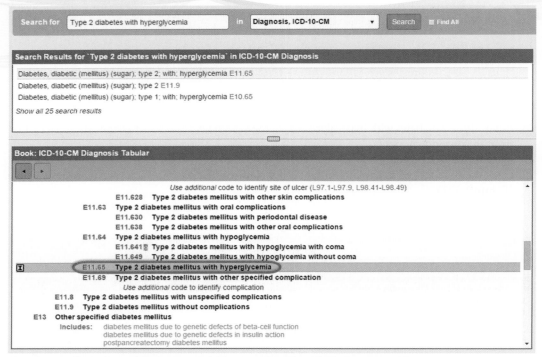

Figure 3-122 Populating the code in the ICD-10 field of the Add Problem window.

Now use the Back to Assignment link to complete the Post-Case Quiz found on the Info Panel for this assignment.

52. Document a Phone Encounter and Order for Charles Johnson

■ Objectives

- Search for a patient record.
- Document a phone encounter.
- Document an order.
- Create a lab requisition.

■ Overview

Charles Johnson had a lipid profile during his visit last week. The results of the test are total cholesterol: 136, HDL: 45, LDL: 80. Triglycerides of 140. Dr. Martin reviewed the results and documented "Normal results. Repeat lipid profile in one year." Charles Johnson calls the office today to ask about the results. Document the phone consultation, enter the order for the cholesterol screening (include the ICD-10 code), and complete the requisition form for the lab order for Charles Johnson.

■ Competencies

- Demonstrate professional telephone techniques, CAAHEP V.P-6, ABHES 7-g
- Demonstrate sensitivity to patients' rights, CAAHEP X.A-1, ABHES 4-g, 5-h
- Differentiate between normal and abnormal test results, CAAHEP II.P-2, ABHES 2-c
- Document telephone messages accurately, CAAHEP V.P-7, ABHES 7-g
- Recognize the impact personal ethics and morals have on the delivery of healthcare, CAAHEP XI.A-1, ABHES 4-g
- Perform patient screening using established protocols, CAAHEP I.P-3, ABHES 2-c, 7-d, 8-c
- Demonstrate appropriate response(s) to ethical issues, CAAHEP XI.P-2

Estimated completion time: 25 minutes

Measurable Steps

1. Click on the Find Patient icon (Figure 3-123).

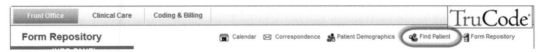

Figure 3-123 Find Patient icon.

2. Using the Patient Search fields, search for Charles Johnson's patient record. Once you locate his patient record in the List of Patients, confirm his date of birth.

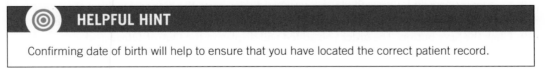

> **HELPFUL HINT**
>
> Confirming date of birth will help to ensure that you have located the correct patient record.

3. Select the radio button for Charles Johnson and click the Select button. Confirm the auto-populated details in the Patient Header.
4. Create a phone encounter for Charles Johnson by clicking Phone Encounter in the Info Panel to the left (Figure 3-124).
5. In the Create New Encounter window, document "Charles Johnson" in the Caller field.

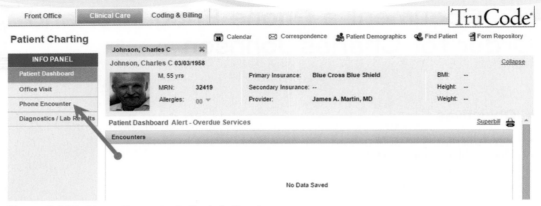

Figure 3-124 Phone Encounter in the Info Panel.

6. Select James A. Martin, MD from the Provider dropdown menu.
7. Document "Patient informed about normal lipid profile results. Will repeat lipid profile in one year." in the Message field.
8. Click the Save button.
9. Select Order Entry from the Record dropdown menu.
10. Select the TruCode encoder link in the top right corner. The encoder tool will open in a new tab (Figure 3-125).

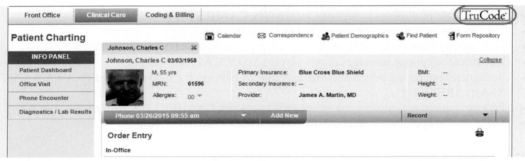

Figure 3-125 TruCode encoder tool.

11. Enter "Cholesterol screening" in the Search field and select Diagnosis, ICD-10-CM from the corresponding dropdown menu.
12. Click the Search button.
13. Click the Z13.9 code to expand this code and confirm that it is the most specific code available (Figure 3-126). Scroll up through the codes to find "Encounter for screening for cholesterol level."
14. Copy the Z13.220 code for "Encounter for screening for lipoid disorders" that populates in the search results (Figure 3-127).
15. Click the Add button below the Out-of-Office grid to add an order.
16. In the Add Order window, select Requisitions from the Order dropdown menu.
17. Select Laboratory from the Requisition Type dropdown menu.
18. Document "repeat lipid profile in one year" and then paste the diagnosis within the Notes field so that it is available for documentation and provide any additional information needed.
19. Click the Save button. The order you added will display in the Out-of-Office grid.
20. Click the Form Repository icon.
21. Select the Requisition form from the left Info Panel.
22. Select Laboratory from the Requisition Type dropdown menu.
23. Click the Patient Search button to assign the form to Charles Johnson. Confirm the auto-populated patient demographics.
24. In the Diagnosis field, document "Cholesterol screening."
25. Place the cursor in the Diagnosis Code field to access the encoder (Figure 3-128).

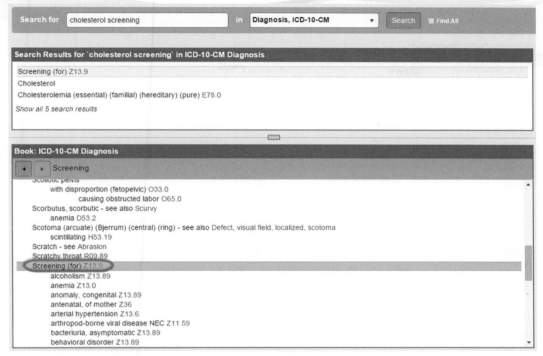

Figure 3-126 Confirm Z13.9 is the most specific code available.

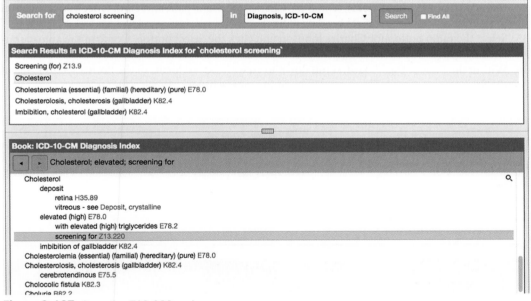

Figure 3-127 Copy the Z13.220 code.

26. Enter "Cholesterol screening" in the Search field and select Diagnosis, ICD-10-CM from the dropdown menu.

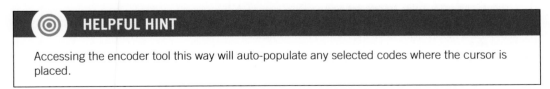

(◎) **HELPFUL HINT**

Accessing the encoder tool this way will auto-populate any selected codes where the cursor is placed.

27. Click the Search button.
28. Click the code Z13.9 to expand this code and confirm that it is the most specific code available.

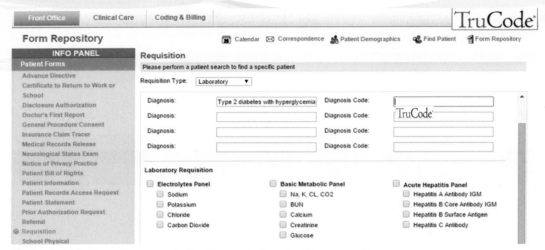

Figure 3-128 Place the cursor in the Diagnosis Code field to access the encoder.

29. Scroll up and click the code Z13.220 for "Cholesterol screening" that appears in the tree. This code will auto-populate in the Diagnosis Code field (Figure 3-129).
30. Select the Lipid Profile checkbox.
31. Document "Patient should be fasting." in the Patient Preparation field.
32. Document any additional information needed and click the Save to Patient Record button. Confirm today's date and click OK.
33. Click the Clinical Care tab.
34. Using the Patient Search fields, search for Charles Johnson's patient record. Once you locate him in the List of Patients, confirm his date of birth.
35. Select the radio button for Charles Johnson and click the Select button. Confirm the auto-populated details.
36. Within the Patient Dashboard, scroll down to view the saved forms in the Forms section. Select the form you prepared. The form will open in a new window, allowing you to print.

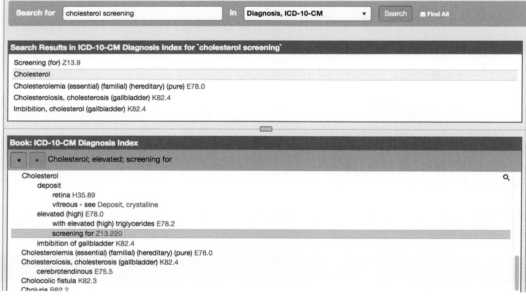

Figure 3-129 Click the code to auto-populate in the Diagnosis Code field.

Now use the Back to Assignment link to complete the Post-Case Quiz found on the Info Panel for this assignment.

53. Document Phone Encounter for Ella Rainwater

■ Objectives

- Search for a patient record.
- Document a phone encounter.

■ Overview

Dr. Martin conducted a bone density test during Ella Rainwater's last appointment and she is now calling to find out the results. Dr. Martin has not reviewed the test results yet, so the medical assistant takes a message. Ella Rainwater says the best time to return her call is after 1:00 pm today at 123-232-5690. Document this phone encounter in Ella Rainwater's patient record and prepare a message for Dr. Martin using the Correspondence section.

■ Competencies

- Define the principles of self-boundaries, CAAHEP V.C-11, ABHES 5-f
- Demonstrate professional telephone techniques, CAAHEP V.P-6, ABHES 7-g
- Document telephone messages accurately, CAAHEP V.P-7, ABHES 5-f, 7-g
- Relate assertive behavior to professional communication, CAAHEP V.C-14a, ABHES 5-f, 5-h
- Report relevant information concisely and accurately, CAAHEP V.P-11, ABHES 7-g

Estimated completion time: 25 minutes

Measurable Steps

1. Click on the Find Patient icon (Figure 3-130).

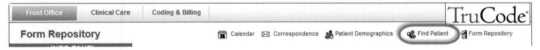

Figure 3-130 Find Patient icon.

2. Using the Patient Search fields, search for Ella Rainwater's patient record. Once you locate her in the List of Patients, confirm her date of birth.
3. Select the radio button for Ella Rainwater and click the Select button. Confirm the auto-populated details in the Patient Header.
4. Create a phone encounter for Ella Rainwater by clicking Phone Encounter in the left Info Panel (Figure 3-131).
5. In the Create New Encounter window, document "Ella Rainwater" in the Caller field.
6. Select James A. Martin, MD from the Provider dropdown.
7. Document "Patient calling for bone density examination results. Ella can be reached after 1:00 PM today at 123-232-5690." in the Message field.
8. Click the Save button.
9. Click on the Correspondence icon (Figure 3-132).
10. Select the Phone Message template from the left Info Panel.
11. Click the Patient Search button to perform a patient search and assign the phone message to Ella Rainwater. Confirm the auto-populated details.
12. Document the current date in the Date field.

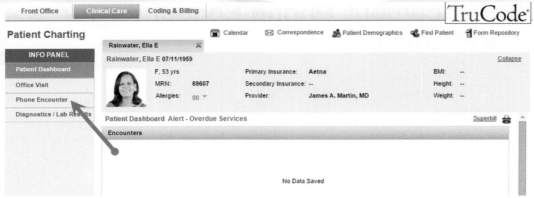

Figure 3-131 Phone Encounter in the Info Panel.

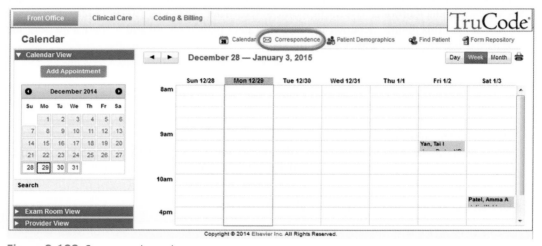

Figure 3-132 Correspondence icon.

13. Document the current time of the call in the Time field.
14. Document "Ella Rainwater" in the Caller field.
15. Document "Dr. Martin" in the Provider field.
16. Select the Please Call checkbox.
17. Document "Patient calling for bone density examination results. Ella can be reached after 1:00 PM today at 123-232-5690." in the Message field.
18. Click the Save to Patient Record button. Confirm the date and click OK.
19. Click on the Find Patient icon.
20. Using the Patient Search fields, search for Ella Rainwater's patient record. Once you locate her in the List of Patients, confirm her date of birth.
21. Select the radio button for Ella Rainwater and click the Select button. Confirm the auto-populated details.
22. Scroll down to view the Correspondence section of the Patient Dashboard.
23. Select the phone message you prepared. The phone message will open in a new window, allowing you to print (Figure 3-133).

WALDEN-MARTIN
FAMILY MEDICAL CLINIC
1234 ANYSTREET | ANYTOWN, ANYSTATE 12345
PHONE 123-123-1234 | FAX 123-123-5678

Phone Message

Date:	January 14, 2015	**Time:**	10:45 am
Caller:	Ella Rainwater	**Provider:**	Dr. Martin
Regarding Patient:	Rainwater, Ella E	**Patient Date of Birth:**	07/11/1959

PLEASE CALL

Message: Patient calling for bone density examination results. Ella can be reached after 1:00 PM today at 123-232-5690.

Pharmacy: --

Provider Recommendation: --

Action Documentation: --

Completed By:	Kate Gilliam	**Date/Time:**	January 14, 2015/10:45 am

Figure 3-133 The phone message will open in a new window for printing.

 Now use the Back to Assignment link to complete the Post-Case Quiz found on the Info Panel for this assignment.

54. Document Preventative Services and Immunizations for Ella Rainwater

■ Objectives

- Search for a patient record.
- Document preventative services.
- Document immunizations.

■ Overview

The medical assistant must add Ella Rainwater's bone density test performed seven days ago to her patient record as a preventative service. After receiving the results from Anytown Bones, Dr. Martin determined that the results are a normal study. Dr. Martin also notices that Ella Rainwater is due for a tetanus booster and she decides to have the vaccination today. She has no adverse reaction. The label displays the following information:

0.5 mL, given IM in the right deltoid, Manufacturer: Sanofi-Pasteur, Lot#: 774521, Expiration: 01/15.*

---

* The year of expiration displayed on the labels should reflect an expiration date of three years past the current year.

■ Competencies

- Administer parenteral (excluding IV) medications, CAAHEP I.P-7, ABHES 8-f
- Define and use medical abbreviations when appropriate and acceptable, ABHES 3-d
- Define coaching a patient, CAAHEP V.C-6, ABHES 5-c, 8-h
- Document patient care accurately in the medical record, CAAHEP X.P-3, ABHES 4-a
- Identify body systems, CAAHEP I.C-2, ABHES 2-a
- Define personal protective equipment, CAAHEP III.C-6, ABHES 8-a
- Organize a patient's medical record, CAAHEP VI.P-4, ABHES 7-a, 7-b
- Report relevant information concisely and accurately, CAAHEP V.P-11, ABHES 4-a, 7-g
- Use proper body mechanics, CAAHEP XII.P-3, ABHES 1-d
- Document telephone messages accurately, CAAHEP V.P-7

Estimated completion time: 15 minutes

Measurable Steps

1. Click on the Find Patient icon (Figure 3-134).

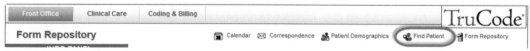

Figure 3-134 Find Patient icon.

2. Using the Patient Search fields, search for Ella Rainwater's patient record. Once you locate her in the List of Patients, confirm her date of birth.

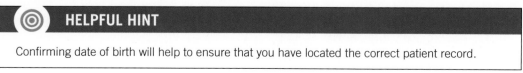

HELPFUL HINT

Confirming date of birth will help to ensure that you have located the correct patient record.

3. Select the radio button for Ella Rainwater and click the Select button.
4. Create a new encounter by clicking Office Visit in the left Info Panel (Figure 3-135).

Clinical Care

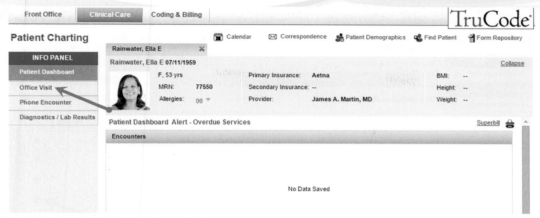

Figure 3-135 Office Visit in the Info Panel.

5. In the Create New Encounter window, select Follow-Up/Established Visit from the Visit Type dropdown.
6. Select James A. Martin, MD from the Provider dropdown.
7. Click the Save button.
8. Select Preventative Services from the Record dropdown menu.
9. Click the Add button in the Procedures section (Figure 3-136).

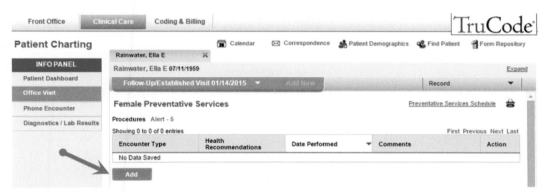

Figure 3-136 Add button in the Procedures section.

10. Select Bone Density from the Health Recommendation dropdown menu.
11. Document the date performed using the calendar picker.
12. Document "Normal study" in the Comments field.
13. Click the Save button. The preventative service you added will display in the Preventative Services table.
14. Select Immunizations from the Record dropdown menu.
15. Locate the row for the "DTap (Diphtheria, Tetanus, Pertussis)" vaccine and click on the green plus sign to the far right of that row. That row will become active so you can add an immunization to Ella Rainwater's record (Figure 3-137).
16. Within the Type column, select DTaP.
17. Within the Dose column, document "0.5 mL".
18. Within the Date column, use the calendar picker to select the date administered.
19. Within the Provider column, document "James A. Martin, MD" in the text box.
20. Within the Route/Site column, document "IM R deltoid" in the text box.
21. Within the Manufacturer/Lot# column, document "Sanofi-Pasteur/774521" in the text box.
22. Within the Exp column, document "01/15/20XX" in the text box.
23. Within the Reaction column, document "Patient has no reaction" in the text box.
24. Click the Save button. The Immunizations table will display the new immunization.

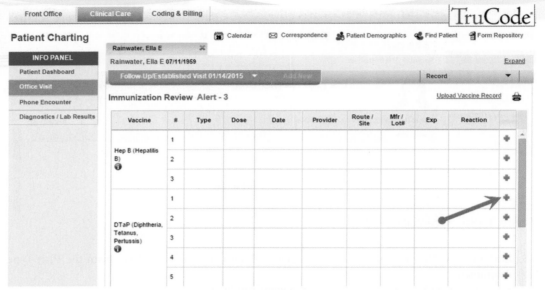

Figure 3-137 Activating a row to add an immunization.

⭐ Now use the Back to Assignment link to complete the Post-Case Quiz found on the Info Panel for this assignment.

55. Document Vital Signs, Allergies, Medications, and Order for Maude Crawford

■ Objectives

- Search for a patient record.
- Document vital signs.
- Document allergies.
- Document medications.
- Document an order.

■ Overview

Maude Crawford is three weeks post right hip replacement (status post hip replacement) after slipping on ice in front of her grocery store. Her stepson, Mark Melley, has brought her in to see Dr. Martin for a post-op visit. Maude Crawford states that she has less pain while walking and her mobility is improving with physical therapy. Penicillin makes her nauseous and her current medications are Dicalcium Phosphate, St. John's Wort, and Acetaminophen/Hydrocodone 300mg/5mg po q4-6hr prn. The medical assistant obtains her vital signs as HT: 66 in, WT: 155 pounds (standing scale), T: 99.0°F (tympanic), P: 100 reg, bounding (radial), R: 20 reg, BP: 122/80 (right arm, sitting, manual with cuff). Dr. Martin recommends that Maude Crawford continue physical therapy (S/P R hip replacement; CPT 27110) for two more weeks, three times per week.

Document Maude Crawford's vital signs, allergies, medications, and order for continuation of physical therapy.

    Range of Motion Physical Therapy
    565 Rehab Avenue
    Anytown, AL 12345

■ Competencies

- Incorporate critical thinking skills when performing patient assessment, CAAHEP I.A-1, ABHES 5-f
- Incorporate critical thinking skills when performing patient care, CAAHEP I.A-2, ABHES 5-f
- Maintain medication and immunization records, ABHES 4-a, 4-f
- Measure and record vital signs, CAAHEP I.P-1, ABHES 8-b
- Perform procedural coding, CAAHEP IX.P-1, ABHES 7-d
- Recognize elements of fundamental writing skills, CAAHEP V.C-7, ABHES 7-g
- Verify the rules of medication administration, CAAHEP I.P-4, ABHES 8-f
- Define a patient-centered medical home (PCMH), CAAHEP VIII.C-4

Estimated completion time: 50 minutes

Measurable Steps

1. Click on the Find Patient icon (Figure 3-138).

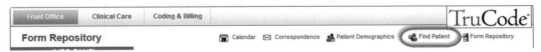

Figure 3-138 Find Patient icon.

2. Using the Patient Search fields, search for Maude Crawford's patient record. Once you locate her in the List of Patients, confirm her date of birth.

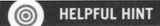
3. Select the radio button for Maude Crawford and click the Select button.
4. Create a new encounter by clicking Office Visit in the left Info Panel (Figure 3-139). Click the Add New button to create a new encounter.

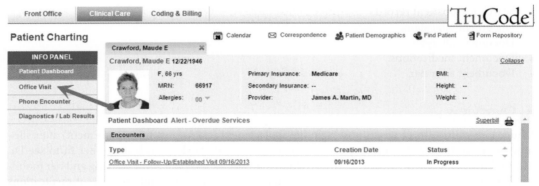

Figure 3-139 Office Visit in the Info Panel.

5. In the Create New Encounter window, select Follow-Up/Established Visit from the Visit Type dropdown.
6. Select James A. Martin, MD from the Provider dropdown.
7. Click the Save button.
8. Select Vital Signs from the Record dropdown menu.
9. In the Vital Signs tab, click the Add button.
10. Document "99.0°F" in the Temperature field and select Tympanic from the Site dropdown.
11. Document "100" in the Pulse field and select Radial from the Site dropdown.
12. Document "20" in the Respiration field.
13. Document "122" in the Systolic field.
14. Select Right arm from the Site dropdown menu.
15. Document the "80" in the Diastolic field.
16. Select Manual with Cuff in the Mode dropdown menu.
17. Select Sitting from the Position dropdown menu.
18. Click the Save button. The Vital Signs table will display the vital signs for this encounter (Figure 3-140).

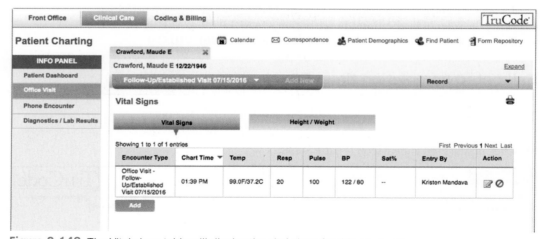

Figure 3-140 The Vital signs table will display the vital signs for this encounter.

19. In the Height/Weight tab, click the Add button.
20. Document "5" as the feet and "6" as the inches for the Height field.
21. Document "155" in the Weight field.
22. Select Standing scale from the Method dropdown menu.
23. Click the Save button. The Height/Weight table will display the height and weight for this encounter.
24. Select Allergies from the Record dropdown menu.
25. Click the Add Allergy button.
26. Select the Medication radio button in the Allergy Type field.
27. Document "penicillin" in the Allergen field.
28. Select the Nausea checkbox in the Reactions field.
29. Select Self in the Informant field.
30. Click the Save button. The Allergies table will display the new allergy.
31. Select Medications from the Record dropdown menu.
32. Within the Prescription Medications tab, click the Add Medication button to add Acetaminophen to Maude Crawford's medications.
33. Select Acetaminophen/Hydrocodone 300mg/5mg Tablet - (Xodol 5/300) from the Medication dropdown menu.
34. Select Tablet from the Form dropdown menu.
35. Select Oral from the Route dropdown menu.
36. Select Every 4 Hours PRN from the Frequency menu.
37. Document any additional information needed and select the Active radio button in the Status field.
38. Click the Save button. The Medications table will display the new medication.
39. Within the Over-the-Counter Medications tab, click the Add Medication button to add calcium to Maude Crawford's medications.
40. Select Dicalcium Phosphate from the Generic Name dropdown menu.
41. Select Vitamins/Minerals – Calcium Supplements from the Product Type dropdown menu.
42. Select Tablet from the Form dropdown menu.
43. Document "once daily" in the Frequency field.
44. Select Oral from the Route dropdown menu.
45. Document any additional information needed and select the Active radio button in the Status field.
46. Click the Save button. The Medications table will display the new medication.
47. Within the Herbal and Natural Remedy Products tab, click the Add Medication button to add St. John's Wort to Maude Crawford's medications.
48. Select St. John's wort from the Product dropdown menu.
49. Select Capsule from the Preparation dropdown menu.
50. Document "once daily" in the Frequency field.
51. Select Oral from the Route field.
52. Document any additional information needed and select the Active radio button in the Status field.
53. Click the Save button. The Medications table will display the new medication (Figure 3-141).
54. Select Order Entry from the Record dropdown menu.
55. Select the TruCode encoder link in the top right corner. The encoder tool will open in a new tab (Figure 3-142).
56. Enter "status post hip replacement" in the Search field and select Diagnosis, ICD-10-CM from the corresponding dropdown menu.
57. Click the Search button.
58. Click Presence, hip joint implant, and then the Z96.64 code that appears in red to expand this code and confirm that it is the most specific code available (Figure 3-143).
59. Copy the code Z96.641 for "Presence of right artificial hip joint" that populates in the search results (Figure 3-144).
60. Click the Add button below the Out-of-Office grid to add an order.
61. In the Add Order window, select Blank Prescription from the Order dropdown menu.
62. Select the checkbox to indicate that Dr. Martin is the physician.

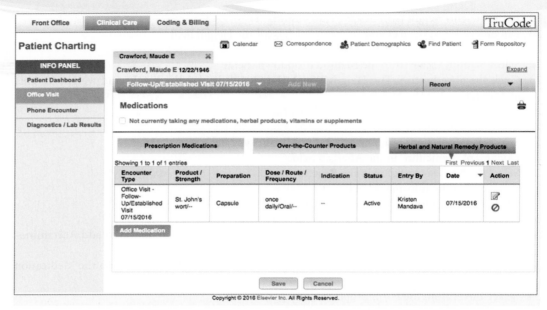

Figure 3-141 The Medications table will update with the new medication.

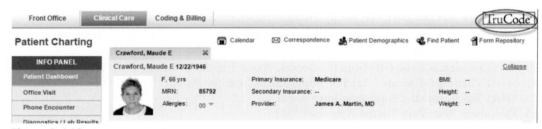

Figure 3-142 TruCode encoder tool.

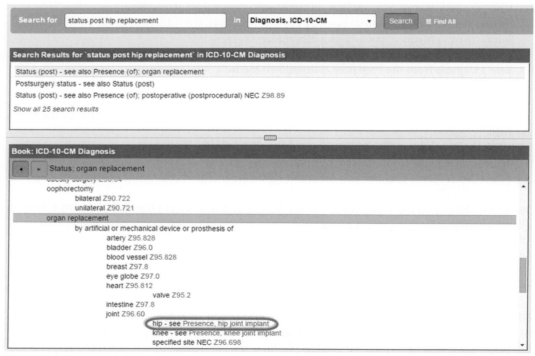

Figure 3-143 Confirm Z96.64 is the most specific code available.

63. Paste the diagnosis within the body of the blank prescription template so that it is available for documentation.

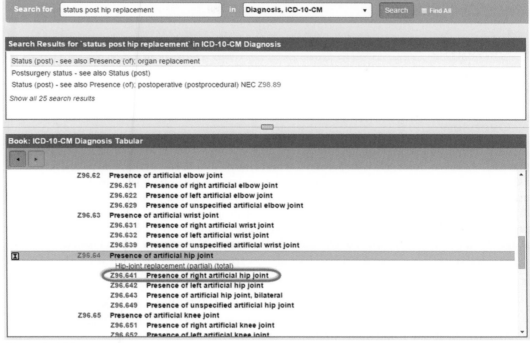

Figure 3-144 Copy the Z96.641 code.

64. Document "S/P R hip replacement (27110). Continue PT evaluation and treatment." in the text field.
65. Document "Physical therapy" in the Notes field.
66. Document any additional information provided and click the Save button. The Out-of-Office table will display the new order.

 Now use the Back to Assignment link to complete the Post-Case Quiz found on the Info Panel for this assignment.

56. Document Health History for Al Neviaser

■ Objectives

- Search for a patient record.
- Document health history.

■ Overview

Al Neviaser moved into a condo five months ago after getting a divorce. He now lives alone and states that he feels safe at home. He is an accountant and enjoys his job. He smokes one pack of cigarettes a day and occasionally has a glass of wine with dinner but has never had problems with illegal drug use. He enjoys walking his dog in the park for exercise. He does not follow any particular diet and drinks a cup of coffee every morning. Al Neviaser had an appendectomy in 1978 and a hernia repair procedure in 1985. His mother died from a stroke at age 70 and his father died from stomach cancer at age 78. Al Neviaser is a patient of Dr. Martin's. Document Al Neviaser's health history.

■ Competencies

- Administer parenteral (excluding IV) medications, CAAHEP I.P-7, ABHES 8-f
- Document patient care accurately in the medical record, CAAHEP X.P-3, ABHES 4-a
- Maintain medication and immunization records, ABHES 4-a, 4-f
- Use medical terminology correctly and pronounced accurately to communicate information to providers and patients, CAAHEP V.P-3, ABHES 3-a, 5-f
- Utilize an EMR, CAAHEP VI.P-6, ABHES 7-b
- Create a patient's medical record, CAAHEP VI.P-3

Estimated completion time: 25 minutes

Measurable Steps

1. Click on the Find Patient icon.
2. Using the Patient Search fields, search for Al Neviaser's patient record. Once you locate him in the List of Patients, confirm his date of birth.

 HELPFUL HINT

Confirming date of birth will help to ensure that you have located the correct patient record.

3. Select the radio button for Al Neviaser and click the Select button.
4. Create a new encounter by clicking Office Visit in the left Info Panel (Figure 3-145).
5. In the Create New Encounter window, select Follow-Up/Established Visit from the Visit Type dropdown.
6. Select James A. Martin, MD from the Provider dropdown.
7. Click the Save button.
8. Select Health History from the Record dropdown menu.
9. Within the Medical History tab, click the Add New button beneath the Past Surgeries section (Figure 3-146).
10. In the Add Past Surgery window, document "1978" in the Date field.
11. Document "Appendectomy" in the Type of Surgery field, along with any additional information needed.

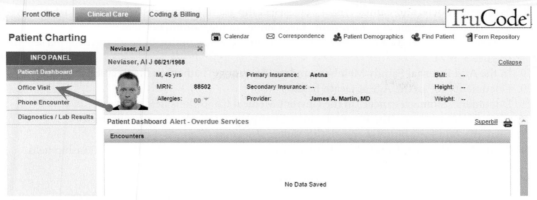

Figure 3-145 Office Visit in the Info Panel.

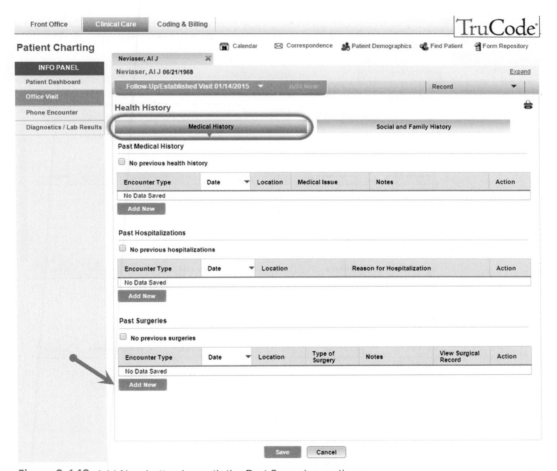

Figure 3-146 Add New button beneath the Past Surgeries section.

12. Click the Save button. The Past Surgeries table will display the newly added health history.
13. Click the Add New button beneath the Past Surgeries section.
14. In the Add Past Surgery window, document "1985" in the Date field.
15. Document "Hernia repair" in the Type of Surgery field, along with any additional information needed.
16. Click the Save button. The Past Surgeries table will display the newly added health history.

17. Within the Social and Family History tab, select the Yes radio button to document that Al Neviaser feels safe at home and document "Lives alone" in the Comments field.
18. Within the Social and Family History tab, click the Add New button beneath the Paternal section (Figure 3-147).
19. In the Add Paternal Family Member window, document "Father" in the Relationship field.
20. Document "78" in the Age at Death field.
21. Document "Stomach cancer" in the Current Medical Conditions field.
22. Click the Save button. The Paternal table will display the newly added health history.
23. Click the Add New button beneath the Maternal section (Figure 3-148).
24. In the Add Maternal Family Member window, document "Mother" in the Relationship field.
25. Document "70" in the Age at Death field.
26. Document "Stroke" in the Current Medical Conditions field.
27. Click the Save button. The Maternal table will display the newly added health history.
28. Select Divorced from the Marital Status dropdown menu.

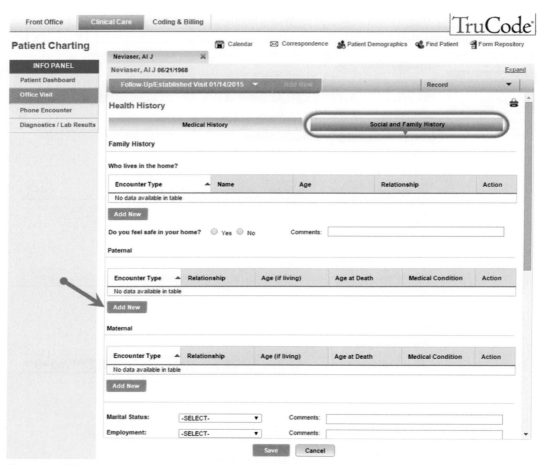

Figure 3-147 Add New button beneath the Paternal section.

29. Select Satisfied with job from the Employment dropdown menu and document "Accountant" in the Comments field.
30. Within the Tobacco section, select the Regularly radio button to indicate how often Al Neviaser smokes. Document "one pack of cigarettes a day" in the Comments field.
31. Within the Alcohol/Drugs section, select the Occasionally radio button to indicate how often Mr. Neviaser drinks alcohol. Document "glass of wine with dinner" in the Comments field.
32. Within the Alcohol/Drugs section, select the Never button to indicate that Mr. Neviaser does not use illegal drugs or substances.

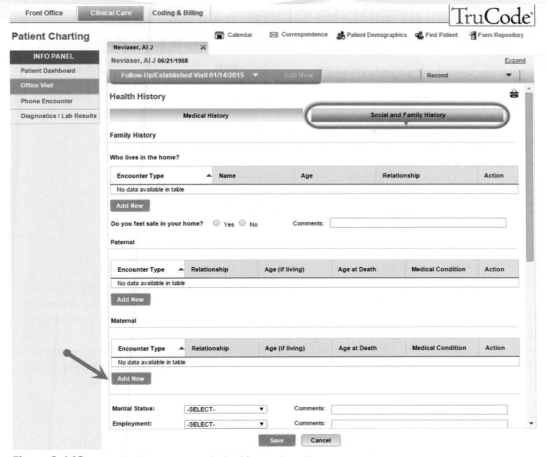

Front Office | Clinical Care | Coding & Billing

Patient Charting

Calendar   Correspondence   Patient Demographics   Find Patient   Form Repository

INFO PANEL
Patient Dashboard
Office Visit
Phone Encounter
Diagnostics / Lab Results

Neviaser, Al J   ✕

Neviaser, Al J 06/21/1968   Expand

Follow-Up/Established Visit 01/14/2015   ▼   Add New   Record   ▼

Health History

Medical History	Social and Family History

Family History

Who lives in the home?

Encounter Type ▲	Name	Age	Relationship	Action
No data available in table				

Add New

Do you feel safe in your home?   ○ Yes   ○ No   Comments: [_____]

Paternal

Encounter Type ▲	Relationship	Age (if living)	Age at Death	Medical Condition	Action
No data available in table					

Add New

Maternal

Encounter Type ▲	Relationship	Age (if living)	Age at Death	Medical Condition	Action
No data available in table					

Add New

Marital Status: [-SELECT-　▼]   Comments: [_____]

Employment: [-SELECT-　▼]   Comments: [_____]

Save   Cancel

Figure 3-148 Add New button beneath the Maternal section.

33. Within the Activities/Exposures/Habits section, select the Yes radio button and document "walks dog in park" in the Comments field.
34. Within the Nutrition section, select the No radio button to indicate that Al Neviaser does not follow a diet.
35. Within the Nutrition section, select the Yes radio button to indicate that Al Neviaser does consume caffeine. Document "one cup of coffee every morning" in the Comments field.
36. Click the Save button.

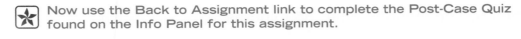

Now use the Back to Assignment link to complete the Post-Case Quiz found on the Info Panel for this assignment.

Clinical Care

57. Document Problem List, Chief Complaint, Medications, and Allergies for Carl Bowden

■ Objectives

- Search for a patient record.
- Document in the problem list.
- Document chief complaint.
- Document medications.
- Document allergies.

■ Overview

Three weeks ago, Carl Bowden tripped over some gardening tools and cut his left foot. He finished a course of antibiotics Dr. Walden prescribed one week ago, but his foot is still tender and swollen. He states the pain is a 5 on a scale of 1-10. Carl Bowden also has Type 2 diabetes (without complications) and is being treated for alcohol dependence. Dr. Walden states that Carl Bowden still has a local wound infection. He takes Actos 30 mg daily and does not have any allergies. Document the problem list (for diabetes type 2, local wound infection, and alcohol dependence) using ICD-10, chief complaint, medications, and allergies for Carl Bowden.

■ Competencies

- Collect, label, and process specimens: Perform wound collection procedures, ABHES 9-d
- Comply with safety signs, symbols, and labels, CAAHEP XII.P-1, ABHES 4-e
- Describe the process in compliance reporting for errors in patient care, CAAHEP X.C-11b, ABHES 4-e
- Define the principles of standard precautions, CAAHEP III.C-5, ABHES 8-a
- Document patient care accurately in the medical record, CAAHEP X.P-3, ABHES 4-a
- Identify safety signs, symbols, and labels, CAAHEP XII.C-1, ABHES 4-e
- Report relevant information concisely and accurately, CAAHEP V.P-11, ABHES 4-a, 7-d
- Use medical terminology correctly and pronounced accurately to communicate information to providers and patients, CAAHEP V.P-3, ABHES 3-a
- Utilize an EMR, CAAHEP VI.P-6, ABHES 7-b

Estimated completion time: 35 minutes

Measurable Steps

1. Click on the Find Patient icon.
2. Using the Patient Search fields, search for Carl Bowden's patient record. Once you locate him in the List of Patients, confirm his date of birth.

HELPFUL HINT

Confirming date of birth will help to ensure that you have located the correct patient record.

3. Select the radio button for Carl Bowden and click the Select button.
4. Create a new encounter by clicking Office Visit in the left Info Panel (Figure 3-149).

Clinical Care

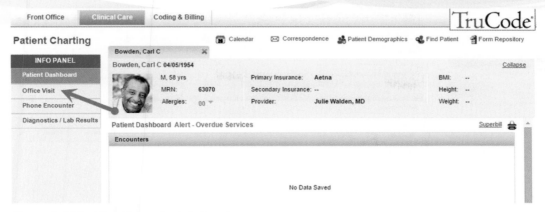

Figure 3-149 Office Visit in the Info Panel.

5. In the Create New Encounter window, select Follow-Up/Established Visit from the Visit Type dropdown.
6. Select Julie Walden, MD from the Provider dropdown.
7. Click the Save button.
8. Select Problem List from the Record dropdown menu.
9. Click the Add Problem button to add a problem (Figure 3-150).

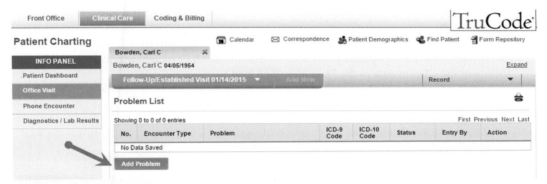

Figure 3-150 Add Problem button.

10. In the Add Problem window, select Diabetes mellitus, Type 2 without complications from the Diagnosis dropdown menu.
11. Select the ICD-10 Code radio button and place the cursor in the text box to access the TruCode encoder (Figure 3-151).
12. Enter "Type 2 diabetes mellitus without complications" in the Search field and select Diagnosis, ICD-10-CM from the dropdown menu.
13. Click the Search button.

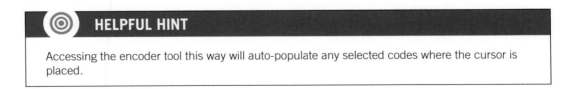

HELPFUL HINT

Accessing the encoder tool this way will auto-populate any selected codes where the cursor is placed.

Clinical Care

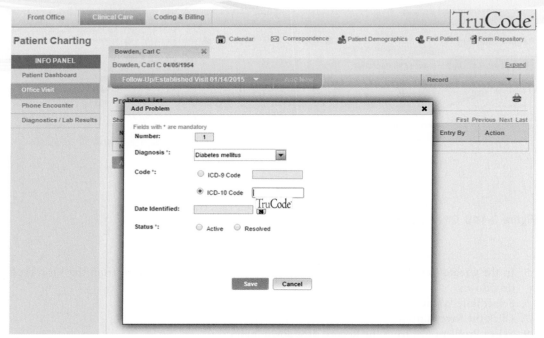

Figure 3-151 ICD-10 radio button to access TruCode encoder.

14. Click the code E11.9 to expand this code and confirm that it is the most specific code available (Figure 3-152).
15. Click the code E11.9 for "Type 2 diabetes mellitus without complications" that appears in the tree. This code will auto-populate in the ICD-10 field of the Add Problem window (Figure 3-153).
16. Document the current date in the Date Identified field.

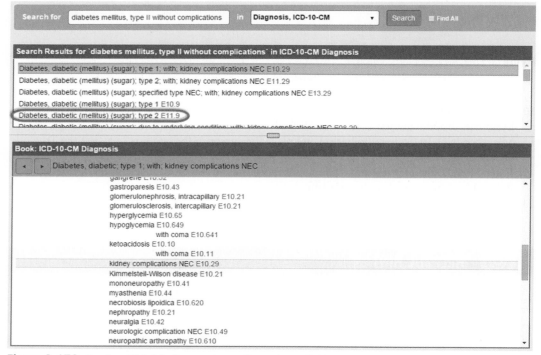

Figure 3-152 Confirm E11.9 is the most specific code available.

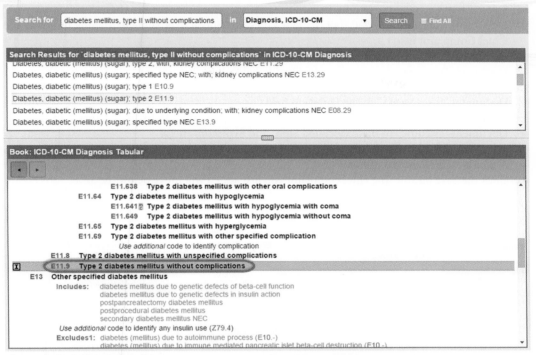

Figure 3-153 Populating the code in the ICD-10 field of the Add Problem window.

17. Select the Active radio button in the Status field.
18. Click the Save button. The Problem List table will display the newly added problem.
19. Click the Add Problem button.
20. In the Add Problem window, select Infection, wound from the Diagnosis dropdown menu.
21. Select the ICD-10 radio button and place the cursor in the text box to access the TruCode encoder.
22. Enter "Local wound infection" in the Search field and select Diagnosis, ICD-10-CM from the dropdown menu.
23. Click the Search button.
24. Click the code L08.9 to expand this code and confirm that it is the most specific code available.
25. Click the code L08.9 for "Local infection of the skin and subcutaneous tissue, unspecified" that appears in the tree. This code will auto-populate in the ICD-10 field of the Add Problem window.
26. Document the current date in the Date Identified field.
27. Select the Active radio button in the Status field.
28. Click the Save button. The Problem List table will display the newly added problem.
29. Click the Add Problem button.
30. In the Add Problem window, select Alcohol dependence from the Diagnosis dropdown menu.
31. Select the ICD-10 radio button and place the cursor in the text box to access the TruCode encoder.
32. Enter "Alcohol dependence" in the Search field and select Diagnosis, ICD-10-CM from the dropdown menu.
33. Click the Search button.
34. Click the code F10.20 to expand this code and confirm that it is the most specific code available.
35. Click the code F10.20 for "Alcohol dependence, uncomplicated" that appears in the tree. This code will auto-populate in the ICD-10 field of the Add Problem window.
36. Document the current date in the Date Identified field.
37. Select the Active radio button in the Status field.
38. Click the Save button. The Problem List table will display the newly added problem.

39. Select Chief Complaint from the Record dropdown menu.
40. Document "Laceration to left foot. Patient states he tripped over some gardening tools." in the Chief Complaint field.
41. Document "left foot" in the Location field.
42. Document "tender and swollen" in the Quality field.
43. Document "5/10" in the Severity field.
44. Document "three weeks" in the Duration field.
45. Document "finished course of antibiotics one week ago" in the Modifying Factors field.
46. Document "swelling" in the Associated Signs and Symptoms field.
47. Select the No radio button at the top of the column in each section to indicate that Carl Bowden denies having these symptoms.
48. Click the Save button. The chief complaint you just added will move below the Saved tab (Figure 3-154).

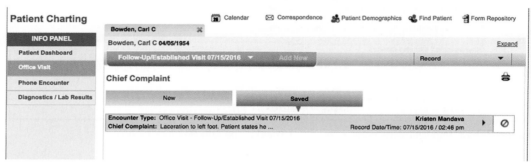

Figure 3-154 The chief complaint will be added to the Saved tab.

49. Select Medications from the Record dropdown menu.
50. Within the Prescription Medications tab, click the Add Medication button to add Actos to Carl Bowden's medications. An Add Prescription Medication window will appear.
51. Select Pioglitazone Tablet - (Actos) from the Medication dropdown menu.
52. Select 30 from the Strength dropdown menu.
53. Select Tablet from the Form dropdown menu.
54. Select Oral from the Route dropdown menu.
55. Select Daily from the Frequency dropdown menu.
56. Document any additional information needed and select the Active radio button in the Status field.
57. Click the Save button. The Medications table will display the new medication.
58. Select Allergies from the Record dropdown menu.
59. Select the No known allergies checkbox to indicate that Mr. Bowden does not have any current allergies.
60. Click the Save button.

 Now use the Back to Assignment link to complete the Post-Case Quiz found on the Info Panel for this assignment.

58. Document Chief Complaint and Order for Carl Bowden

■ Objectives

- Search for a patient record.
- Document chief complaint.
- Document ECG administration.

■ Overview

Carl Bowden has a follow-up appointment with Dr. Walden after a hospitalization for a myocardial infarction one month ago. He continues to experience fatigue, mild chest pain he describes as "pressure," shortness of breath with activity, and palpitations at night. He states his pain is a 4 on a scale of 1-10. Dr. Walden orders a 12 lead ECG test. Document the chief complaint and ECG test for Carl Bowden.

■ Competencies

- Analyze pathology for each body system including diagnostic and treatment measures, CAAHEP I.C-9, ABHES 2-c
- Coach patients regarding treatment plan, CAAHEP V.P-4d, ABHES 8-h
- Define the principles of standard precautions, CAAHEP III.C-5, ABHES 8-a
- Describe the purpose of Safety Data Sheets (SDS) in a healthcare setting, CAAHEP XII.C- 5, ABHES 9-a
- Identify methods of controlling the growth of microorganisms, CAAHEP III.C- 4, ABHES 8-a, 9-a
- Perform electrocardiography, CAAHEP I.P-2a, ABHES 8-d
- Perform hand washing, CAAHEP III.P-3, ABHES 8-a
- Select appropriate barrier/personal protective equipment (PPE), CAAHEP III.P-2, ABHES 8-a
- Show awareness of a patient's concerns related to the procedure being performed, CAAHEP I.A-3, ABHES 5-h
- Discuss the theories of Maslow, Erikson, and Kubler-Ross, CAAHEP V.C-17

Estimated completion time: 25 minutes

Measurable Steps

1. Click on the Find Patient icon (Figure 3-155).

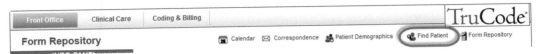

Figure 3-155 Find Patient icon.

2. Using the Patient Search fields, search for Carl Bowden's patient record. Once you locate him in the List of Patients, confirm his date of birth.

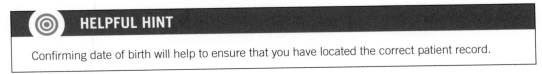

> ◎ **HELPFUL HINT**
>
> Confirming date of birth will help to ensure that you have located the correct patient record.

3. Select the radio button for Carl Bowden and click the Select button.
4. Create a new encounter by clicking Office Visit in the left Info Panel (Figure 3-156).

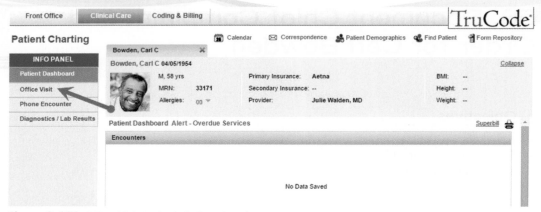

Figure 3-156 Office Visit in the Info Panel.

5. In the Create New Encounter window, select Follow-Up/Established Visit from the Visit Type dropdown.
6. Select Julie Walden, MD from the Provider dropdown.
7. Click the Save button.
8. Select Chief Complaint from the Record dropdown menu.
9. Document "fatigue, mild chest pain, shortness of breath with activity, palpitations at night" in the Chief Complaint field.
10. Document "chest" in the Location field.
11. Document "chest pressure" in the Quality field.
12. Document "4/10" in the Severity field.
13. Document "one month" in the Duration field.

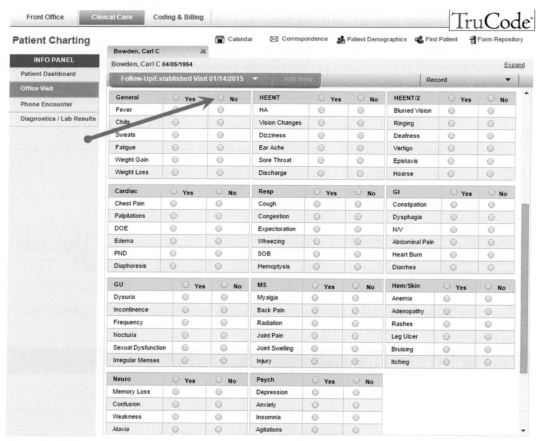

Figure 3-157 No radio button at the top of the column in each section.

14. Select the No radio button at the top of the column in each section to indicate that Carl Bowden denies having these symptoms (Figure 3-157).
15. After indicating that Carl Bowden does not have most of the symptoms in the General section, select the Fatigue, Palpitations, and SOB radio buttons in the Yes column of the Cardiac section to indicate that he is experiencing those symptoms.
16. Click the Save button. The chief complaint you just added will move below the Saved tab.
17. Select Order Entry from the Record dropdown menu.
18. Click the Add button below the In-Office table to add an order.
19. In the Add Order window, select ECG from the Order dropdown menu.
20. Document "12 lead" in the Method field.
21. Document any additional information provided and click the Save button. The In-Office table will display the new order.

 Now use the Back to Assignment link to complete the Post-Case Quiz found on the Info Panel for this assignment.

59. Document Problem List, Allergies, Vital Signs, Medications, and Order for Robert Caudill

■ Objectives

- Search for a patient record.
- Update medications.
- Update the problem list.
- Document allergies.
- Document vital signs.
- Prepare a prescription refill for the physician's approval.

■ Overview

Robert Caudill has a history of Alzheimer's disease and Diabetes Mellitus, Type 2 (without complications). Robert Caudill's daughter, Carol, scheduled an appointment with Dr. Walden because she says her father has been confused and agitated for the past three nights. She thinks his medication might need to be adjusted. In addition to his history of Alzheimer disease and diabetes, Robert Caudill is being treated for hypertension and coronary artery disease. He has no known allergies and takes the following medications: Avandamet 500 mg/4 mg twice daily, Toprol XL 100 mg daily, Diovan 80 mg daily, Aricept 10 mg daily. Robert Caudill's vital signs are measured as H: 5 feet and 9 inches, W: 172 (standing scale), T: 97.9°F (oral), P: 88 reg, thready (radial); R: 24 reg; BP: 144/84 (right arm, sitting, manual with cuff). Dr. Walden increases his Aricept dosage from 10 mg daily to 20 mg daily. Document the problem list (using the ICD-10 codes), allergies, vital signs, medications, and enter a new order for Aricept (using electronic transfer) in Mr. Caudill's patient record.

■ Competencies

- Define basic units of measurement in metric and household systems, CAAHEP II.C-3, ABHES 6-b
- Describe components of the Health Information Portability & Accountability Act (HIPAA), CAAHEP X.C-3, ABHES 4-h
- Prepare proper dosages of medication for administration, CAAHEP II.P-1, ABHES 6-b
- Define a patient-centered medical home (PCMH), CAAHEP VIII.C-4

Estimated completion time: 40 minutes

Measurable Steps

1. Click on the Find Patient icon.
2. Using the Patient Search fields, search for Robert Caudill's patient record. Once you locate him in the List of Patients, confirm his date of birth.

 HELPFUL HINT

Confirming date of birth will help to ensure that you have located the correct patient record.

Clinical Care

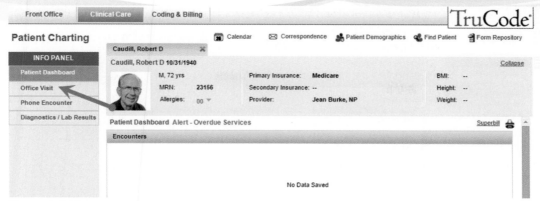

Figure 3-158 Office Visit in the Info Panel.

3. Select the radio button for Robert Caudill and click the Select button.
4. Create a new encounter by clicking Office Visit in the left Info Panel (Figure 3-158).
5. In the Create New Encounter window, select Urgent Visit from the Visit Type dropdown.
6. Select Julie Walden, MD from the Provider dropdown.
7. Click the Save button.

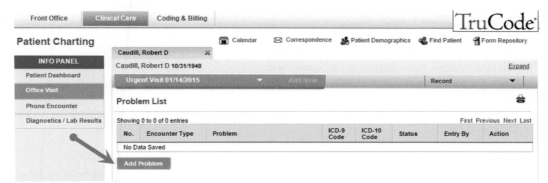

Figure 3-159 Add Problem button.

8. Select Problem List from the Record dropdown menu.
9. Click the Add Problem button to add a problem (Figure 3-159).
10. In the Add Problem window, document "Alzheimer disease" in the Diagnosis field.
11. Select the ICD-10 radio button and place the cursor in the text box to access the TruCode encoder (Figure 3-160).

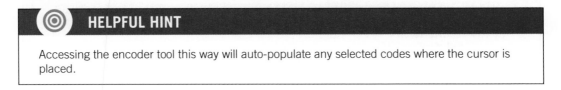

HELPFUL HINT

Accessing the encoder tool this way will auto-populate any selected codes where the cursor is placed.

12. Enter "Alzheimer disease" in the Search field and select Diagnosis, ICD-10-CM from the dropdown menu.
13. Click the Search button.
14. Click the code G30.9 to expand this code and confirm that it is the most specific code available (Figure 3-161).
15. Click the code G30.9 for "Alzheimer disease, unspecified" that appears in the tree. This code will auto-populate in the ICD-10 field of the Add Problem window (Figure 3-162).

Clinical Care

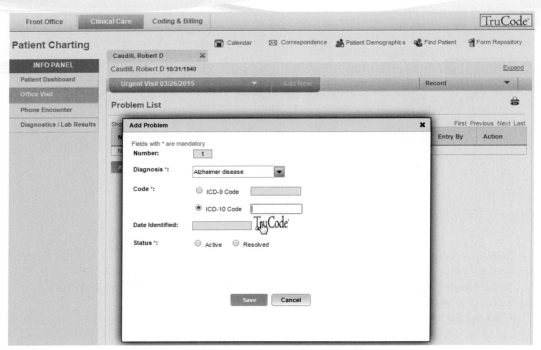

Figure 3-160 TruCode encoder tool.

16. Document the current date in the Date Identified field.
17. Select the Active radio button in the Status field.
18. Click the Save button. The Problem List table will display the new problem.
19. Click the Add Problem button.
20. In the Add Problem window, document "Diabetes mellitus, Type 2 without complications" in the Diagnosis field.

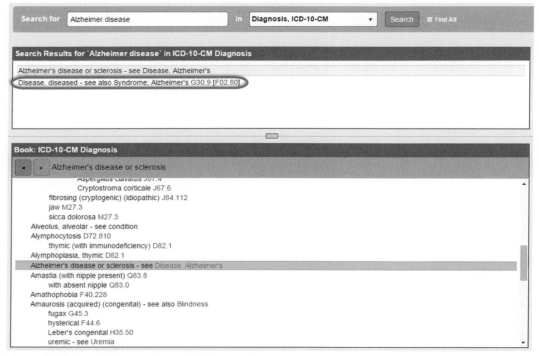

Figure 3-161 Confirm G30.9 is the most specific code available.

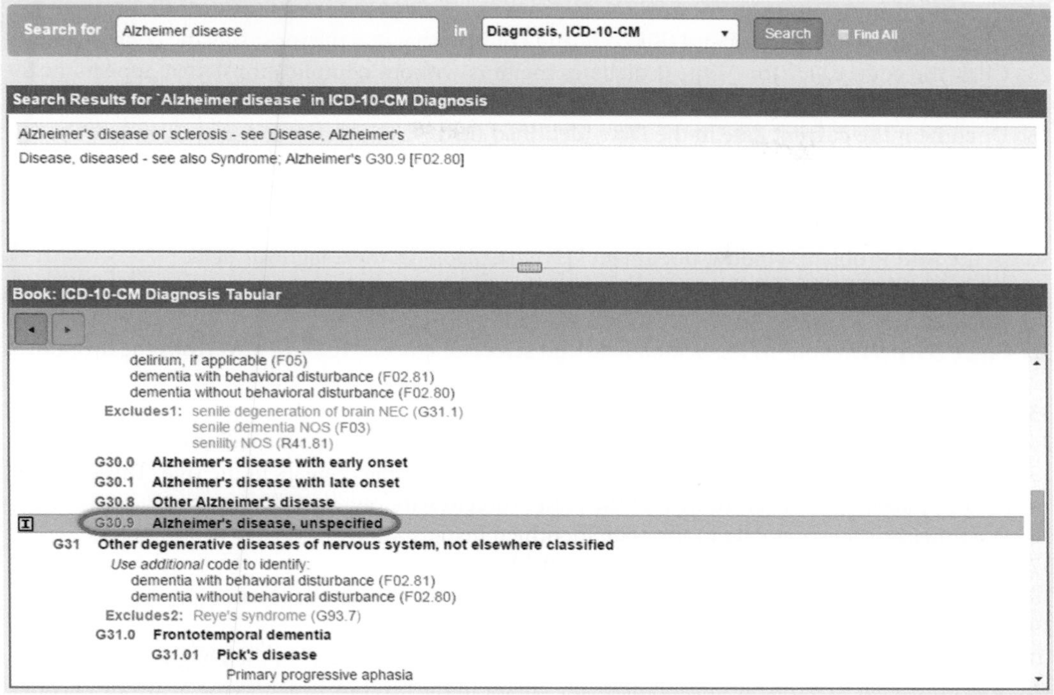

Figure 3-162 Populating the code in the ICD-10 field of the Add Problem window.

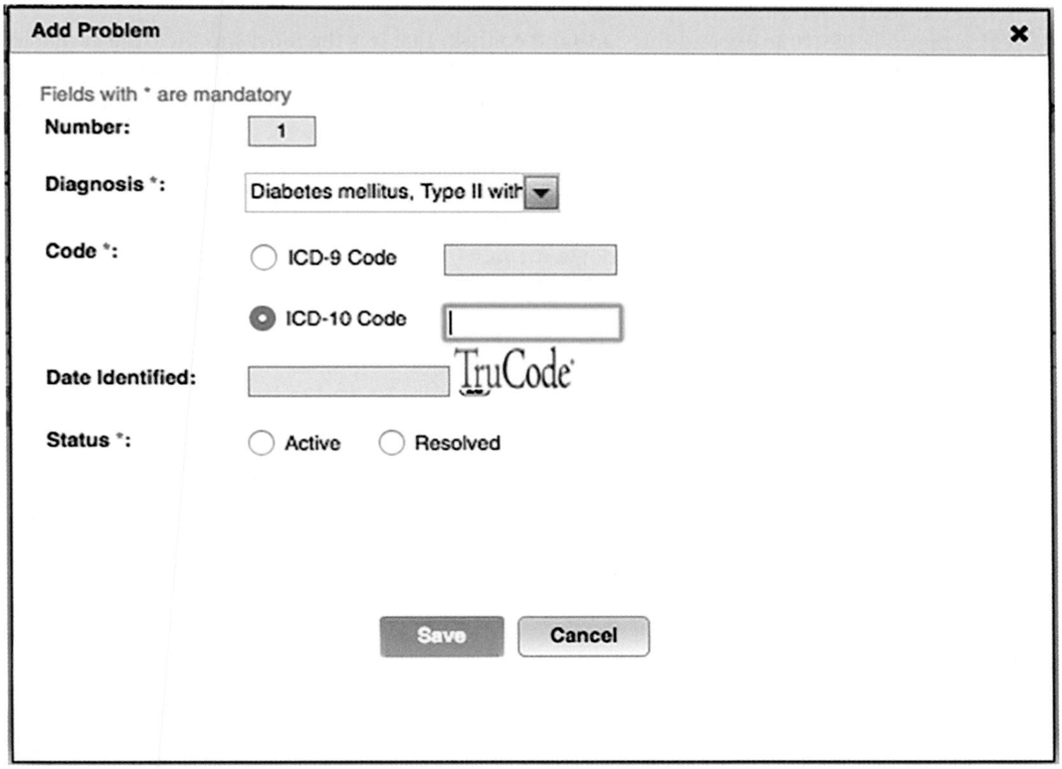

Figure 3-163 In the Add Problem window, type in the Diagnosis, select the ICD-10 radio button, and place the cursor in the text box to access the TruCode encoder.

21. Select the ICD-10 radio button and place the cursor in the text box to access the TruCode encoder (Figure 3-163).
22. Enter "Diabetes mellitus, Type 2 without complications" in the Search field and select Diagnosis, ICD-10-CM from the dropdown menu.

23. Click the Search button.
24. Click the code E11.9 to expand this code and confirm that it is the most specific code available.
25. Click the code E11.9 for "Type 2 diabetes mellitus without complications" that appears in the tree. This code will auto-populate in the ICD-10 field of the Add Problem window.
26. Document the current date in the Date Identified field.
27. Select the Active radio button in the Status field.
28. Click the Save button. The Problem List table will display the new problem.
29. Click the Add Problem button.
30. In the Add Problem window, document "Hypertension" in the Diagnosis field.
31. Select the ICD-10 radio button and place the cursor in the text box to access the TruCode encoder.
32. Enter "Hypertension" in the Search field and select Diagnosis, ICD-10-CM from the dropdown menu.
33. Click the Search button.
34. Click the code I10 to expand this code and confirm that it is the most specific code available.
35. Click the code I10 for "Essential (primary) hypertension" that appears in the tree. This code will auto-populate in the ICD-10 field of the Add Problem window.
36. Document the current date in the Date Identified field.
37. Select the Active radio button in the Status field.
38. Click the Save button. The Problem List table will display the new problem.
39. Click the Add Problem button.
40. In the Add Problem window, document "Coronary Artery Disease" in the Diagnosis field.
41. Select the ICD-10 radio button and place the cursor in the text box to access the TruCode encoder.
42. Enter "Coronary Artery Disease" in the Search field and select Diagnosis, ICD-10-CM from the dropdown menu.
43. Click the Search button.
44. Click the code I25.10 to expand this code and confirm that it is the most specific code available.
45. Click the code I25.10 for "Atherosclerotic heart disease of native coronary artery without angina pectoris" that appears in the tree. This code will auto-populate in the ICD-10 field of the Add Problem window.
46. Document the current date in the Date Identified field.
47. Select the Active radio button in the Status field.
48. Click the Save button. The Problem List table will display the new problem.
49. Select Allergies from the Record dropdown menu.
50. Select the No known allergies checkbox to indicate that Robert Caudill does not have any current allergies (Figure 3-164).
51. Click the Save button.
52. Select Vital Signs from the Record dropdown menu.
53. In the Vital Signs tab, click the Add button.
54. Document "97.9°F" in the Temperature field and select Oral from the Site dropdown menu.
55. Document "88, reg, thready" in the Pulse field and select Radial from the Site dropdown.

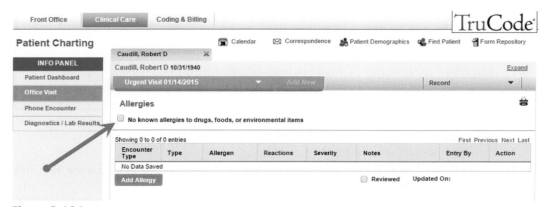

Figure 3-164 No known allergies checkbox.

56. Document "24" in the Respiration field.
57. Document "144" in the Systolic field and select Right arm from the Site dropdown menu.
58. Document "84" in the Diastolic field and Manual with cuff from the Mode dropdown menu.
59. Select Sitting from the Position dropdown menu.
60. Click the Save button. The Vital Signs table will display the vital signs for this encounter.
61. In the Height/Weight tab, click the Add button.
62. Document "5" in the 'ft' text box and "9" in the 'in' text box of the Height field.
63. Document "172" in the Weight field.
64. Select Standing scale from the Method dropdown menu.
65. Click the Save button. The Height/Weight table will display the height and weight for this encounter.
66. Select Medications from the Record dropdown menu.
67. Within the Prescription Medications tab, click the Add Medication button to add Avandamet to Robert Caudill's medications. An Add Prescription Medication window will appear.
68. Select Metformin/Rosiglitazone 500 mg/4mg tablet - (Avandamet) from the Medication dropdown menu.
69. Select Tablet from the Form dropdown menu.
70. Select Oral from the Route dropdown menu.
71. Select 2 Times/Day from the Frequency dropdown menu.
72. Document any additional information needed and select the Active radio button in the Status field.
73. Click the Save button. The Medications table will display the new medication (Figure 3-165).

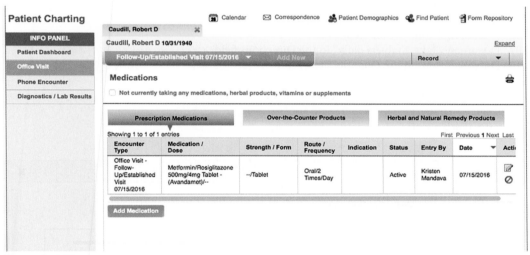

Figure 3-165 The Medications table will display the new medication.

74. Within the Prescription Medications tab, click the Add Medication button to add Toprol to Robert Caudill's medications. An Add Prescription Medication window will appear.
75. Select Metoprolol Extended Release Tablet - (Toprol-XL) from the Medication dropdown menu.
76. Select 100 from the Strength dropdown menu.
77. Select Tablet ER from the Form dropdown menu.
78. Select Oral from the Route dropdown menu.
79. Select Daily from the Frequency dropdown menu.
80. Document any additional information needed and select the Active radio button in the Status field.
81. Click the Save button. The Medications table will display the new medication.
82. Click the Add Medication button.
83. Select Valsartan Tablet - (Diovan) from the Medication dropdown menu.
84. Select 80 from the Strength dropdown menu.
85. Select Tablet from the Form dropdown menu.
86. Select Oral from the Route dropdown menu.

87. Select Daily from the Frequency dropdown menu.
88. Document any additional information needed and select the Active radio button in the Status field.
89. Click the Save button. The Medications table will display the new medication.
90. Click on the Add Medication button.
91. Select Donepezil Tablet - (Aricept) from the Medication dropdown menu.
92. Document "10" in the Strength field.
93. Select Tablet from the Form dropdown menu.
94. Select Oral from the Route dropdown menu.
95. Select Daily from the Frequency dropdown menu. Document "take 2 tablets daily" in the Dose field.
96. Document any additional information needed and select the Active radio button in the Status field.
97. Select the Refill requested checkbox.
98. Click the Save button. The Medications table will display the new medication.
99. Select Order Entry from the Record dropdown menu.
100. Click the Add button below the Out-of-Office grid.
101. Select Medication Prescription from the Order dropdown menu.
102. Select the checkbox for Dr. Walden.
103. Document "Increased agitation and confusion due to Alzheimer disease" in the Diagnosis field.
104. Document "Aricept" in the Drug field (Figure 3-166).
105. Document "20 mg" in the Strength field.
106. Document "oral" in the Route field.
107. Document "tablet" in the Form field.
108. Document "none" in the Refills field.
109. Document "take 2 tablets daily" in the Directions field.
110. Document "60" in the Quantity field.
111. Document "30" in the Days Supply field.
112. Select the Electronic transfer radio button in the Issue Via field.

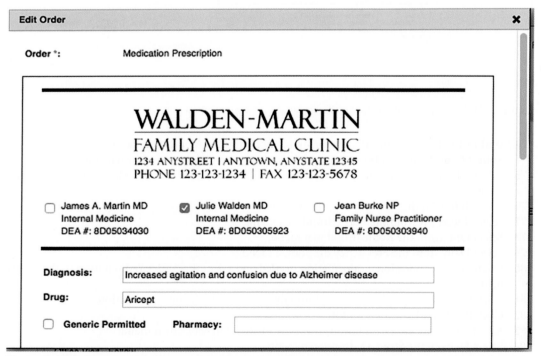

Figure 3-166 Select the Medication Prescription form from the Order dropdown menu, and begin to fill out all the necessary information.

113. Provide any additional information needed and click the Save button. The order you added will display in the Out-of-Office table (Figure 3-167).

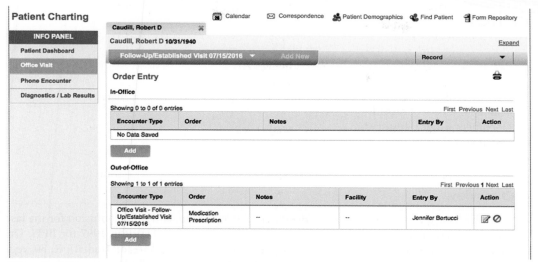

Figure 3-167 The order will display in the Out-of-Office table.

⭐ Now use the Back to Assignment link to complete the Post-Case Quiz found on the Info Panel for this assignment.

Clinical Care

60. Document Chief Complaint, Vital Signs, and Surgical History for Walter Biller

■ Objectives

- Search for a patient record.
- Document surgical history.
- Document chief complaint.
- Document vital signs.

■ Overview

Walter Biller has been experiencing some dizziness, blurred vision, and mild confusion for the last three days. He reports a left eye cataract removal two years ago and TURP in 1997 for BPH. Dr. Walden obtains the following vital signs: T: 98.0°F (oral); P: 116 reg, thready (radial); R: 30, reg, shallow; BP: 90/58 (left arm, sitting, manual with cuff). Document Mr. Biller's chief complaint, vital signs, and surgical history.

■ Competencies

- Differentiate between normal and abnormal test results, CAAHEP II.P-2, ABHES 2-c
- Identify body systems, CAAHEP I.C-2, ABHES 2-a
- Measure and record vital signs, CAAHEP I.P-1, ABHES 8-b
- Prepare items for autoclaving, CAAHEP III.P-4, ABHES 8-a

Estimated completion time: 30 minutes

Measurable Steps

1. Click on the Find Patient icon (Figure 3-168).

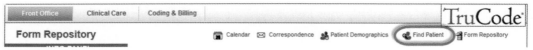

Figure 3-168 Find Patient icon.

2. Using the Patient Search fields, search for Walter Biller's patient record. Once you locate him in the List of Patients, confirm his date of birth.

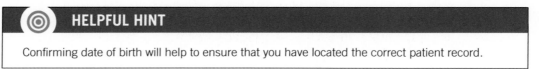

> ◎ **HELPFUL HINT**
>
> Confirming date of birth will help to ensure that you have located the correct patient record.

3. Select the radio button for Walter Biller and click the Select button.
4. Create a new encounter by clicking Office Visit in the left Info Panel (Figure 3-169).
5. In the Create New Encounter window, select Urgent Visit from the Visit Type dropdown.
6. Select Julie Walden, MD from the Provider dropdown.
7. Click the Save button.
8. Select Chief Complaint from the Record dropdown menu.
9. Document "dizziness, blurred vision, and mild confusion" in the Chief Complaint field.

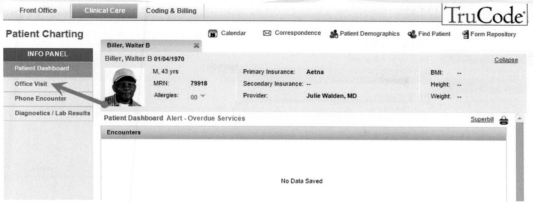

Figure 3-169 Office Visit in the Info Panel.

10. Document "3 days" in the Duration field.
11. Select the No radio button at the top of the column in the sections containing symptoms Walter Biller denies having.
12. Select the Yes radio button at the top of the column for the HEENT, HEENT/2, and Neuro sections to indicate that Walter Biller is experiencing those symptoms.
13. Click the Save button. The chief complaint you just added will move below the Saved tab.
14. Select Vital Signs from the Record dropdown menu.
15. In the Vital Signs tab, click the Add button (Figure 3-170).

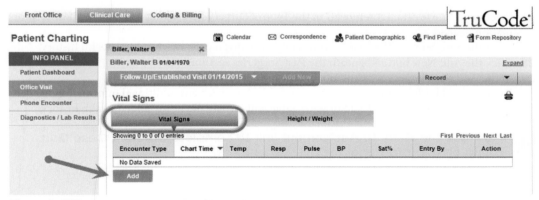

Figure 3-170 Add button in the Vital Signs tab.

16. Document "98.0°F" in the Temperature field and select Oral from the Site dropdown menu.
17. Document "116 reg, thready" in the Pulse field and select Radial from the Site dropdown.
18. Document "30 reg, shallow" in the Respiration field.
19. Document "90" in the Systolic field and select Left arm from the Site dropdown menu.
20. Document "58" in the Diastolic field and select Manual with cuff from the Mode dropdown menu.
21. Select Sitting from the Position dropdown menu.
22. Click the Save button. The Vital Signs table will display the vital signs for this encounter.
23. Select Health History from the Record dropdown menu.
24. Within the Medical History tab, click the Add New button beneath the Past Surgeries section (Figure 3-171).
25. In the Add Past Surgery window, document the date as two years ago.

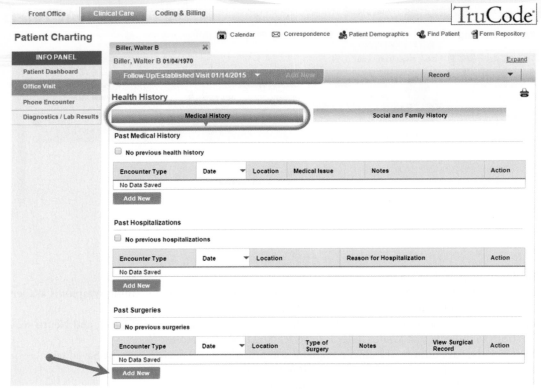

Figure 3-171 Add New button beneath the Past Surgeries section.

26. Document "L eye cataract removal" in the Type of Surgery field, along with any additional information needed.
27. Click the Save button. The Past Surgeries table will display the newly added health history.
28. Click the Add New button beneath the Past Surgeries section.
29. In the Add Past Surgery window, document the date as 1997.
30. Document "TURP" in the Type of Surgery field, along with any additional information needed.
31. Click the Save button. The Past Surgeries table will display the newly added health history.

Now use the Back to Assignment link to complete the Post-Case Quiz found on the Info Panel for this assignment.

61. Document Chief Complaint, Problem List, and Order for Robert Caudill

■ Objectives

- Search for a patient record.
- Document chief complaint.
- Document a glucose screening.

■ Overview

Robert Caudill has been experiencing dizziness and blurred vision for the past few hours. His skin is cool and clammy. Dr. Walden orders a finger stick glucose test and the result is a random blood sugar of 52 mg/dL. Dr. Walden diagnoses Robert Caudill with hypoglycemia. Document the chief complaint and order for Robert Caudill. Then update his problem list using the ICD-10 code.

■ Competencies

- Assist provider with a patient exam, CAAHEP I.P-9, ABHES 8-c, 8-d
- Demonstrate the proper use of sharps disposal containers, CAAHEP XII.P-2c, ABHES 8-a
- Describe personal protective equipment, CAAHEP III.C-6, ABHES 8-a
- Obtain specimens and perform CLIA-waived chemistry test, CAAHEP I.P- 11b, ABHES 9-b
- Perform capillary puncture, CAAHEP I.P-2c, ABHES 9-d
- Use feedback techniques to obtain patient information including reflection, restatement, and clarification, CAAHEP V.P-1, ABHES 5-h
- Respond to nonverbal communication, CAAHEP V.P-2, ABHES 5-h
- Coach patients appropriately considering cultural diversity, developmental life stage, and communication barriers, CAAHEP V.P- 5, ABHES 5-h, 7-g
- Demonstrate proper disposal of biohazardous material, CAAHEP III.P-10
- Utilize medical necessity guidelines, CAAHEP IX.P-3

Estimated completion time: 35 minutes

Measurable Steps

1. Click on the Find Patient icon (Figure 3-172).

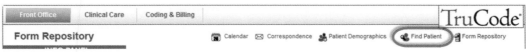

Figure 3-172 Find Patient icon.

2. Using the Patient Search fields, search for Robert Caudill's patient record. Once you locate him in the List of Patients, confirm his date of birth.

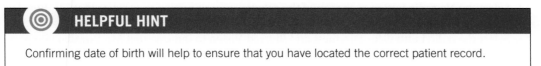

HELPFUL HINT

Confirming date of birth will help to ensure that you have located the correct patient record.

3. Select the radio button for Robert Caudill and click the Select button.
4. Create a new encounter by clicking Office Visit in the left Info Panel (Figure 3-173).

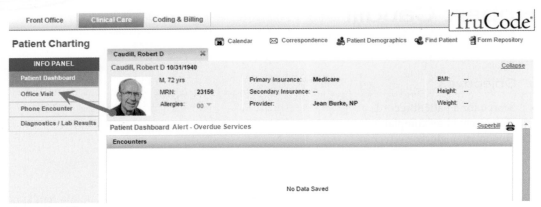

Figure 3-173 Office Visit in the Info Panel.

5. In the Create New Encounter window, select Urgent Visit from the Visit Type dropdown.
6. Select Julie Walden, MD from the Provider dropdown.
7. Click the Save button.
8. Select Chief Complaint from the Record dropdown menu.
9. Document "Dizziness and blurred vision" in the Chief Complaint field.
10. Document "past few hours" in the Duration field.
11. Document "skin is cold and clammy" in the Associated Signs and Symptoms field (Figure 3-174).

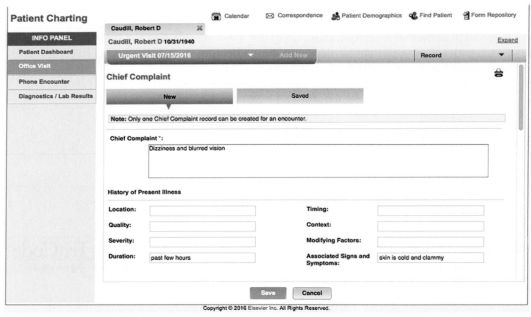

Figure 3-174 Document necessary information in the Chief Complaint section.

12. Select the No radio button at the top of the column in each section to indicate that Mr. Bowden denies having these symptoms.
13. Select the radio buttons for Dizziness and Blurred Vision to indicate that Mr. Bowden is experiencing these symptoms.
14. Click the Save button. The chief complaint you just added will move below the Saved tab.

15. Select Order Entry from the Record dropdown.
16. Click the Add button below the In-Office table to add an order.
17. In the Add Order window, select Glucometer Reading from the Order dropdown menu.
18. Document "52 mg/dL" in the Results field.
19. Select the RBS radio button.
20. Document any additional information provided and click the Save button. The In-Office table will display the new order.
21. Select Problem List from the Record dropdown menu.
22. Click the Add Problem button to add a problem.
23. In the Add Problem window, document "Hypoglycemia" in the Diagnosis field.
24. Select the ICD-10 Code radio button and place the cursor in the text box to access the TruCode encoder (Figure 3-175).

> ### ⊚ HELPFUL HINT
>
> Accessing the encoder tool this way will auto-populate any selected codes where the cursor is placed.

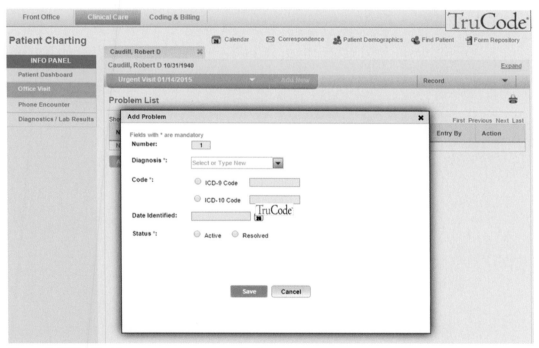

Figure 3-175 ICD-10 radio button to access TruCode encoder.

25. Enter "Hypoglycemia" in the Search field and select Diagnosis, ICD-10-CM from the dropdown menu.
26. Click the Search button.
27. Click the code E16.2 to expand this code and confirm that it is the most specific code available.
28. Click the code E16.2 for "Hypoglycemia, unspecified" that appears in the tree. This code will auto-populate in the ICD-10 field of the Add Problem window.
29. Document the current date in the Date Identified field.
30. Select the Active radio button in the Status field.
31. Click the Save button. The Problem List table will display the new problem.

 Now use the Back to Assignment link to complete the Post-Case Quiz found on the Info Panel for this assignment.

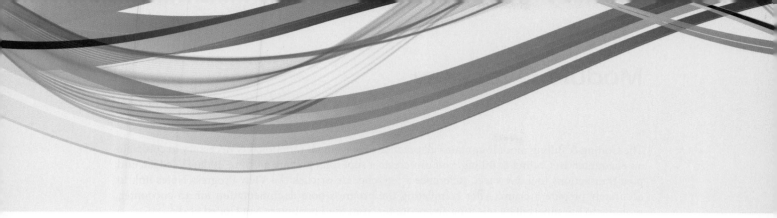

Unit 4 | Coding & Billing

Objectives

- Search for a patient record.
- Document patient information and education in the patient record.
- Order a procedure and document orders in the patient record.
- Document and update the problem list.
- Post charges, payments, and adjustments to a ledger.
- Complete a claim and an insurance claim tracer.
- Create a bank deposit slip.
- Generate referrals, orders, requisitions, and prior authorizations.
- Prepare a patient statement.
- Complete and review a superbill.
- Using the encoder, update the problem list and locate ICD-10 codes.
- Complete a medical records release.
- Document and update daily transactions on a day sheet.
- Update the medication record and prepare a prescription for electronic transmission.
- Review a claim.
- Use a fee schedule.

Module Overview

The Coding & Billing module contains all practice management functionality necessary to complete an encounter. In Coding & Billing, you can create a superbill, prepare a claim, update a ledger, and post transactions to a day sheet. Reference a fee schedule or click the View Progress Notes link to accurately prepare a claim. After completing the progress note documentation for an encounter, progress to the superbill by selecting an encounter from the Encounters Not Coded grid.

HELPFUL HINT

Once you submit a claim electronically by clicking the Submit Claim button, review the submitted claim by clicking the Output Claim button. You can also use the Back to List of Superbills link and select the desired encounter from the grid using the edit icon in the Action column.

HELPFUL HINT

To resubmit a claim, click the edit icon in the Action column for the desired encounter, make any necessary changes within the claim, and then click the Submit Claim button.

See the following pages for assignments related to the Coding & Billing module.

Coding & Billing

62. Document Progress Note and Submit Superbill for Walter Biller

■ **Objectives**

- Search for a patient record.
- Document in the progress note.
- Complete a superbill.

■ **Overview**

Walter Biller is back to see Dr. Walden for his diabetes mellitus type 2 follow-up appointment. He has been taking metformin 500 mg PO bid and is checking his blood sugar at home daily. He states he is feeling much better and learning to take better control of his blood sugar. His vital signs are T: 98.2°F (tympanic); P: 78, reg; R: 14, reg; BP: 126/84 (right arm, sitting), and a random glucose reading done in the office today is 120 mg/dL. Dr. Walden determines a diagnosis of diabetes mellitus type 2 without complications. She instructs Walter Biller to continue his current medications and revisit Walden-Martin in three months. Walter Biller has a previous balance of $25.00 and a copay of $25.00, which he paid for both during his visit. Dr. Walden indicated that there was a problem-focused history, problem-focused examination, and straightforward medical decision making. Document the progress note for Mr. Biller. Add the 10-minute office visit and glucose screening (with a monitoring device) to the superbill and submit with the appropriate CPT code for the office visit.

■ **Competencies**

- Define statute of limitations, CAAHEP X.C-7c, ABHES 4-f
- Discuss the effects of upcoding and downcoding, CAAHEP IX.C-4, ABHES 7-d
- Perform accounts receivable procedures to patient accounts including posting charges, payments, and adjustments, CAAHEP VII.P-1, ABHES 7-c
- Perform diagnostic coding, CAAHEP IX.P-2, ABHES 7-d
- Perform procedural coding, CAAHEP IX.P-1, ABHES 7-d
- Identify types of information contained in the patient's billing record, CAAHEP VII.C-5
- Differentiate between fraud and abuse, CAAHEP VIII.C-5

Estimated completion time: 25 minutes

Measurable Steps

1. Click on the Find Patient icon.
2. Using the Patient Search fields, search for Walter Biller's patient record. Once you locate his patient record in the List of Patients, confirm his date of birth.

 HELPFUL HINT

Confirming date of birth will help to ensure that you have located the correct patient record.

3. Select the radio button for Walter Biller and click the Select button.
4. Create a new encounter by clicking Office Visit in the left Info Panel (Figure 4-1).
5. In the Create New Encounter window, select Follow-Up/Established Visit from the Visit Type dropdown.
6. Select Julie Walden, MD from the Provider dropdown.
7. Click the Save button.

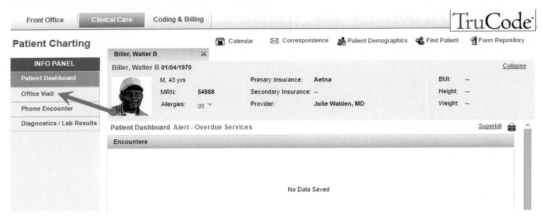

Figure 4-1 Office Visit in the Info Panel.

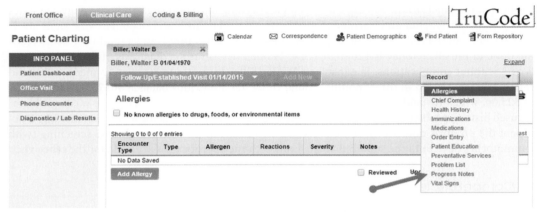

Figure 4-2 Progress Notes in the Record dropdown menu.

8. Select Progress Notes from the Record dropdown menu (Figure 4-2).
9. Document the date using the calendar picker.
10. Document "CC: DM Type 2 follow-up. Patient reports feeling much better and has better control of his BS." in the Subjective field.
11. Document "T: 98.2°F tympanic; P: 78, reg; R: 14, reg; BP: 126/84 right arm, sitting" in the Objective field.
12. Document "Diabetes Mellitus Type 2 without complications" in the Assessment field.
13. Document "Continue current medications and recheck in 3 months." in the Plan field.
14. Click the Save button.
15. Click the Coding & Billing tab.
16. You will land on the Superbill page. Perform a patient search to locate Walter Biller. (Figure 4-3).
17. Select the correct encounter from the Encounters Not Coded table and confirm the auto-populated details.
18. On page one of the superbill, Select the ICD-10 radio button.
19. In the Rank 1 row of the Diagnoses box, place the cursor in the Diagnosis field to access the encoder (Figure 4-4).
20. Enter "Type 2 diabetes mellitus without complications" in the Search field and select Diagnosis ICD-10-CM from the dropdown menu. Click the Search button.
21. Click the code E11.9 to expand this code and confirm that it is the most specific code available.
22. Click the code E11.9 for "Type 2 diabetes mellitus without complications" that appears in the tree. This code will auto-populate in the Rank 1 row of the Diagnoses box.
23. Document "1" in the Rank column for problem focused office visit.
24. Place the cursor in the Est field for problem-focused office visit to access the encoder.
25. Enter "Office Visit" in the Search for field and click CPT Tabular from the corresponding dropdown menu. Click the Search button, and then click the link in the Search Results pane to show all 15 search results.
26. Click Office Outpatient Visit 10 Minutes 99212 that appears in blue to expand this code (Figure 4-5).

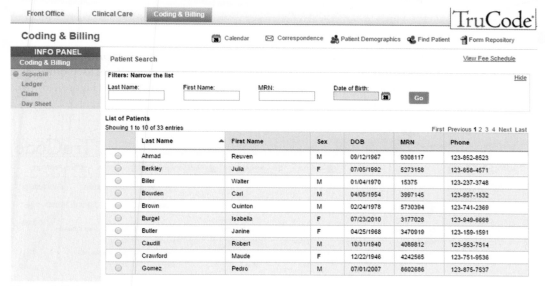

Figure 4-3 Superbill in the left Info Panel.

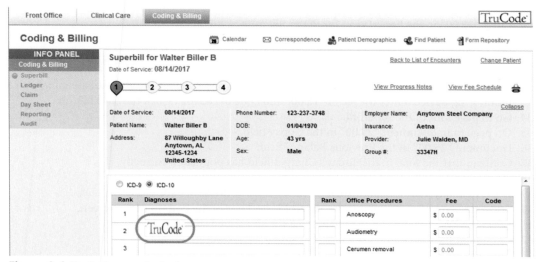

Figure 4-4 TruCode encoder tool.

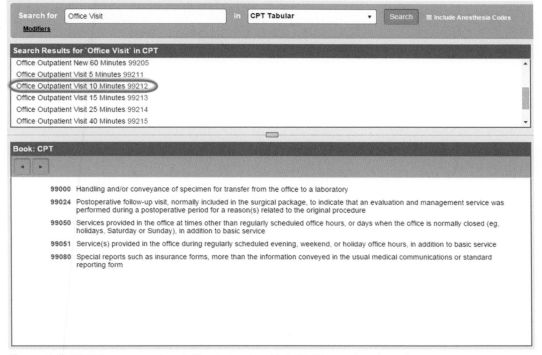

Figure 4-5 99212 appears when Office Outpatient Visit 10 Minutes is selected.

27. Review the information to determine if this is the correct code for the service provided. Click the code for 99212. This code will auto-populate in the Est field for the Problem focused office visit.
28. Click the View Fee Schedule link to obtain the charges for the office visit 99212 (Figure 4-6). This document will open in a new tab.

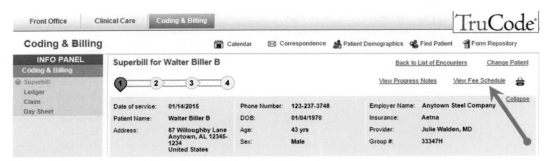

Figure 4-6 Click the View Fee Schedule link to obtain the charges.

29. Enter "32.00" in the Fee column for the problem-focused office visit.
30. Click the Save button.
31. Go to page three of the superbill.
32. Document "2" in the Rank column for Blood glucose, monitoring device.
33. Click the View Fee Schedule link to obtain the charges and code for the glucose screening with a monitoring device. Enter the fee of "16.00" and code of "82962". Click the Save button.
34. Go to page four of the superbill.
35. On page four, document "25.00" in the Copay field.
36. Document "25.00" in the Previous Balance field.
37. Confirm that the total in the Today's Charges field has populated correctly.
38. Document "48.00" in the Balance Due field.
39. Document any additional information needed. Click the Save button (Figure 4-7).
40. Select the I am ready to submit the Superbill checkbox at the bottom of the screen.
41. Select the Yes radio button to indicate that the signature is on file.
42. Document the date in the Date field.
43. Click the Submit Superbill button.

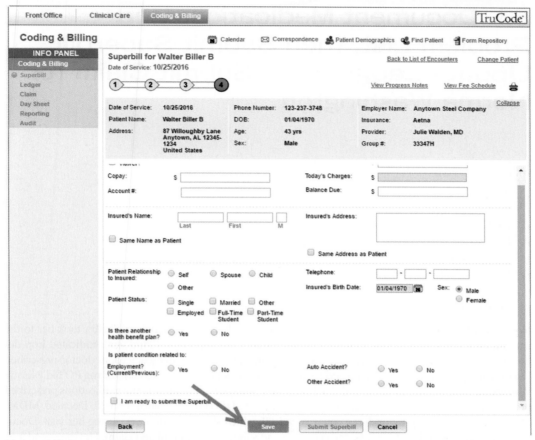

Figure 4-7 Saving documentation.

> ⊞ Now use the Back to Assignment link to complete the Post-Case Quiz found on the Info Panel for this assignment.

63. Document Medications and Problem List, then Submit Superbill, Update Ledger, and Submit Claim for Norma Washington

■ Objectives

- Search for a patient record.
- Document medications.
- Update a problem list.
- Complete a superbill.
- Complete a claim.
- Update a patient ledger.

■ Overview

Norma Washington had a right knee replacement two weeks ago. Her daughter, Shelby, took her to the emergency room last night due to fever, extreme fatigue, and weakness. Blood work indicated iron deficiency anemia and localized skin infection at the surgical site. The emergency room doctor prescribed Keflex 500 mg twice daily for 10 days and Ferrous Sulfate (extended release tablet) 325 mg PO bid. Norma Washington is following up today with Dr. Martin, who suggests she continue the medications prescribed in the ER. Dr. Martin documents the following office visit: HISTORY: Detailed, EXAM: Detailed, MDM: Moderate. Norma Washington has a copay of $25.00, which she paid with cash during her visit. Document medications and problem list, and complete and submit the superbill and claim. Use the encoder to determine the appropriate CPT code for the 25-minute office visit. Update the patient ledger to reflect the copay paid during the visit.

■ Competencies

- Complete insurance claim forms, CAAHEP VIII.P-4, ABHES 7-d
- Define medical terms and abbreviations related to all body systems, CAAHEP V.C-10, ABHES 3-a, 3-c, 3-d
- Identify common pathology related to each body system including signs, symptoms, and etiology, CAAHEP I.C-8, ABHES 2-b, 2-c
- Identify and define common abbreviations that are accepted in prescription writing, ABHES 6-c
- Report relevant information concisely and accurately, CAAHEP V.P-11, ABHES 7-g
- Perform diagnostic coding, CAAHEP IX.P-2, ABHES 7-d
- Perform procedural coding, CAAHEP IX.P-1, ABHES 7-d
- Differentiate between fraud and abuse, CAAHEP VIII.C-5
- Interact professionally with third party representatives, CAAHEP VIII.A-1

Estimated completion time: 50 minutes

Measurable Steps

1. Click on the Find Patient icon.
2. Using the Patient Search fields, search for Norma Washington's patient record. Once you locate her patient record in the List of Patients, confirm her date of birth.

 HELPFUL HINT

Confirming date of birth will help to ensure that you have located the correct patient record.

Coding & Billing

3. Select the radio button for Norma Washington and click the Select button.
4. Create a new encounter by clicking Office Visit in the left Info Panel (Figure 4-8). Click the Add New button.

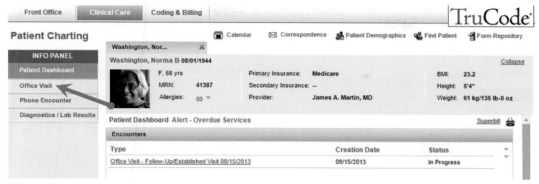

Figure 4-8 Office Visit in the Info Panel.

5. In the Create New Encounter window, select Urgent Visit from the Visit Type dropdown.
6. Select James A. Martin, MD from the Provider dropdown.
7. Click the Save button.
8. Select Medications from the Record dropdown menu (Figure 4-9).

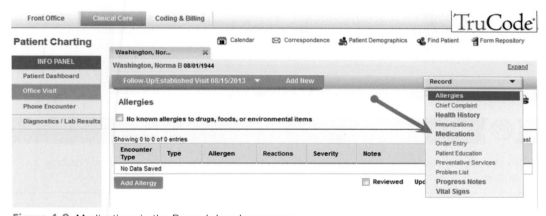

Figure 4-9 Medications in the Record dropdown menu.

9. Within the Prescription Medications tab, click the Add Medication button to add Keflex to Norma Washington's medications. An Add Prescription Medication window will appear.
10. Select Cephalexin Capsule - (Keflex) from the Medication dropdown menu.
11. Select 500 from the Strength dropdown.
12. Select Capsule from the Form dropdown.
13. Select Oral from the Route dropdown.
14. Document "Twice daily for 10 days" in the Frequency field.
15. Select the Active radio button in the Status field.
16. Click the Save button. The Medications table will display the new medication.
17. Within the Prescription Medications tab, click the Add Medication button to add Ferrous Sulfate to Norma Washington's medications. An Add Prescription Medication window will appear.
18. Select Ferrous Sulfate Extended Release Tablet (iron sulfate) - (Slow-Fe) from the Medication dropdown menu.
19. Document "325 mg" in the Strength field.
20. Select Tablet ER from the Form dropdown.
21. Select Oral from the Route dropdown.
22. Document "Twice daily" in the Frequency field.
23. Select the Active radio button in the Status field.

24. Click the Save button.
25. Select Problem List from the Record dropdown menu and click the Add Problem button.
26. In the Add Problem window, document "Anemia, iron deficiency" in the Diagnosis field.
27. Select the ICD-10 code radio button and place the cursor in the text box to access the TruCode encoder (Figure 4-10).

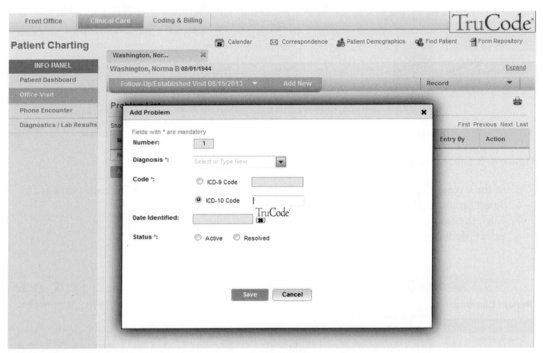

Figure 4-10 ICD-10 radio button to access TruCode encoder.

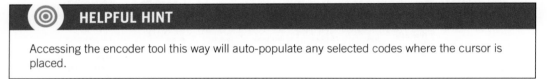

HELPFUL HINT

Accessing the encoder tool this way will auto-populate any selected codes where the cursor is placed.

28. Enter "Iron Deficiency Anemia" in the Search field and select Diagnosis, ICD-10-CM from the dropdown menu.
29. Click the Search button.
30. Click the code D50.9 to expand this code and confirm that it is the most specific code available (Figure 4-11).
31. Click the code D50.9 for "Iron deficiency anemia, unspecified" that appears in the tree. This code will auto-populate in the ICD-10 field of the Add Problem window (Figure 4-12).
32. Document the current date in the Date Identified field.
33. Select the Active radio button in the Status field.
34. Click the Save button. The Problem List table will display the new problem.
35. Click the Add Problem button.
36. In the Add Problem window, document "Localized skin infection at surgical site" in the Diagnosis field.
37. Select the ICD-10 code radio button and place the cursor in the text box to access the TruCode encoder. Accessing the encoder tool this way will auto-populate any selected codes where the cursor is placed.
38. Enter "localized skin infection" in the Search field and select Diagnosis, ICD-10-CM from the dropdown menu.
39. Click the Search button.
40. Click the code L08.9 to expand this code and confirm that it is the most specific code available.

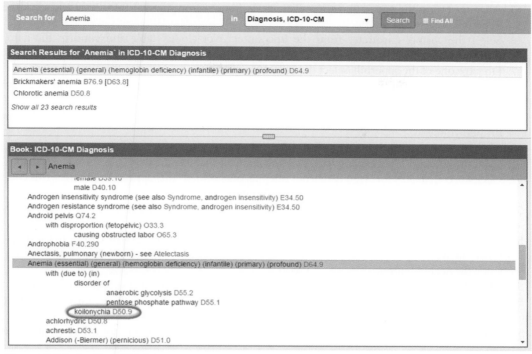

Figure 4-11 Confirm D50.9 is the most specific code available.

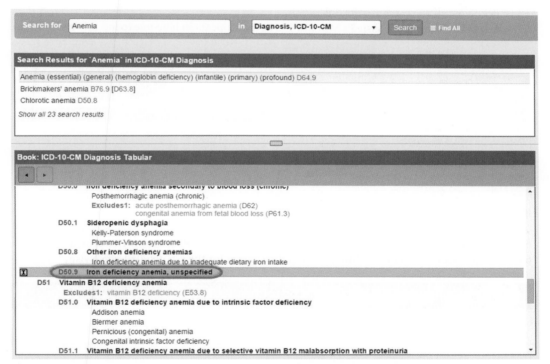

Figure 4-12 Populating the code in the ICD-10 field of the Add Problem window.

41. Click the code L08.9 for "Local infection of the skin and subcutaneous tissue, unspecified" that appears in the tree. This code will auto-populate in the ICD-10 field of the Add Problem window.
42. Document the current date in the Date Identified field.
43. Select the Active radio button in the Status field.
44. Click the Save button. The Problem List table will display the new problem.

45. After reviewing the encounter, select Patient Dashboard from the left Info Panel and click the Superbill link.
46. Select the correct encounter from the Encounters Not Coded table and confirm the auto-populated details.
47. On page one of the superbill, select the ICD-10 radio button.
48. In the Rank 1 row of the Diagnoses box, place the cursor in the Diagnosis Code field to access the encoder.
49. Enter "Iron deficiency anemia" in the Search field and select Diagnosis ICD-10-CM from the dropdown menu.
50. Click the Search button.
51. Click the code D50.9 to expand this code and confirm that it is the most specific code available.
52. Click the code D50.9 for "Iron deficiency anemia, unspecified" that appears in the tree. This code will auto-populate in the Rank 1 row of the Diagnoses box.
53. In the Rank 2 row of the Diagnoses box, place the cursor in the Diagnosis Code field to access the encoder.
54. Enter "Local skin infection" in the Search field and select Diagnosis ICD-10-CM from the dropdown menu.
55. Click the Search button.
56. Click the code L08.9 to expand this code and confirm that it is the most specific code available.
57. Click the code L08.9 for "Local infection of the skin and subcutaneous tissue, unspecified" that appears in the tree. This code will auto-populate in the Rank 2 row of the Diagnoses box.
58. Select the TruCode encoder button in the top right corner. The encoder tool will open in a new tab.
59. Enter "Office Visit" in the Search for field and click CPT Tabular from the corresponding dropdown menu. Click Search.
60. Click Show all 15 search results link.
61. Click Office Outpatient Visit 25 Minutes 99214 that appears in blue to expand this code (Figure 4-13).

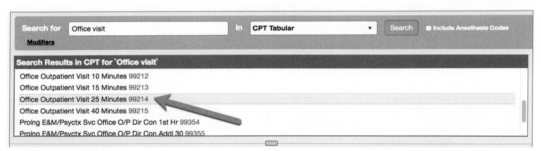

Figure 4-13 Click the code 99214 that appears in blue.

62. Review the information to determine if this is the correct code for the service provided.
63. Click the View Fee Schedule link to obtain the charges for the est. detailed office visit.

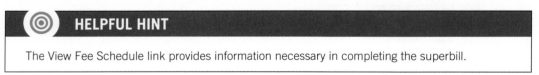

HELPFUL HINT

The View Fee Schedule link provides information necessary in completing the superbill.

64. Document "1" in the Rank column for Detailed office visit.
65. Document "99214" in the Est field for detailed office visit. Enter "65.00" in the Fee column for the detailed office visit.
66. Click the Save button.
67. Go to page four of the superbill.
68. On page four, document "25.00" in the Copay field.
69. Confirm that the total in the Today's Charges field has populated correctly.
70. Document "40.00" in the Balance Due field.
71. Document any additional information needed.

Coding & Billing

72. Click the Save button.
73. Select the I am ready to submit the Superbill checkbox at the bottom of the screen.
74. Select the Yes radio button to indicate that the signature is on file.
75. Document the date in the Date field.
76. Click the Submit Superbill button. A confirmation message will appear.
77. Select Claim from the left Info Panel (Figure 4-14) and perform a patient search to locate the claim for Norma Washington.

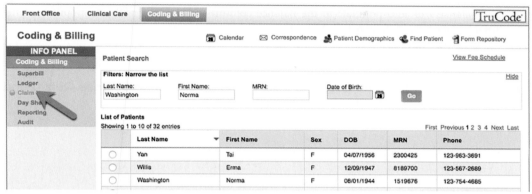

Figure 4-14 Select Claim from the left Info Panel.

78. Select the correct encounter and confirm the auto-populated details. Click the Edit icon in the Action column. Seven tabs appear within the claim: Patient Info, Provider Info, Payer Info, Encounter Notes, Claim Info, Charge Capture, and Submission. Certain patient demographic and encounter information is auto-populated in the claim.
79. Review the auto-populated information in the Patient Info tab and document any additional information needed. Click the Save button.
80. Click the Provider Info tab.
81. Review the auto-populated information in the Patient Info tab and document any additional information needed. Click the Save button.
82. Click the Payer Info tab.
83. Review the auto-populated information and document any additional information needed. Click the Save button.
84. Click the Encounter Notes tab.
85. Review the auto-populated information and select the Yes radio button to indicate that the HIPAA form is on file for Norma Washington and document the current date in the Dated field.
86. Document any additional information needed and click the Save button.
87. Click the Claim Info tab.
88. Review the auto-populated information and document any additional information needed. Click the Save button.
89. Click the Charge Capture tab.
90. Document the encounter date in the DOS From and DOS To columns.
91. Document "99214" in the CPT/HCPCS columns.
92. Document "11" in the POS column.
93. Document "12" in the DX column.
94. Document "65.00" in the Fee column.
95. Document any additional information needed and click the Save button.
96. Click the Submission tab. Click in the I am ready to submit the Claim box. Click on the Yes radio button to indicate that there a signature on file and enter today's date in the Date field.
97. Click the Submit Claim button.
98. Select Ledger from the left Info Panel and perform a patient search to locate the ledger for Norma Washington.
99. Select the radio button for Norma Washington and click the Select button.
100. Confirm the auto-populated details in the header.
101. Select the arrow to expand the ledger for Norma Washington.

102. All charges submitted on the claim will auto-populate the ledger. Document the copay made at the time of the visit.
103. Click Add Row.
104. Document the current date in the Transaction Date column using the calendar picker.
105. Document the date of service in the DOS column using the calendar picker.
106. Select James A. Martin, MD using the dropdown in the Provider field.
107. Select PTPYMTCSH from the Service column dropdown.
108. Document $25.00" in the Payment column.
109. The balance will auto-populate in the Balance column and the total will auto-populate in the Total Ledger Balance field below the table.
110. Click the Save button.

 Now use the Back to Assignment link to complete the Post-Case Quiz found on the Info Panel for this assignment.

64. Document Chief Complaint and Progress Note, then Submit Superbill, Update Ledger, and Submit Claim for Talibah Nasser

▪ Objectives

- Search for a patient record.
- Document a chief complaint.
- Document in the progress note.
- Complete a superbill.
- Complete a claim.
- Review a patient ledger.

▪ Overview

Established patient Talibah Nasser is here to see Jean Burke, NP because she has acute lower abdominal pain and is very nauseated all day long. She states the symptoms began about a week ago. In the review of symptoms, Talibah Nasser admits fatigue, weight gain, abdominal pain, and nausea and vomiting. Jean Burke orders a urinalysis by dipstick (no microscopy) and a urine pregnancy test. The pregnancy test is positive and the urinalysis is within normal limits. The plan is to start Talibah Nasser on prenatal vitamins and refer her to an OB. Jean Burke has indicated that the visit is routine, involved straightforward decision-making, and took approximately 15 minutes to complete. Document the chief complaint and progress note. Complete and submit the superbill and claim using ICD-10 coding. Review the patient ledger to see all charges for the patient visit.

▪ Competencies

- Identify information required to file a third party claim, types of third party plans, and the steps for filing a third party claim, CAAHEP VIII.C-1, ABHES 7-d
- Instruct patients in the collection of a clean-catch mid-stream urine specimen, ABHES 9-e
- Instruct patients in the collection of a fecal specimen, ABHES 9-e
- Obtain specimens and perform CLIA-waived microbiologic test, CAAHEP I.P-11e, ABHES 9-b
- Obtain specimens and perform CLIA-waived urinalysis, CAAHEP I.P-11c, ABHES 9-b
- Perform diagnostic coding, CAAHEP IX.P-2, ABHES 7-d
- Perform procedural coding, CAAHEP IX.P-1, ABHES 7-d
- Perform selected CLIA-waived tests that assist with diagnosis and treatment: kit testing dip stick, ABHES 9-b
- Perform selected CLIA-waived tests that assist with diagnosis and treatment: kit testing pregnancy, ABHES 9-b
- Perform quality control, CAAHEP I.P-10, ABHES 9-a
- Interact professionally with third party representatives, CAAHEP VIII.A-1

Estimated completion time: 50 minutes

Measurable Steps

1. Click on the Find Patient icon.
2. Using the Patient Search fields, search for Talibah Nasser's patient record. Once you locate her patient record in the List of Patients, confirm her date of birth.

 HELPFUL HINT

Confirming date of birth will help to ensure that you have located the correct patient record.

3. Select the radio button for Talibah Nasser and click the Select button.
4. Create a new encounter by clicking Office Visit in the left Info Panel (Figure 4-15).

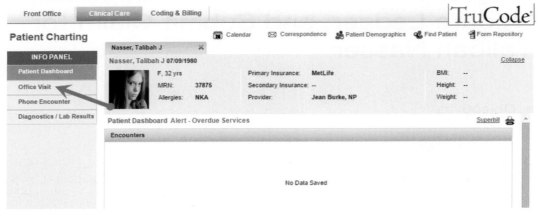

Figure 4-15 Office Visit in the Info Panel.

5. In the Create New Encounter window, select Urgent Visit from the Visit Type dropdown. If the New Encounter window does not appear, select Add New and follow previous instructions.
6. Select Jean Burke, NP from the Provider dropdown.
7. Click the Save button.
8. Select Chief Complaint from the Record dropdown menu that is already open (Figure 4-16).

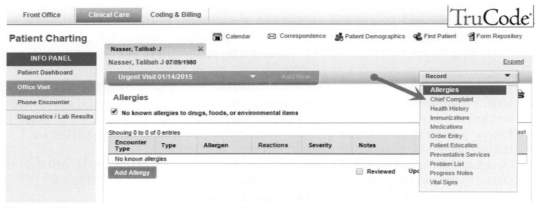

Figure 4-16 Chief Complaint in the Record dropdown menu.

9. Document "Abdominal pain" in the Chief Complaint field.
10. Document "Lower abdomen" in the Location field.
11. Document "1 week" in the Duration field.
12. Document "All day" in the Timing field.
13. Document "Nausea" in the Associated Signs and Symptoms field.
14. Select the Yes radio buttons for Fatigue and Weight Gain in the General section.
15. Select the Yes radio buttons for N/V and Abdominal Pain in the GI section.
16. Document any additional information needed and click the Save button.
17. Select Progress Notes from the Record dropdown menu.
18. Document the Date of Service using the calendar picker.
19. Document "Acute lower abdominal pain, nausea, fatigue" in the Subjective field.
20. Document "HCG positive, UA negative/WNL, weight gain 5lbs in one week" in the Objective field.
21. Document "Normal pregnancy" in the Assessment field.
22. Document "Begin prenatal vitamins and refer to an OB" in the Plan field.
23. Click the Save button.
24. Click the Coding & Billing tab at the top of the screen (Figure 4-17).

Coding & Billing

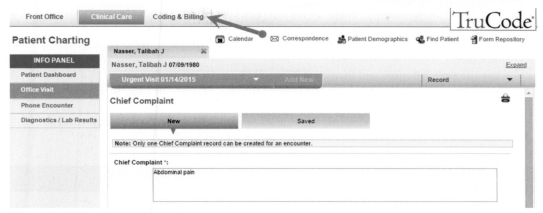

Figure 4-17 Coding & Billing tab.

25. Using the Patient Search fields, search for Talibah Nasser. Once you locate her, confirm her date of birth.
26. Select the correct encounter from the Encounters Not Coded grid and confirm the auto-populated details in the patient header.
27. On page one of the superbill, select the ICD-10 radio button.
28. In the Rank 1 row of the Diagnoses box, place the cursor in the text field to access the encoder (Figure 4-18).

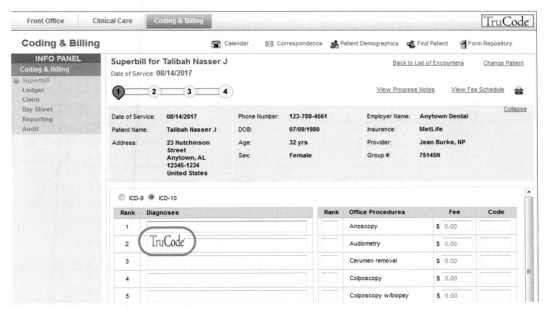

Figure 4-18 TruCode encoder tool.

29. Enter "Abdominal pain" in the Search field and select Diagnosis ICD-10-CM from the drop-down menu.
30. Click the Search button.
31. Click the code R10.9 to confirm that it is the most specific code available.
32. Click the code R10.30 for "Lower abdominal pain, unspecified" that appears in the tree. This code will auto-populate in the Rank 1 row of the Diagnoses box.
33. In the Rank 2 row of the Diagnoses box, place the cursor in the text field to access the encoder.
34. Enter "Encounter for positive pregnancy test" in the Search field and select Diagnosis, ICD-10-CM from the dropdown menu.
35. Click the Search button.
36. Click the code Z32.01 to expand this code and confirm that it is the most specific code available.
37. Click the code Z32.01 for "Encounter for pregnancy test, result positive" that appears in the tree. This code will auto-populate in the Rank 2 row of the Diagnoses box.

38. Select the TruCode encoder button in the top right corner. The encoder tool will open in a new tab.
39. Enter "Office Visit" in the Search for field and click CPT Tabular from the corresponding drop-down menu.
40. Click the Search button, and then click Show all 15 search results.
41. Click Office Outpatient Visit 15 Minutes 99213 that appears in blue to expand this code (Figure 4-19).
42. Review the information to determine if this is the correct code for the service provided.
43. Click the View Fee Schedule link to determine the office visit charge (Figure 4-20).

> ◎ **HELPFUL HINT**
>
> The View Fee Schedule link provides information necessary in completing the superbill.

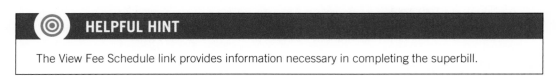

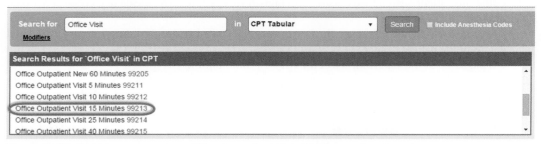

Figure 4-19 99213 appears when Office Outpatient Visit 15 Minutes is selected.

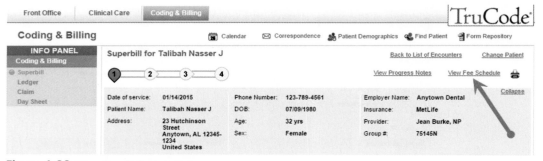

Figure 4-20 View Fee Schedule link.

44. Document "1" in the Rank column for Expanded problem-focused office visit with the corresponding fee of "43.00" and code of "99213" in the Est column (Figure 4-21).
45. Click the Save button.
46. Go to page three of the superbill.
47. Document "2" in the Rank column for Pregnancy, urine.
48. Click the View Fee Schedule link to determine the corresponding code and fee. Document "18.00" in the Fee column and "81025" in the Code column.
49. Document "3" in the Rank column for UA, w/o micro, non-automated.
50. Click the View Fee Schedule link to determine the corresponding code and fee. Document "22.00" in the Fee column and "81002" in the Code column.
51. Click the Save button and then click Next to move to page four of the superbill.
52. Confirm that the total in the Today's Charges field has populated correctly. Document 83.00 in the Balance Due field.
53. Document any additional information needed.
54. Click the Save button.
55. Select the I am ready to submit the Superbill checkbox at the bottom of the screen.
56. Select the Yes radio button to indicate that the signature is on file.
57. Document the date in the Date field.

58. Click the Submit Superbill button. A confirmation message will appear.
59. Select Claim from the left Info Panel and perform a patient search to locate the claim for Talibah Nasser (Figure 4-22).
60. Select the correct encounter and click the Edit icon in the Action column. Seven tabs appear within the claim: Patient Info, Provider Info, Payer Info, Encounter Notes, Claim Info, Charge

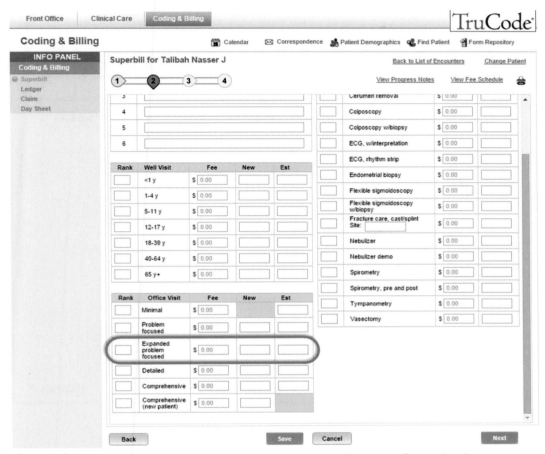

Figure 4-21 Documenting an Expanded problem-focused visit with its rank, fee, and code.

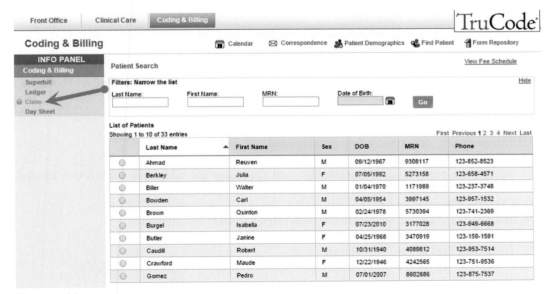

Figure 4-22 Claim in the Info Panel.

Capture, and Submission (Figure 4-23). Certain patient demographic and encounter information is auto-populated in the claim.

61. Within the Patient Info tab, review the auto-populated information and document any additional information needed. Click the Save button.
62. Click the Provider Info tab.
63. Within the Provider Info tab, review the auto-populated information and document any additional information needed. Click the Save button.

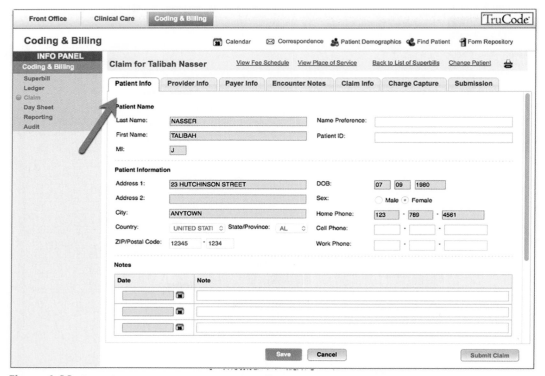

Figure 4-23 Once the correct encounter is clicked, seven tabs appear within the claim.

64. Click the Payer Info tab.
65. Review the auto-populated information and document any additional information needed. Click the Save button.
66. Click the Encounter Notes tab.
67. Review the auto-populated information and Document "HCG urine" in the Lab Orders table.
68. Click the Add button below the Lab Orders table to document "UA, w/o micro, non-automated" in the Lab Orders table.
69. Select the Yes radio button to indicate that the HIPAA form is on file for Talibah Nasser and document the current date in the Dated field.
70. Confirm that R10.30 appears in the first row of the DX column.
71. Confirm that Z32.01 appears in the second row of the DX column.
72. Document any additional information needed and click the Save button.
73. Click the Claim Info tab.
74. Review the auto-populated information and document any additional information needed. Click the Save button.
75. Click the Charge Capture tab.
76. Document the encounter date in the DOS From and DOS To columns.
77. Document "99213" in the CPT/HCPCS column.
78. Document "11" in the POS column.
79. Document "12" in the DX column.
80. Document "43.00" in the Fee column.
81. Document the encounter date in the DOS From and DOS To columns.

82. Document "81002" in the CPT/HCPCS column.
83. Document "11" in the POS column.
84. Document "12" in the DX column.
85. Document "22.00" in the Fee column.
86. Document the encounter date in the DOS From and DOS To columns.
87. Document "81025" in the CPT /HCPCS column.
88. Document "11" in the POS column.
89. Document "12" in the DX column.
90. Document "18.00" in the Fee column.
91. Document any additional information needed and click the Save button (Figure 4-24).

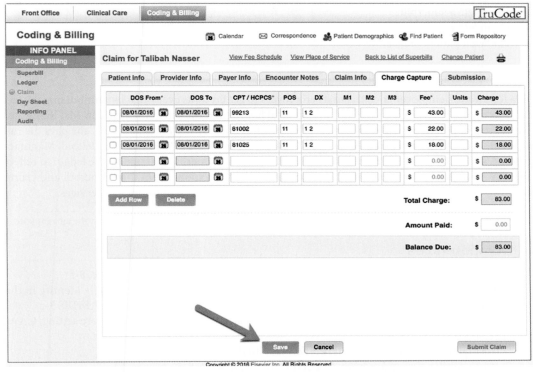

Figure 4-24 Document all applicable and necessary information, then click the Save button.

92. Click the Submission tab. Click in the I am ready to submit the Claim box. Click on the Yes radio button to indicate that there a signature on file and enter today's date in the Date field.
93. Click the Submit Claim button.
94. Select Ledger from the left Info Panel and perform a patient search to locate the claim for Talibah Nasser.
95. Select the arrow to expand the ledger for Talibah Nasser.
96. All charges submitted on the claim will auto-populate on the ledger. Review the ledger to see all charges for the patient visit.

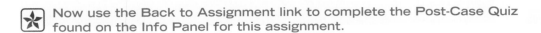 Now use the Back to Assignment link to complete the Post-Case Quiz found on the Info Panel for this assignment.

65. Document Immunization, Submit Superbill, and Post Payment to Ledger for Ella Rainwater

■ Objectives

- Search for a patient record.
- Document immunizations.
- Complete a superbill.
- Complete a claim.
- Update a patient ledger.

■ Overview

Ella Rainwater's employer encourages its employees to get flu shots every year by reimbursing the fee. Dr. Martin approves the vaccine and the medical assistant administers the flu shot. Ms. Rainwater has no reaction. Since Ms. Rainwater's employer will reimburse her for the vaccine, she pays the full amount for the procedure with a check. IIV, Dosage: 0.5 mL, given IM in the right deltoid. Manufacturer: AS Lab. Lot#: 342B, Expiration: 03/18.* Complete the superbill and update the ledger to reflect these two services and the payment. Document the immunization, submit the superbill and claim, and then update the patient ledger to reflect Ella Rainwater's payment for today's services.

*The year of expiration displayed on the labels should reflect an expiration date of three years past the current year.

■ Competencies

- Administer parenteral (excluding IV) medications, CAAHEP I.P-7, ABHES 2-c, 8-f
- Define and use entire basic structure of medical words and be able to accurately identify in the correct context, i.e. root, prefix, suffix, combinations, spelling and definitions, ABHES 3-a
- Define medical asepsis and surgical asepsis as practiced within an ambulatory care setting, CAAHEP III.C-3, ABHES 3-a, 8-a
- Perform diagnostic coding, CAAHEP IX.P-2, ABHES 7-d
- Perform sterilization procedures, CAAHEP III.P-5, ABHES 8-a
- Prepare a sterile field, CAAHEP III.P-6
- Perform within a sterile field, CAAHEP III.P-7

Estimated completion time: 35 minutes

Measurable Steps

1. Click on the Find Patient icon.
2. Using the Patient Search fields, search for Ella Rainwater's patient record. Once you locate her patient record in the List of Patients, confirm her date of birth.

> **HELPFUL HINT**
>
> Confirming date of birth will help to ensure that you have located the correct patient record.

3. Select the radio button for Ella Rainwater and click the Select button.
4. Create a new encounter by clicking Office Visit in the left Info Panel (Figure 4-25).
5. In the Create New Encounter window, select Follow-Up/Established Visit from the Visit Type dropdown.
6. Select James A. Martin, MD from the Provider dropdown.
7. Click the Save button.

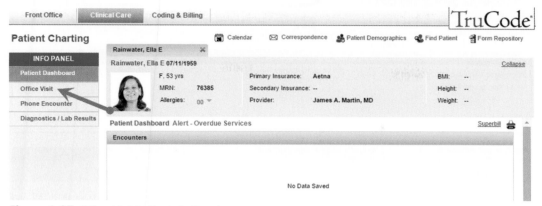

Figure 4-25 Office Visit in the Info Panel.

8. Select Immunizations from the Record dropdown menu (Figure 4-26).
9. Locate the row for the Influenza (Flu) vaccine and click the green plus sign to the far right of that row. That row will become active so you can add an immunization to Ella Rainwater's record.

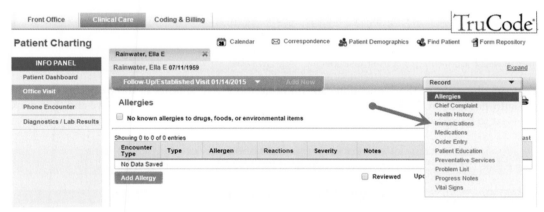

Figure 4-26 Immunizations in the Record dropdown menu.

10. Within the Type column, select IIV.
11. Within the Dose column, document "0.5 mL".
12. Within the Date column, use the calendar picker to select the date administered.
13. Within the Provider column, document "James A. Martin, MD" in the text box.
14. Within the Route/Site column, document "IM, R deltoid" in the text box.
15. Within the Manufacturer/Lot# column, document "AS Lab/342B" in the text box.
16. Document the expiration date in the Exp column.
17. Within the Reaction column, document "No reaction" in the text box.
18. Click the Save button. The immunization you added will display in the Immunization Review table.
19. After reviewing the encounter, select Patient Dashboard from the left Info Panel.
20. Click the Superbill link on the right-hand side.
21. Select the correct encounter from the Encounters Not Coded table and confirm the auto-populated details.
22. On page one of the superbill, select the ICD-10 radio button.
23. In the Rank 1 row of the Diagnoses box, place the cursor in the text field to access the encoder.
24. Enter "Prophylactic vaccination" in the Search field and select Diagnosis ICD-10-CM from the dropdown menu.
25. Click the Search button.
26. Click the code Z23 to expand this code and confirm that it is the most specific code available (Figure 4-27).

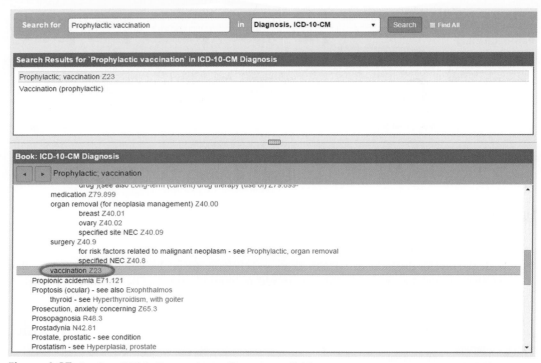

Figure 4-27 Confirm Z23 is the most specific code available.

27. Click the code Z23 for "Encounter for immunization" that appears in the tree. This code will auto-populate in the Rank 1 row of the Diagnoses box (Figure 4-28). Click Save and then click Next to move to page 2 of the Superbill.

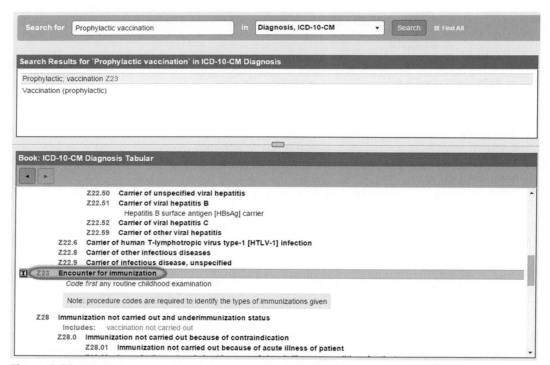

Figure 4-28 Populating the code in the Rank 1 row of the Diagnoses box.

28. On page two, document "1" in the Rank column for Imm admin, one.
29. Click the View Fee Schedule link to determine the corresponding code and fee. Document "10.00" in the Fee column and "90471" in the Code column (Figure 4-29).

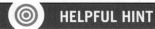
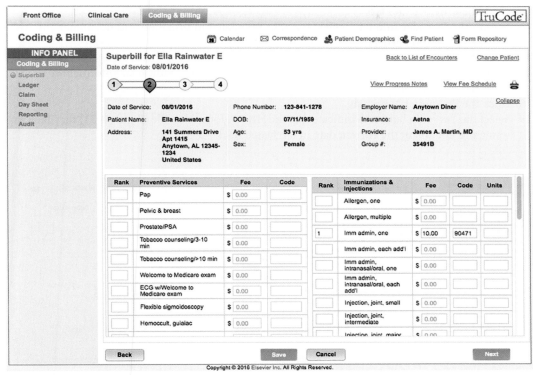

Figure 4-29 Document "10.00" in the Fee column and "90471" in the Code column.

30. Document "2" in the Rank column for Flu, 3 y + with the corresponding fee of "24.00" and code of "90658".
31. Click the Save button.
32. Go to page four of the superbill.
33. Confirm that the total in the Today's Charges field has populated correctly.
34. Document "34.00" in the Balance Due field.
35. Document any additional information needed.
36. Click the Save button.
37. Select the I am ready to submit the Superbill checkbox at the bottom of the screen.
38. Select the Yes radio button to indicate that the signature is on file.
39. Document the date in the Date field.
40. Click the Submit Superbill button. A confirmation message will appear (Figure 4-30).

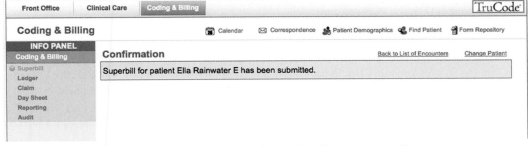

Figure 4-30 Click the Submit Superbill button and a confirmation message will appear.

41. Select Claim from the left Info Panel and perform a patient search to locate the claim for Ella Rainwater.
42. Click the Edit icon in the Action column. Seven tabs appear within the claim: Patient Info, Provider Info, Payer Info, Encounter Notes, Claim Info, Charge Capture, and Submission. Certain patient demographic and encounter information is auto-populated on the claim.
43. Within the Patient Info tab, review the auto-populated information and document any additional information needed. Click the Save button.
44. Click the Provider Info tab.
45. Within the Provider Info tab, review the auto-populated information and document any additional information needed. Click the Save button.
46. Click the Payer Info tab.
47. Review the auto-populated information and document any additional information needed. Click the Save button.
48. Click the Encounter Notes tab.
49. Select the Yes radio button to indicate that the HIPAA form is on file (Figure 4-31) for Ella Rainwater and document the current date in the Dated field.

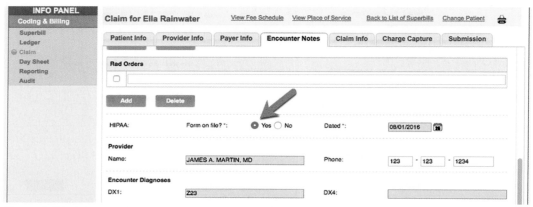

Figure 4-31 Select the Yes radio button to indicate the HIPAA form is on file for Ella Rainwater.

50. Confirm that Z23 appears in the first row of the DX column.
51. Document any additional information needed and click the Save button.
52. Click the Claim Info tab.
53. Review the auto-populated information and document any additional information needed. Click the Save button.
54. Click the Charge Capture tab.
55. Document the encounter date in the DOS From and DOS To columns.
56. Document "90471" in the CPT/HCPCS column.
57. Document "11" in the POS column.
58. Document "1" in the DX column.
59. Document "10.00" in the Fee column.
60. Document the encounter date in the DOS From and DOS To columns.
61. Document "90658" in the CPT/HCPCS column.
62. Document "11" in the POS column.
63. Document "1" in the DX column.
64. Document "24.00" in the Fee column.
65. Document any additional information needed and click the Save button.
66. Click the Submission tab. Click in the I am ready to submit the Claim box. Click on the Yes radio button to indicate that there a signature on file and enter today's date in the Date field.
67. Click the Submit Claim button.
68. Select Ledger from the left Info Panel and perform a patient search to locate the claim for Ella Rainwater.
69. Select the arrow to expand the ledger for Ella Rainwater.

70. All charges submitted on the claim will auto-populate on the ledger.
71. Click Add Row to enter the payment made by Ella Rainwater.
72. Document the current date in the Transaction Date column using the calendar picker.
73. Document the date of service in the DOS column using the calendar picker.
74. Select James A. Martin, MD using the dropdown in the Provider field.
75. Select PTPYMTCK in the Service column.
76. Document "34.00" in the Payment column.
77. The balance will auto-populate in the Balance column and the total will auto-populate in the Total Ledger Balance field below the table.
78. Click the Save button.

 Now use the Back to Assignment link to complete the Post-Case Quiz found on the Info Panel for this assignment.

66. Submit Insurance Claim Tracer for Amma Patel

■ Objectives

- Search for a patient record.
- Review a superbill.
- Review a claim.
- Create an insurance claim tracer form.

■ Overview

Walden-Martin has not received payment for Amma Patel's OB/GYN consultation performed August 9. Submit an insurance claim tracer to check the status of the claim payments. Review the claim (claim #132455) to determine the information needed on the insurance claim tracer form.

■ Competencies

- Demonstrate respect for individual diversity, CAAHEP V.A-3, ABHES 5-i, 10-b
- Describe filing indexing rules, CAAHEP VI.C-7, ABHES 7-a
- Describe how to use the most current HCPCS level II coding system, CAAHEP IX.C-3, ABHES 7-d
- Display tactful behavior when communicating with medical providers regarding third party requirements, CAAHEP VIII.A-2, ABHES 5-h, 7-d, 7-g
- Outline managed care requirements for patient referral, CAAHEP VIII.C-2, ABHES 7-d
- Perform accounts receivable procedures to patient accounts including posting charges, payments, and adjustments CAAHEP VII.P-1, ABHES 7-c
- Interact professionally with third party representatives, CAAHEP VIII.A-1

Estimated completion time: 15 minutes

Measurable Steps

1. Click on the Coding & Billing tab at the top of the screen.
2. Select Claim in the Info Panel on the left-hand side.
3. Using the Patient Search fields, search for Amma Patel's patient record. Once you locate her patient record, confirm her date of birth.
4. Select the radio button for Amma Patel and click the select button.
5. Select the Edit icon in the Action column to view the submitted claim.
6. Gather the following information from the claim.
7. Insurance carrier can be found in the Payer Info tab: Blue Cross Blue Shield.
8. Date of Service can be found in the Encounter Notes tab: 08/09/2013.
9. Diagnosis can be found in the Encounter Notes tab: N87.1.
10. Procedure code can be found in the Charge Capture tab: 99242.
11. Procedure cost can be found in the Charge Capture tab: $60.00.
12. Click on the Form Repository icon.
13. Select Insurance Claim Tracer from the Patient Forms section of the left Info Panel (Figure 4-32).
14. Click the Patient Search button to perform a patient search and assign the form to Ms. Patel. Confirm the auto-populated details.

 HELPFUL HINT

Performing a patient search before completing a form helps to ensure accurate documentation.

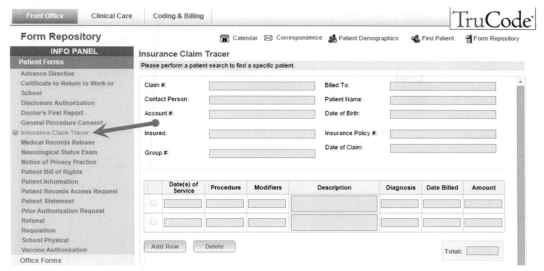

Figure 4-32 Insurance Claim Tracer in the Patient Forms section of the Info Panel.

15. Select the radio button for Amma Patel and click the Select button.
16. Document "132455" in the Claim # field.
17. Document "Blue Cross Blue Shield" in the Billed To field.
18. Document your name in the Contact Person field.
19. Document "August 9" and the correct year in the Date(s) of Service column.
20. Document "99242" in the Procedure column.
21. Document "N87.1" in the Diagnosis column.
22. Document "August 9" and the correct year in the Date Billed column.
23. Document "60.00" in the Amount column.
24. Document "60.00" in the Total field.
25. Click the Save to Patient Record button. Confirm the date and click the OK button.
26. Click the Find Patient icon.
27. Using the Patient Search fields, search for Amma Patel's patient record. Once you locate her in the List of Patients, confirm her date of birth.
28. Select the radio button for Amma Patel and click the Select button. Confirm the auto-populated details.
29. Select the form you prepared from the Forms section of the Patient Dashboard (Figure 4-33). The form will open in a new window, allowing you to print.

Coding & Billing

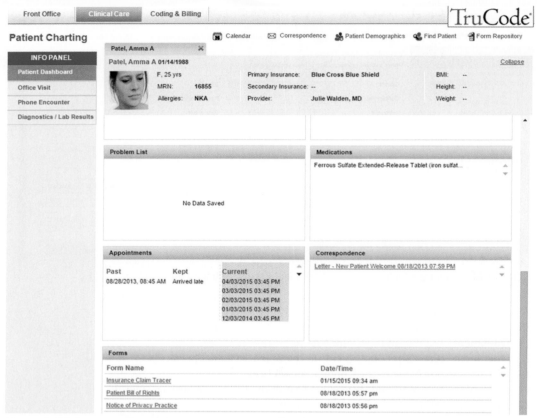

Figure 4-33 Forms section of the Patient Dashboard.

Now use the Back to Assignment link to complete the Post-Case Quiz found on the Info Panel for this assignment.

67. Submit Superbill and Post Charges to Ledger for Amma Patel

■ Objectives

- Search for a patient record.
- Use a fee schedule.
- Complete a superbill.
- Complete a claim.
- Post charges to a patient ledger.

■ Overview

Amma Patel had a colposcopy (entire vagina, with cervix), with biopsies during today's visit. A previous pap smear showed moderate cervical dysplasia. Amma Patel has a $25.00 copay, which she paid during the visit with a check. Complete and submit the superbill and claim for Amma Patel. Review the patient ledger and post the payment for today's copay.

■ Competencies

- Define medical terms and abbreviations related to all body systems, CAAHEP V.C-10, ABHES 3-a, 3-d
- Define medical legal terms, CAAHEP X.C-13, ABHES 3-a
- Identify types of third party plans, CAAHEP VIII.C-1a, ABHES 7-d
- Perform diagnostic coding, CAAHEP IX.P-2, ABHES 7-d
- Show sensitivity when communicating with patients regarding third party requirements, CAAHEP VIII.A-3, ABHES 5-h, 7-d
- Utilize an EMR, CAAHEP VI.P-6, ABHES 7-b

Estimated completion time: 25 minutes

Measurable Steps

1. Click on the Find Patient icon.
2. Using the Patient Search field, search for Amma Patel's patient record.
3. Select the radio button for Amma Patel and click the select button.

 HELPFUL HINT

Confirming patient demographics helps to ensure you have located the correct patient record.

4. Confirm the auto-populated details in the patient header.
5. After reviewing the encounter, click the Superbill link below the patient header.
6. Select the correct encounter from the Encounters Not Coded table and confirm the auto-populated details.
7. On page one of the superbill, select the ICD-10 radio button.
8. In the Rank 1 row of the Diagnoses box, place the cursor in the text field to access the encoder.
9. Enter "Moderate cervical dysplasia" in the Search field and select Diagnosis ICD-10-CM from the dropdown menu.
10. Click the Search button.
11. Click the code N87.1 to expand this code and confirm that it is the most specific code available.

Coding & Billing

12. Click the code N87.1 for "Moderate cervical dysplasia" that appears in the tree. This code will auto-populate in the Rank 1 row of the Diagnoses box (Figure 4-34).

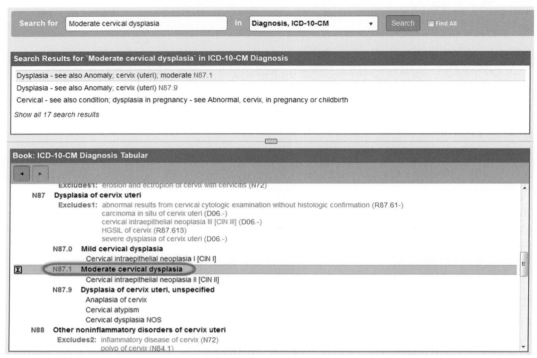

Figure 4-34 Populating the code in the Rank 1 row of the Diagnoses box.

13. Click the View Fee Schedule link to obtain the charges and code for the colposcopy.
14. Document "1" in the Rank column for Colposcopy w/biopsy with the corresponding fee of "178.00" and code of "57455".
15. Click the Save button.
16. Go to page four of the superbill.
17. On page four, document "25.00" in the Copay field.
18. Confirm that the total in the Today's Charges field has populated correctly.
19. Document "153.00" in the Balance Due field (Figure 4-35).

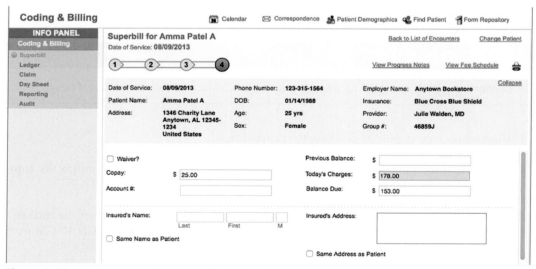

Figure 4-35 Document the Copay and the Balance Due.

20. Document any additional information needed.
21. Click the Save button.
22. Select the I am ready to submit the Superbill checkbox at the bottom of the screen.
23. Select the Yes radio button to indicate that the signature is on file.
24. Document the date in the Date field.
25. Click the Submit Superbill button. A confirmation message will appear.
26. Select Claim from the left Info Panel and perform a patient search to locate the claim for Amma Patel.
27. Select the correct encounter and click the Edit icon in the Action column. Seven tabs appear within the claim: Patient Info, Provider Info, Payer Info, Encounter Notes, Claim Info, Charge Capture, and Submission.
28. Within the Patient Info tab, review the auto-populated information and document any additional information needed. Click the Save button.
29. Click the Provider Info tab.
30. Within the Provider Info tab, review the auto-populated information and document any additional information needed. Click the Save button.
31. Click the Payer Info tab.
32. Review the auto-populated information and document any additional information needed. Click the Save button.
33. Click the Encounter Notes tab.
34. Select the Yes radio button to indicate that the HIPAA form is on file for Amma Patel and document the current date in the Dated field.
35. Confirm that N87.1 appears in the first row of the DX column.
36. Document any additional information needed and click the Save button.
37. Click the Claim Info tab.
38. Review the auto-populated information and document any additional information needed. Click the Save button.
39. Click the Charge Capture tab.
40. Document the encounter date in the DOS From and DOS To columns.
41. Document "57455" in the CPT/HCPCS column.
42. Document "11" in the POS column.
43. Document "1" in the DX column.
44. Document "178.00" in the Fee column.
45. Click the Save button.
46. Click the Submission tab. Click the I am ready to submit the Claim box (Figure 4-36). Click on the Yes radio button to indicate that there a signature on file and enter today's date in the Date field.

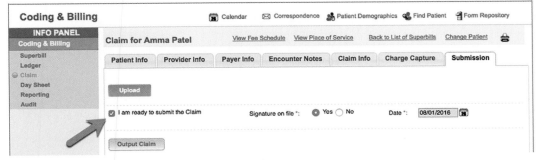

Figure 4-36 Click the "I am ready to submit the Claim" box.

47. Click the Submit Claim button.
48. Select Ledger from the left Info Panel and perform a patient search to locate the claim for Amma Patel.
49. Select the arrow to expand the ledger for Amma Patel.
50. All charges submitted on the claim will auto-populate on the ledger.
51. Click Add Row to enter the payment made by Amma Patel.

52. Document the current date in the Transaction Date column using the calendar picker.
53. Document the date of service in the DOS column using the calendar picker.
54. Select Julie Walden, MD using the dropdown in the Provider field.
55. Select PTPYMTCK in the Service column.
56. Document "25.00" in the Payment column.
57. The balance will auto-populate in the Balance column and the total will auto-populate in the Total Ledger Balance field below the table (Figure 4-37).
58. Click the Save button.

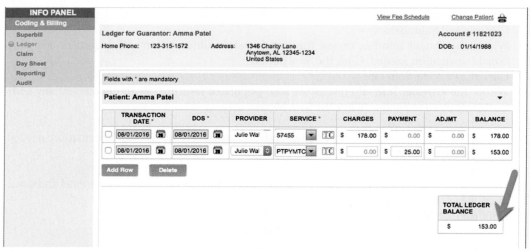

Figure 4-37 The balance will auto-populate in the Balance column and the total will auto-populate in the Total Ledger Balance field below the table.

Now use the Back to Assignment link to complete the Post-Case Quiz found on the Info Panel for this assignment.

68. Complete Superbill, Ledger, and Claim for Diego Lupez

■ Objectives

- Search for a patient record.
- Use a fee schedule.
- Complete a superbill.
- Complete a claim.
- Update a patient ledger.

■ Overview

During Diego Lupez's encounter, Dr. Martin performed an established patient expanded problem-focused office visit for iron deficiency anemia, as well as a complete blood count with automated differential. Diego Lupez paid his copay of $25.00 with a credit card. Complete and submit the superbill and claim. Post Mr. Lupez's copay to the patient ledger.

■ Competencies

- Describe types of adjustments made to patient accounts, CAAHEP VII.C-4, ABHES 7-c
- Explain patient financial obligations for services rendered, CAAHEP VII.C-6, ABHES 5-c, 7-c
- Identify types of information contained in the patient's billing record, CAAHEP VII.C-5, ABHES 7-a, 7-b, 7-c
- Obtain specimens and perform CLIA-waived hematology test, CAAHEP I.P-11a, ABHES 9-b
- Perform accounts receivable procedures to patient accounts including posting charges, payments, and adjustments, CAAHEP VII.P-1, ABHES 7-c
- Perform diagnostic coding, CAAHEP IX.P-2, ABHES 7-d
- Utilize an EMR, CAAHEP VI.P-6, ABHES 7-b

Estimated completion time: 1 hour

Measurable Steps

1. Click on the Find Patient icon.
2. Using the Patient Search field, search for Diego Lupez's patient record.
3. Select the radio button for Diego Lupez and click the select button.

 HELPFUL HINT

Confirming patient demographics helps to ensure you have located the correct patient record.

4. After reviewing the encounter, click the Superbill link below the patient header on the Patient Dashboard (Figure 4-38).
5. Select the correct encounter from the Encounters Not Coded table and confirm the auto-populated details.
6. On page one of the superbill, select the ICD-10 radio button.
7. In the Rank 1 row of the Diagnoses box, place the cursor in the text field to access the encoder.
8. Enter "Iron deficiency anemia" in the Search field and select Diagnosis ICD-10-CM from the dropdown menu.
9. Click the Search button.
10. Click the code D50.9 to expand this code and confirm that it is the most specific code available (Figure 4-39).

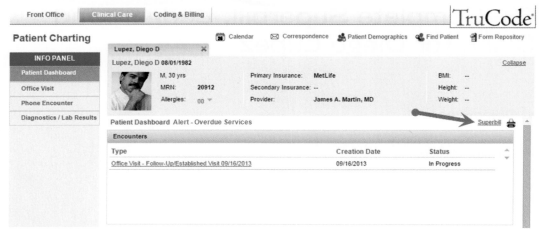

Figure 4-38 Superbill link below the patient header.

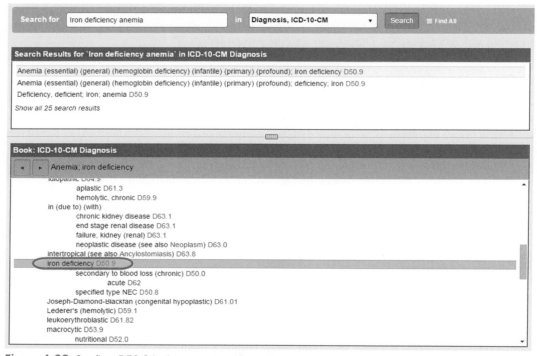

Figure 4-39 Confirm D50.9 is the most specific code available.

11. Click the code D50.9 for "Iron deficiency anemia, unspecified" that appears in the tree. This code will auto-populate in the Rank 1 row of the Diagnoses box (Figure 4-40).
12. Click on the View Fee Schedule link to determine the correct code and fee for the office visit.
13. Document "1" in the Rank column for Expanded problem-focused office visit with the corresponding fee of "43.00" and CPT code of "99213" in the Est column.
14. Click the Save button.
15. Go to page three of the superbill.
16. Click on the View Fee Schedule link to determine the correct code and fee for CBC with auto differential and Venipuncture.

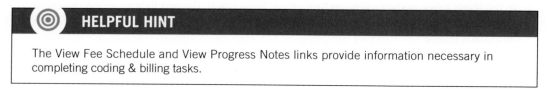

HELPFUL HINT

The View Fee Schedule and View Progress Notes links provide information necessary in completing coding & billing tasks.

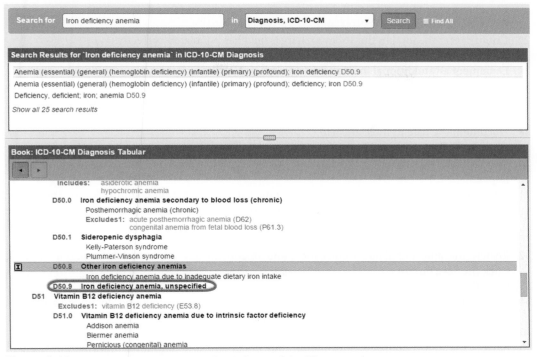

Figure 4-40 Populating the code in the Rank 1 row of the Diagnoses box.

17. Document "2" in the Rank column for CBC w/ auto differential with the corresponding fee of "35.00" and CPT code of "85025".
18. Document "3" in the Rank column for Venipuncture with the corresponding fee of "10.00" CPT code of "36415".
19. Click the Save button (Figure 4-41).

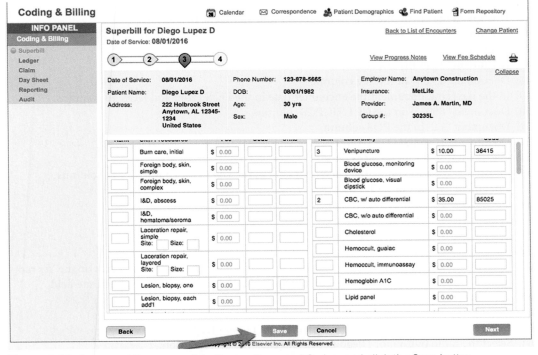

Figure 4-41 Document the appropriate Ranks, Fees, and Codes, and click the Save button.

20. Go to page four of the superbill.
21. On page four, document "25.00" in the Copay field.
22. Confirm that the total in the Today's Charges field has populated correctly.
23. Document "63.00" in the Balance Due field.
24. Document any additional information needed.
25. Click the Save button.
26. Select the I am ready to submit the Superbill checkbox at the bottom of the screen.
27. Select the Yes radio button to indicate that the signature is on file.
28. Document the date in the Date field.
29. Click the Submit Superbill button. A confirmation message will appear.
30. Select Claim from the left Info Panel and perform a patient search to locate the claim for Diego Lupez.
31. Select the correct encounter and click the Edit icon in the Action column. Seven tabs appear within the claim: Patient Info, Provider Info, Payer Info, Encounter Notes, Claim Info, Charge Capture, and Submission. Certain patient demographic and encounter information is auto-populated in the claim.
32. Review the auto-populated information and document any additional information needed. Click the Save button.
33. Click the Provider Info tab.
34. Within the Provider Info tab, review the auto-populated information and document any additional information needed. Click the Save button.
35. Click the Payer Info tab.
36. Review the auto-populated information and document any additional information needed. Click the Save button.
37. Click the Encounter Notes tab.
38. Review the auto-populated information and document "CBC w/ auto differential" in the Lab Orders table.
39. Select the Yes radio button to indicate that the HIPAA form is on file for Diego Lupez and document the current date in the Date field.
40. Document any additional information needed and click the Save button.
41. Click the Claim Info tab.
42. Review the auto-populated information and document any additional information needed. Click the Save button.
43. Click the Charge Capture tab.
44. Document the encounter date in the DOS From and DOS To columns.
45. Document "99213" in the CPT/HCPCS column.
46. Document "11" in the POS column.
47. Document "1" in the DX column.
48. Document "43.00" in the Fee column.
49. In the next row, document the encounter date in the DOS From and DOS To columns.
50. Document "85025" in the CPT/HCPCS columns.
51. Document "11" in the POS column.
52. Document "1" in the DX column.
53. Document "35.00" in the Fee column.
54. In the next row, document the encounter date in the DOS From and DOS To columns.
55. Document "36415" in CPT/HCPCS column.
56. Document "11" in the POS column.
57. Document "1" in the DX column.
58. Document "10.00" in the Fee column.
59. Click the Save button.
60. Click the Submission tab. Click in the I am ready to submit the Claim box. Click on the Yes radio button to indicate that there is a signature on file and enter today's date in the Date field.
61. Click the Submit Claim button.
62. Select Ledger from the left Info Panel.
63. Using the Patient Search fields, search for Diego Lupez's ledger.
64. Select the radio button for Diego Lupez and click the Select button.
65. Confirm the auto-populated details in the header.

66. Select the arrow to expand the ledger for Diego Lupez.
67. All charges submitted on the claim will auto-populate on the ledger.
68. Click Add Row to enter the payment made by Diego Lupez.
69. Document the current date in the Transaction Date column using the calendar picker.
70. Document the date of service in the DOS column using the calendar picker.
71. Select James A. Martin, MD using the dropdown in the Provider field.
72. Select PTPYMTCC in the Service column.
73. Document "25.00" in the Payment column.
74. The balance will auto-populate in the Balance column and the total will auto-populate in the Total Ledger Balance field below the table (Figure 4-42).
75. Click the Save button.

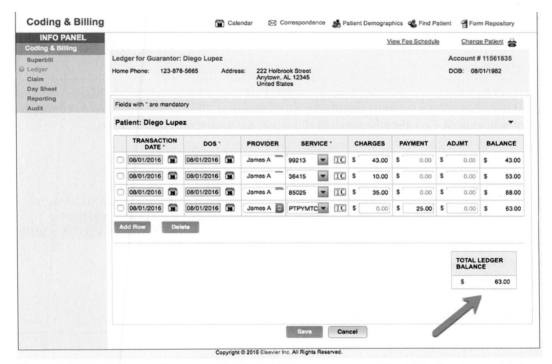

Figure 4-42 The balance will auto-populate in the Balance column and the total will auto-populate in the Total Ledger Balance field below the table.

Now use the Back to Assignment link to complete the Post-Case Quiz found on the Info Panel for this assignment.

69. Complete Superbill, Post Payment to Ledger, and Complete Claim for Ella Rainwater

■ Objectives

- Search for a patient record.
- Complete a superbill.
- Complete a claim.
- Update a patient ledger.

■ Overview

During Ella Rainwater's established patient detailed office visit for bronchitis, Dr. Martin administered Rocephin 250 mg IM, and ordered a handheld nebulizer. Ella Rainwater paid her $25.00 copayment with a check. Complete the superbill and claim, and update the patient ledger.

■ Competencies

- Complete insurance claim forms, CAAHEP VIII.P-4, ABHES 7-d
- Explain patient financial obligations for services rendered, CAAHEP VII.C-6, ABHES 5-c, 7-c
- Identify information required to file a third party claim, CAAHEP VIII.C-1b, ABHES 7-d
- Identify types of information contained in the patient's billing record, CAAHEP VII.C-5, ABHES 7-b, 7-c
- Perform diagnostic coding, CAAHEP IX.P-2, ABHES 7-d
- Interpret information on an insurance card, CAAHEP VIII.P-1

Estimated completion time: 40 minutes

Measurable Steps

1. Click on the Find Patient icon.
2. Using the Patient Search field, search for Ella Rainwater's patient record.
3. Select the radio button for Ella Rainwater and click the select button.
4. Confirm the auto-populated details in the patient header.

 HELPFUL HINT

Confirming patient demographics helps to ensure you have located the correct patient record.

5. After reviewing the encounter, click the Superbill link below the patient header (Figure 4-43).
6. Select the correct encounter from the Encounters Not Coded table and confirm the auto-populated details.
7. On page one of the superbill, select the ICD-10 radio button.
8. In the Rank 1 row of the Diagnoses box, place the cursor in the text field to access the encoder.
9. Enter "Bronchitis" in the Search field and select Diagnosis ICD-10-CM from the dropdown menu.
10. Click the Search button.
11. Click the code J40 to expand this code and confirm that it is the most specific code available (Figure 4-44).

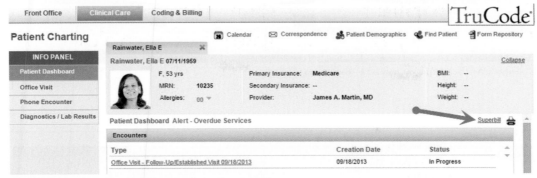

Figure 4-43 Superbill link below the patient header.

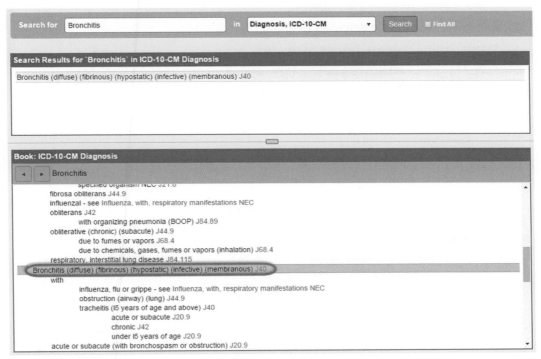

Figure 4-44 Confirm J40 is the most specific code available.

12. Click the code J40 for "Bronchitis, not specific as acute or chronic" that appears in the tree. This code will auto-populate in the Rank 1 row of the Diagnoses box (Figure 4-45).
13. Click on the View Fee Schedule link to determine the correct codes and fees for the detailed office visit (Figure 4-46).

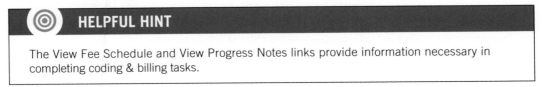

HELPFUL HINT

The View Fee Schedule and View Progress Notes links provide information necessary in completing coding & billing tasks.

14. Document "1" in the Rank column for Detailed office visit with the corresponding fee of "65.00" and code of "99214" in the Est column.
15. Document "2" in the Rank column for Nebulizer with the corresponding fee of "49.22" and code of "94640".
16. Click the Save button and then click the Next button to proceed to page two of the superbill.
17. Document "3" in the Rank column for Injection, ther/proph/diag with the corresponding fee of "25.00" and code of "96372".
18. Document "4" in the Rank column for Rocephin, 250 mg with the corresponding fee of "21.20" and code of "J0696".

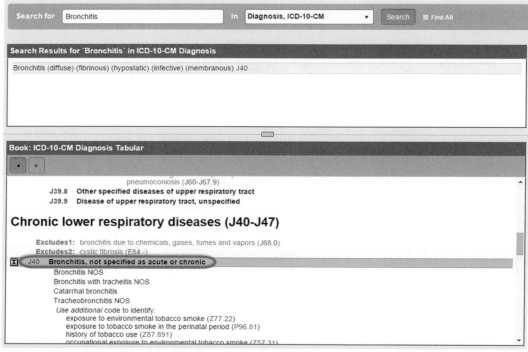

Figure 4-45 Populating the code in the Rank 1 row of the Diagnoses box.

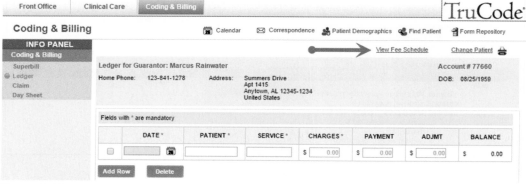

Figure 4-46 View Fee Schedule link.

19. Click the Save button and then click the Next button to proceed to page four of the superbill.
20. On page four, document "25.00" in the Copay field.
21. Confirm that the total in the Today's Charges field has populated correctly.
22. Document "135.42" in the Balance Due field.
23. Document any additional information needed.Click the Save button.
24. Select the I am ready to submit the Superbill checkbox at the bottom of the screen.
25. Select the Yes radio button to indicate that the signature is on file.
26. Document the date in the Date field.
27. Click the Submit Superbill button. A confirmation message will appear.
28. Select Claim from the left Info Panel and perform a patient search to locate the claim for Ella Rainwater.
29. Select the correct encounter and click the Edit icon in the Action column. Seven tabs appear within the claim: Patient Info, Provider Info, Payer Info, Encounter Notes, Claim Info, Charge Capture, and Submission. Certain patient demographic and encounter information is auto-populated in the claim.
30. Review the auto-populated information and document any additional information needed. Click the Save button.

31. Click the Provider Info tab.
32. Within the Provider Info tab, review the auto-populated information and document any additional information needed. Click the Save button.
33. Click the Payer Info tab.
34. Review the auto-populated information and document any additional information needed. Click the Save button.
35. Click the Encounter Notes tab.
36. Review the auto-populated information.
37. Select the Yes radio button to indicate that the HIPAA form is on file for Ella Rainwater and document the current date in the Dated field.
38. Document any additional information needed and click the Save button.
39. Click the Claim Info tab.
40. Review the auto-populated information and document any additional information needed. Click the Save button.
41. Click the Charge Capture tab.
42. Document the encounter date in the DOS From and DOS To columns.
43. Document "99214" in the CPT/HCPCS column (Figure 4-47).

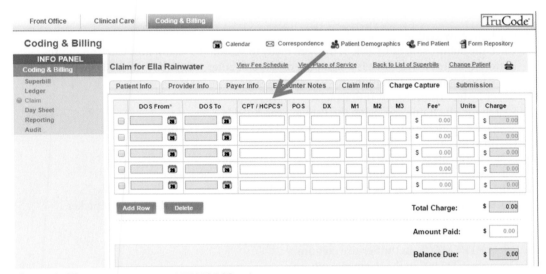

Figure 4-47 Document in the CPT/HCPCS column.

44. Document "11" in the POS column.
45. Document "1" in the DX column.
46. Document "65.00" in the Fee column.
47. In the next row, document the encounter date in the DOS From and DOS To columns.
48. Document "94640" in the CPT/HCPCS columns.
49. Document "11" in the POS column.
50. Document "1" in the DX column.
51. Document "49.22" in the Fee column.
52. In the next row, document the encounter date in the DOS From and DOS To columns.
53. Document "96372" in CPT/HCPCS column.
54. Document "11" in the POS column.
55. Document "1" in the DX column.
56. Document "25.00" in the Fee column.
57. In the next row, document the encounter date in the DOS From and DOS To columns.
58. Document "J0696" in the CPT/HCPCS columns.
59. Document "11" in the POS column.
60. Document "1" in the DX column.
61. Document "21.20" in the Fee column (Figure 4-48).

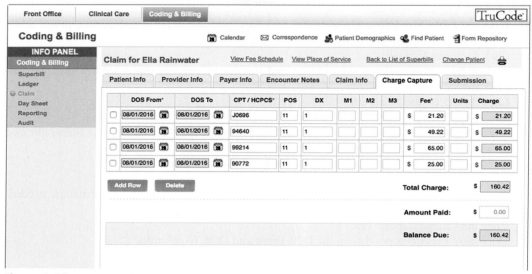

Figure 4-48 Insert all information into the Charge Capture tab.

62. Click the Save button.
63. Click the Submission tab. Click in the I am ready to submit the Claim box. Click on the Yes radio button to indicate that there is a signature on file and enter today's date in the Date field.
64. Click the Submit Claim button.
65. Select Ledger from the left Info Panel.
66. Search for Ella Rainwater using the Patient Search fields.
67. Select the radio button for Ella Rainwater and click the Select button.
68. Confirm the auto-populated details in the header.
69. Select the arrow to expand the ledger for Ella Rainwater.
70. All charges submitted on the claim will auto-populate on the ledger.
71. Click Add Row to enter the payment made by Ella Rainwater.
72. Document the current date in the Transaction Date column using the calendar picker.
73. Document the date of service in the DOS column using the calendar picker.
74. Select James A. Martin, MD using the dropdown in the Provider field.
75. Select PTPYMTCK in the Service column.
76. Document "25.00" in the Payment column.
77. The balance will auto-populate in the Balance column and the total will auto-populate in the Total Ledger Balance field below the table (Figure 4-49).
78. Click the Save button.

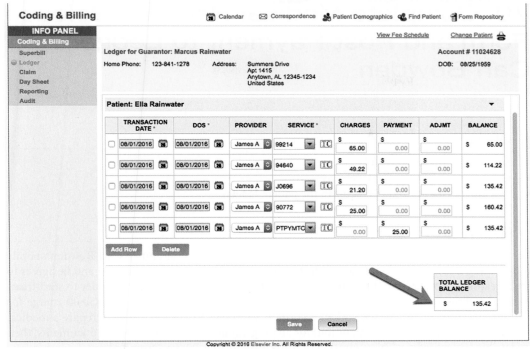

Figure 4-49 The balance will auto-populate in the Balance column and the total will auto-populate in the Total Ledger Balance field below the table.

Now use the Back to Assignment link to complete the Post-Case Quiz found on the Info Panel for this assignment.

70. Complete Medical Records Release Form and Post Payment to Ledger for Carl Bowden

Objectives

- Search for a patient record.
- Complete a medical records release.
- Document charges and payments in the patient ledger.

Overview

Dr. Walden has been following Carl Bowden's increased alcohol abuse. Carl Bowden's family is becoming increasingly concerned with the amount of alcohol he is consuming and he agrees to seek treatment from a rehabilitation clinic, Clean Living Inpatient Services. In order to start treatment, the clinic requests medical records from Dr. Walden's office. There is a $50.00 charge for the retrieval and copying of the patient records. Carl Bowden pays the full fee. Prepare a medical records release form (report preparation) for all progress notes and health history documents, then update his patient ledger. The expiration of the release form is 90 days from today.

Clean Living Inpatient Services:
Marie Alwright
5667 Miller Drive
Anytown, AL 12345
123-897-9777

Competencies

- Apply HIPAA rules in regard to privacy and the release of information, CAAHEP X.P-2, ABHES 4-h
- Describe the role of the medical assistant as a patient navigator, CAAHEP V.C-13, ABHES 5-c
- Perform procedural coding, CAAHEP IX.P-1, ABHES 7-d
- Protect the integrity of the medical record, CAAHEP X.A-2, ABHES 4-a
- Utilize an EMR, CAAHEP VI.P-6, ABHES 7-b
- Define patient navigator, CAAHEP V.C-12

Estimated completion time: 35 minutes

Measurable Steps

1. Click on the Form Repository icon.
2. Select Medical Records Release from the Patient Forms section of the left Info Panel.
3. Click the Patient Search button to perform a patient search and assign the form to Carl Bowden and confirm the auto-populated details.

 HELPFUL HINT

Performing a patient search before completing a form helps to ensure accurate documentation.

4. Document "Clean Living Inpatient Services" in the Name field to designate where to send Carl Bowden's information.
5. Document "5667 Miller Drive Anytown, AL 12345" in the Address field.
6. Document "123-897-9777" in the Phone field.

Coding & Billing

7. Fill out the remaining fields.
8. Click the Save to Patient Record button. Confirm the date and click OK.
9. Click on the Find Patient icon.
10. Using the Patient Search fields, search for Carl Bowden's patient record. Once you locate him in the List of Patients, confirm his date of birth.
11. Select the radio button for Carl Bowden and click the Select button. Confirm the auto-populated details.
12. Scroll down to view the Forms section of the Patient Dashboard (Figure 4-50).

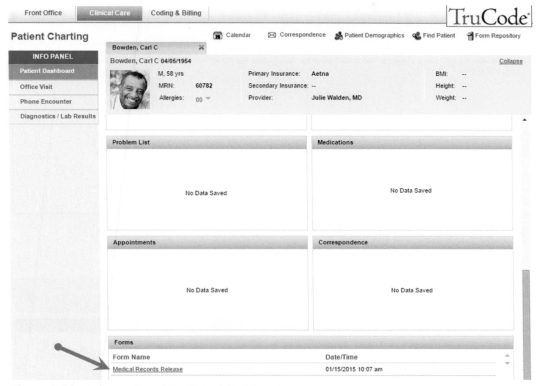

Figure 4-50 Forms section of the Patient Dashboard.

13. Select the form you prepared. The form will open in a new window, allowing you to print.
14. Click the Coding & Billing tab.
15. Select Ledger from the left Info Panel.
16. Search for Carl Bowden using the Patient Search fields.
17. Select the radio button for Carl Bowden and click the Select button.
18. Confirm the auto-populated details in the header.
19. Select the arrow to expand the ledger for Carl Bowden.
20. Document the current date in the Transaction Date column using the calendar picker.
21. Document the date of service in the DOS column using the calendar picker.
22. Select Julie Walden, MD using the dropdown in the Provider field.
23. Place your cursor in the Service column and select the TC button to access the encoder.
24. Enter "report preparation" in the Search field and select CPT Tabular from the dropdown menu.
25. Click the Search button.
26. Click the link in the Search Results pane to show all 16 results and click the 99080 code to expand this code and confirm that it is the most specific code available (Figure 4-51).
27. Click the code 99080 that appears in the tree. This code will auto-populate in the ledger (Figure 4-52).
28. Document "50.00" in the Charges column.
29. Document "50.00" in the Payment column. The balance will auto-populate in the Balance column.
30. Click the Save button.

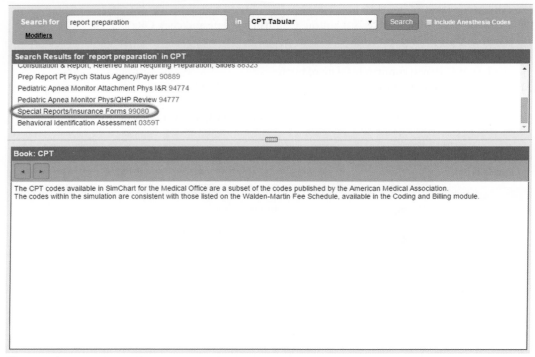

Figure 4-51 Confirm 99080 is the most specific code available.

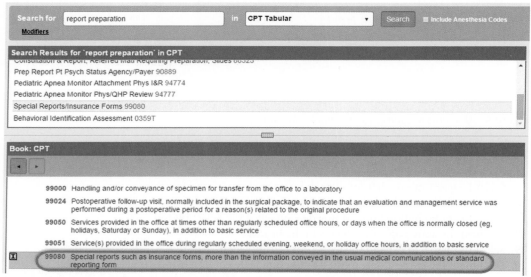

Figure 4-52 Populating the code in the ledger.

Now use the Back to Assignment link to complete the Post-Case Quiz found on the Info Panel for this assignment.

71. Submit Claim for Robert Caudill

■ Objectives

- Search for a patient record.
- Complete a claim.

■ Overview

Robert Caudill has been vomiting for two days and states that the nausea started within 48 hours after taking the first dose of Aricept 10 mg by mouth. He was previously prescribed Aricept, a cholinesterase inhibitor, in order to slow the progression of Robert Caudill's Alzheimer's disease. After assessing Robert Caudill, Dr. Walden identified Aricept as the most likely reason for the nausea and vomiting and discontinues the medication. Dr. Walden assesses the patient and performs a problem-focused history and exam (10-minute exam) with straightforward decision-making. Complete the claim for Robert Caudill's encounter.

■ Competencies

- Complete insurance claim forms, CAAHEP VIII.P-4, ABHES 7-d
- Perform diagnostic coding, CAAHEP IX.P-2, ABHES 7-d
- Interpret information on an insurance card, CAAHEP VIII.P-1
- Interact professionally with third party representatives, CAAHEP VIII.A-1

Estimated completion time: 25 minutes

Measurable Steps

1. Within the Coding & Billing tab, select Claim from the left Info Panel and perform a patient search to locate the claim for Robert Caudill (Figure 4-53).

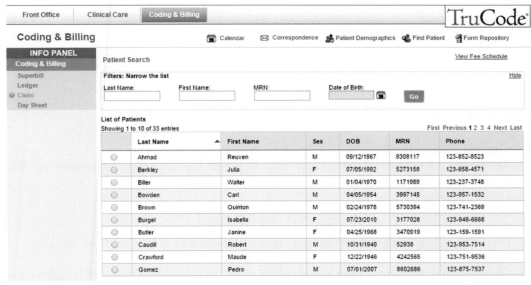

Figure 4-53 Perform a patient search to locate the claim for Robert Caudill.

2. Select the correct encounter and click the Edit icon in the Action column. Seven tabs appear within the claim: Patient Info, Provider Info, Payer Info, Encounter Notes, Claim Info, Charge Capture, and Submission. Certain patient demographic and encounter information is auto-populated in the claim.
3. Within the Patient Info tab, review the auto-populated information and document any additional information needed. Click the Save button.
4. Click the Provider Info tab.
5. Review the auto-populated information and document any additional information needed. Click the Save button.
6. Click the Payer Info tab.
7. Review the auto-populated information and document any additional information needed. Click the Save button.
8. Click the Encounter Notes tab.
9. Review the auto-populated information and document any additional information needed. Click the Save button.
10. Select the Yes radio button to indicate that the HIPAA form is on file for Robert Caudill and document the current date in the Dated field (Figure 4-54). Click the Save button.

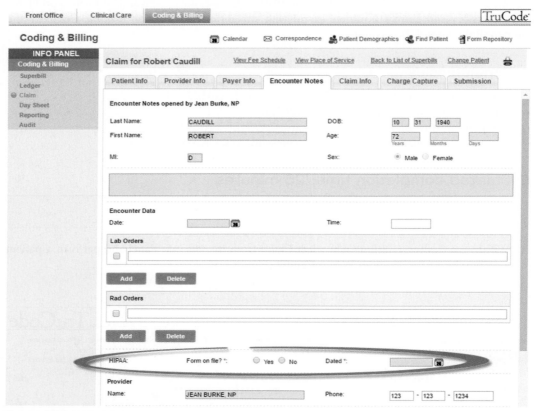

Figure 4-54 The Yes radio button indicates that the HIPAA form is on file.

11. Click the Claim Info tab.
12. Review the auto-populated information and document any additional information needed. Click the Save button.
13. Click the Charge Capture tab.
14. Document the encounter date in the DOS From and DOS To columns.
15. Place your cursor in the CPT/HCPCS column text field to access the encoder.
16. Enter "Office visit" in the Search field and select CPT Tabular from the dropdown menu.
17. Click the Search button.
18. Click the link in the Search Pane to show all 15 results and click the 99212 code to expand this code and confirm that it is the most specific code available (Figure 4-55).
19. Click the code 99212 for "Office or other outpatient visit" that appears in the tree. This code will auto-populate in the Claim (Figure 4-56).

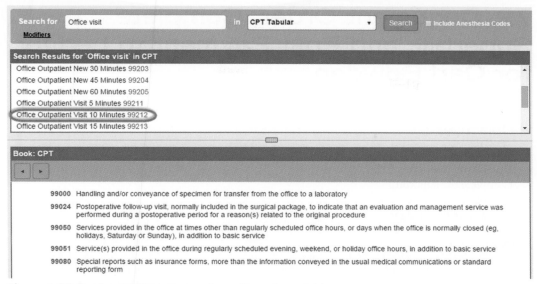

Figure 4-55 Confirm 99212 is the most specific code available.

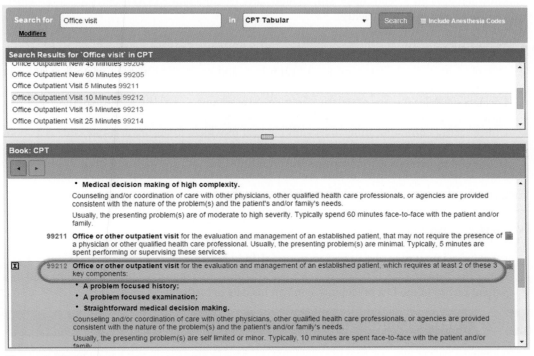

Figure 4-56 Populating the code in the claim.

20. Document "11" in the POS column.
21. Document "1" in the DX column.
22. Click the View Fee Schedule link to determine the fee for the problem-focused office visit.
23. Document "32.00" in the Fee column.
24. Document "1" in the Units column.
25. Click the Save button.
26. Click on the Submission tab. Click in the I am ready to submit the Claim box. Click on the Yes radio button to indicate that there is a signature on file and enter today's date in the Date field.
27. Click the Submit Claim button.

 Now use the Back to Assignment link to complete the Post-Case Quiz found on the Info Panel for this assignment.

72. Document Order, Complete Superbill, and Post Payment to Ledger for Carl Bowden

■ Objectives

- Search for a patient record.
- Document an order.
- Complete the superbill.
- Complete the claim.
- Update a patient ledger.

■ Overview

Carl Bowden is at the Walden-Martin office for an ECG before his bunion removal next week because the podiatrist requires a 12 lead ECG (pre-procedural examination) prior to the procedure. Dr. Walden approves the ECG with interpretation and the medical assistant performs the procedure. Carl Bowden pays his $25.00 copay with a credit card. Document the ECG order, submit the superbill and claim, and update the ledger.

■ Competencies

- Comply with federal, state, and local health laws and regulations as they relate to healthcare settings, ABHES 4-f
- Locate a state's legal scope of practice for medical assistants, CAAHEP X.P-1, ABHES 4-f
- Perform diagnostic coding, CAAHEP IX.P-2, ABHES 7-d
- Utilize tactful communication skills with medical providers to ensure accurate code selection, CAAHEP IX.A-1, ABHES 5-f, 5-g, 5-h, 7-d, 7-g
- Define common medical legal terms, CAAHEP X.C-13

Estimated completion time: 50 minutes

Measurable Steps

1. Click on the Find Patient icon.
2. Using the Patient Search fields, search for Carl Bowden's patient record. Once you locate his patient record in the List of Patients, confirm his date of birth.

> ◎ **HELPFUL HINT**
>
> Confirming date of birth will help to ensure that you have located the correct patient record.

3. Select the radio button for Carl Bowden and click the Select button.
4. Create a new encounter by clicking Office Visit in the left Info Panel (Figure 4-57). If the Create New Encounter window does not appear, select Add New to create a new encounter.

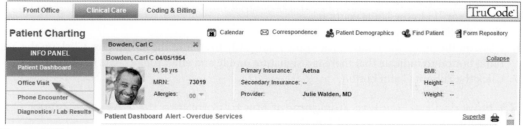

Figure 4-57 Office Visit in the Info Panel.

Coding & Billing

5. In the Create New Encounter window, select Follow-Up/Established Visit from the Visit Type dropdown.
6. Select Julie Walden, MD from the Provider dropdown menu.
7. Click the Save button.
8. Select Order Entry from the Record dropdown menu (Figure 4-58).
9. Click the Add button below the In-Office grid to add an order.

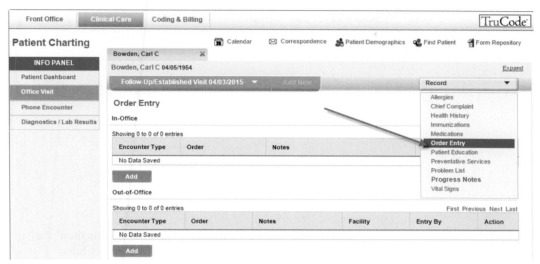

Figure 4-58 Order Entry in the Record dropdown menu.

10. In the Add Order window, select ECG from the Order dropdown menu.
11. Document "12 lead" in the Method field.
12. Document "Pre-op for bunionectomy." in the Notes field.
13. Document any additional information provided and click the Save button. The In-Office table will display the new order (Figure 4-59).

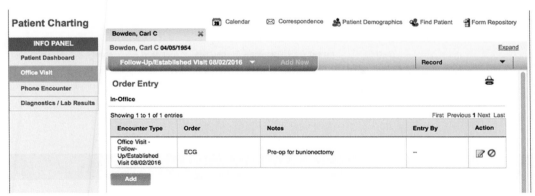

Figure 4-59 The In-Office table will display the new order.

14. After reviewing the encounter, select Patient Dashboard from the Info Panel.
15. Click the Superbill link below the patient header.
16. Select the correct encounter from the Encounters Not Coded table and confirm the auto-populated details.
17. On page one of the superbill, select the ICD-10 radio button (Figure 4-60).
18. In the Rank 1 row of the Diagnoses box, place the cursor in the text field to access the encoder.
19. Enter "Preprocedural examination" in the Search field and select Diagnosis ICD-10-CM from the dropdown menu.
20. Click the Search button.
21. Click the code Z01.810 to expand this code and confirm that it is the most specific code available.

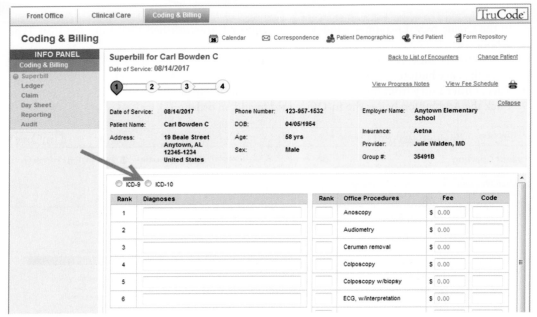

Figure 4-60 The ICD-10 radio button.

22. Click the code Z01.810 for "Encounter for preprocedural cardiovascular examination" that appears in the tree. This code will auto-populate in the Rank 1 row of the Diagnoses box.
23. Click the View Fee Schedule link to determine the correct code and fee for the ECG, w/interpretation (Figure 4-61).

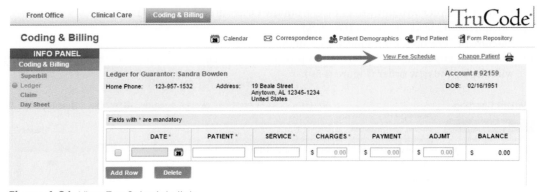

Figure 4-61 View Fee Schedule link.

> **HELPFUL HINT**
>
> The View Fee Schedule and View Progress Notes links provide information necessary in completing coding & billing tasks.

24. Document "1" in the Rank column for ECG, w/interpretation with the corresponding fee of "89.00" and code of "93000".
25. Click the Save button.
26. Go to page four of the superbill.
27. On page four, document "25.00" in the Copay field.
28. Confirm that the total in the Today's Charges field has populated correctly.
29. Document "64.00" in the Balance Due field.
30. Document any additional information needed.
31. Click the Save button.
32. Select the I am ready to submit the Superbill checkbox at the bottom of the screen.

33. Select the Yes radio button to indicate that the signature is on file.
34. Document the date in the Date field.
35. Click the Submit Superbill button. A confirmation message will appear.
36. Select Claim from the left Info Panel and perform a patient search to locate the claim for Carl Bowden.
37. Select the correct encounter and click the Edit icon in the Action column. Confirm the auto-populated details. Seven tabs appear within the claim: Patient Info, Provider Info, Payer Info, Encounter Notes, Claim Info, Charge Capture, and Submission. Certain patient demographic and encounter information is auto-populated in the claim.
38. Within the Patient Info tab, review the auto-populated information and document any additional information needed. Click the Save button.
39. Click the Provider Info tab.
40. Review the auto-populated information and document any additional information needed. Click the Save button.
41. Click the Payer Info tab.
42. Review the auto-populated information and document any additional information needed. Click the Save button.
43. Click the Encounter Notes tab.
44. Review the auto-populated information and document any additional information needed.
45. Select the Yes radio button to indicate that the HIPAA form is on file for Carl Bowden and document the current date in the Dated field. Click the Save button.
46. Click the Claim Info tab.
47. Review the auto-populated information and document any additional information needed. Click the Save button.
48. Click the Charge Capture tab.
49. Document the encounter date in the DOS From and DOS To columns.
50. Document "93000" in the CPT/HCPCS column.
51. Document "11" in the POS column.
52. Document "1" in the DX column.
53. Document "89.00" in the Fee column.
54. Click the Save button.
55. Click on the Submission tab. Click in the I am ready to submit the Claim box. Click on the Yes radio button to indicate that there a signature on file and enter today's date in the Date field.
56. Click the Submit Claim button.
57. Select the Ledger from the left Info Panel.
58. Select the arrow to expand the ledger for Carl Bowden.
59. All charges submitted on the claim will auto-populate on the ledger.
60. Click Add Row to enter the payment made by Carl Bowden.
61. Document the current date in the Transaction Date column using the calendar picker.
62. Document the date of service in the DOS column using the calendar picker.
63. Select PTPYMTCC in the Service column.
64. Document "25.00" in the Payment column.
65. The balance will auto-populate in the Balance column and the total will auto-populate in the Total Ledger Balance field below the table.
66. Click the Save button.

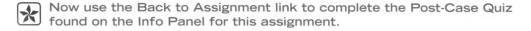 Now use the Back to Assignment link to complete the Post-Case Quiz found on the Info Panel for this assignment.

73. Complete Superbill, Ledger, and Claim for Anna Richardson

■ Objectives

- Search for a patient record.
- Complete a superbill.
- Complete a claim.
- Update a patient ledger.

■ Overview

Anna Richardson delivered her baby two-and-a-half months ago. She had a vaginal delivery with post-partum hemorrhage. She had been feeling fine until last week when she started feeling very tired. She was seen by Dr. Martin for a problem-focused office visit on 08/09 with a CBC with differential. Dr. Martin's diagnosis is iron deficiency anemia secondary to blood loss. She paid her $25.00 copayment with a credit card. Complete the superbill and claim, and update the patient ledger.

■ Competencies

- Describe how to use the most current procedural coding system, CAAHEP IX.C-1, ABHES 7-d
- Perform billing procedures, CAAHEP VII.P-1, ABHES 7-c
- Interact professionally with third party representatives, CAAHEP VIII.A-1

Estimated completion time: 45 minutes

Measurable Steps

1. Click on the Find Patient icon.
2. Using the Patient Search field, search for Anna Richardson's patient record.
3. Select the radio button for Anna Richardson and click the select button.
4. Confirm the auto-populated details in the patient header.

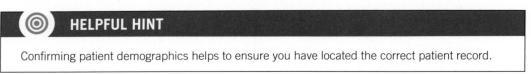

HELPFUL HINT

Confirming patient demographics helps to ensure you have located the correct patient record.

5. After reviewing the encounter, click the Superbill link below the patient header (Figure 4-62).

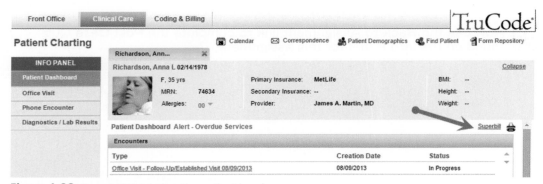

Figure 4-62 Superbill link below the patient header.

6. Select the encounter from the Encounters Not Coded table and confirm the auto-populated details.
7. On page one of the Superbill, select the ICD-10 radio button.
8. In the Rank 1 row of the Diagnoses box, place the cursor in the text field to access the encoder.
9. Enter "Iron deficiency anemia" in the Search field and select Diagnosis ICD-10-CM from the dropdown menu.
10. Click the Search button.
11. Click the code D50.9 to expand this code and confirm that it is the most specific code available (Figure 4-63).

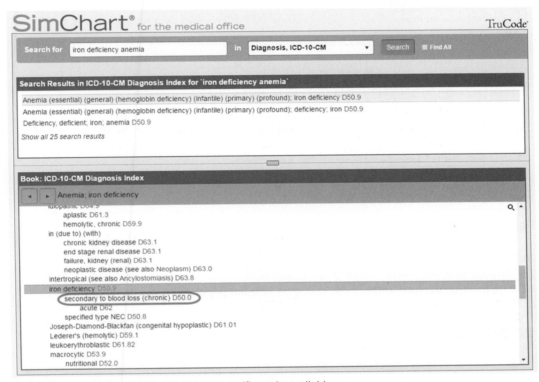

Figure 4-63 Confirm D50.9 is the most specific code available.

12. Click the code D50.9 for "Iron deficiency anemia secondary to blood loss (chronic)" that appears in the tree. This code will auto-populate in the Rank 1 row of the Diagnoses box (Figure 4-64).
13. Click the View Fee Schedule link to determine the charge and code for the problem-focused office visit.
14. Document "1" in the Rank column for a problem-focused office visit with the corresponding fee of "32.00" and code of "99212".

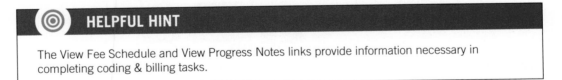

> ⊙ **HELPFUL HINT**
>
> The View Fee Schedule and View Progress Notes links provide information necessary in completing coding & billing tasks.

15. Click the Save button.
16. Go to page three of the superbill.
17. View the Fee Schedule to determine the charge and code for the CBC, w/auto differential and venipuncture.
18. Document "2" in the Rank column for CBC, w/ auto differential with the corresponding fee of "35.00" and code of "85025".
19. Document "3" in the Rank column for venipuncture with the corresponding fee of "10.00" and code of "36415".

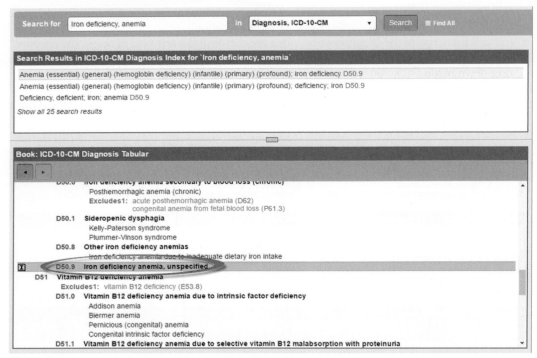

Figure 4-64 Populating the code in the Rank 1 row of the Diagnoses box.

20. Click the Save button and go to page four of the superbill.
21. On page four, document "25.00" in the Copay field.
22. Confirm that the total in the Today's Charges field has populated correctly (Figure 4-65).

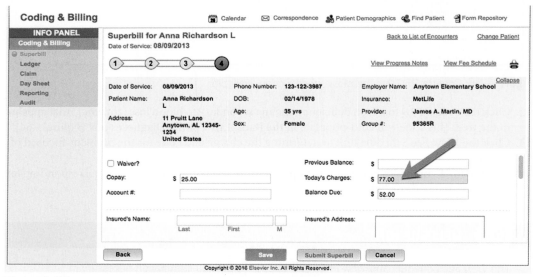

Figure 4-65 Confirm that the total in the Today's Charges field has populated correctly.

23. Document "52.00" in the Balance Due field.
24. Document any additional information needed.
25. Select the I am ready to submit the Superbill checkbox at the bottom of the screen.
26. Select the Yes radio button to indicate that the signature is on file.
27. Document the date in the Date field.
28. Click the Submit Superbill button. A confirmation message will appear.
29. Click Claim from the left Info Panel and perform a patient search to locate Anna Richardson.
30. Select the correct encounter and click the Edit icon in the Action column. Confirm the auto-populated details. Seven tabs appear within the claim: Patient Info, Provider Info, Payer Info,

Encounter Notes, Claim Info, Charge Capture, and Submission. Certain patient demographic and encounter information is auto-populated in the claim.

31. Within the Patient Info tab, review the auto-populated information and document any additional information needed. Click the Save button.
32. Click the Provider Info tab.
33. Review the auto-populated information and document any additional information needed. Click the Save button.
34. Click the Payer Info tab.
35. Review the auto-populated information and document any additional information needed. Click the Save button.
36. Click the Encounter Notes tab.
37. Review the auto-populated information. Select the Yes radio button to indicate that the HIPAA form is on file for Anna Richardson and document the current date in the Dated field. Click the Save button.
38. Click the Claim Info tab.
39. Review the auto-populated information and document any additional information needed. Click the Save button.
40. Click the Charge Capture tab.
41. Document the encounter date in the DOS From and DOS To columns.
42. Document "99212" in the CPT/HCPCS column.
43. Document "11" in the POS column.
44. Document "1" in the DX column.
45. Document "32.00" in the Fee column.
46. Document "1" in the Units column.
47. In the next row, document the Encounter date of service in the DOS From and DOS To columns.
48. Document "36415" in the CPT/HCPCS column.
49. Document "11" in the POS column.
50. Document "1" in the DX column.
51. Document "10.00" in the Fee column.
52. Document "1" in the Units column.
53. Document "85025" in the CPT/HCPCS column.
54. Document "11" in the POS column.
55. Document "1" in the DX column.
56. Document "35.00" in the Fee column.
57. Document "1" in the Units column.
58. Click the Save button (Figure 4-66).
59. Click the Submission tab. Click in the I am ready to submit the Claim box. Click on the Yes radio button to indicate that there a signature on file and enter today's date in the Date field.

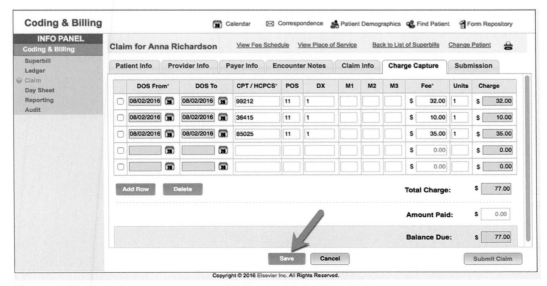

Figure 4-66 After all necessary rows are filled out, click the Save button.

60. Click the Save button. Click the Submit Claim button.
61. Select the Ledger from the left Info Panel.
62. Search for Anna Richardson using the Patient Search fields.
63. Select the radio button for Anna Richardson and click the Select button.
64. Click the arrow to the right of Anna Richardson's name to expand her patient ledger.
65. All charges submitted on the claim will auto-populate on the ledger. Click Add Row to enter the payment made by Anna Richardson.
66. Document the current date in the Transaction Date column using the calendar picker.
67. Document the date of service in the DOS column using the calendar picker.
68. Select PTPYMTCC in the Service column.
69. Document "25.00" in the Payment column.
70. Click the Save button.
71. The balance will auto-populate in the Balance column and the total will auto-populate in the Total Ledger Balance field below the table.

 Now use the Back to Assignment link to complete the Post-Case Quiz found on the Info Panel for this assignment.

74. Post Payment to Ledger and Submit Claim for Al Neviaser

■ Objectives

- Search for a patient record.
- Review a superbill for accuracy.
- Complete a claim.
- Update a patient ledger.

■ Overview

Dr. Martin ordered a flu shot during Al Neviaser's appointment. Al paid his $25.00 copay with a check during his visit. Use the coded superbill to update Al Neviaser's claim and ledger.

■ Competencies

- Complete insurance claim forms, CAAHEP VIII.P-4, ABHES 7-d
- Perform diagnostic coding, CAAHEP IX.P-2, ABHES 7-d
- Perform accounts receivable procedures to patient accounts including posting charges, payments, and adjustments, CAAHEP VII.P-1, ABHES 7-c
- Identify types of information contained in the patient's billing record, CAAHEP VII.C-5
- Obtain accurate patient billing information, CAAHEP VII.P-3

Estimated completion time: 35 minutes

Measurable Steps

1. Within the Coding & Billing tab, select Superbill from the left Info Panel.
2. Search for Al Neviaser using the Patient Search fields.
3. Select the radio button for Al Neviaser and click the Select button.
4. Select the correct encounter from the Encounters Coded table.
5. Review all four pages of the submitted superbill to obtain the charges and codes to be entered on the claim.
6. Select Claim from the left Info Panel and perform a patient search to locate the claim for Al Neviaser (Figure 4-67).

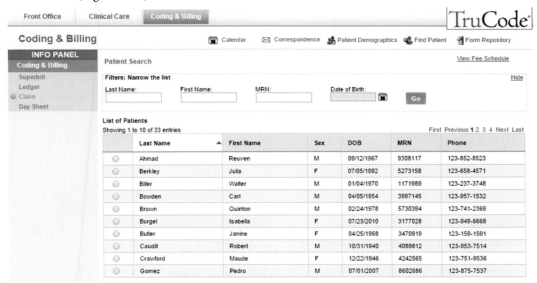

Figure 4-67 Perform a patient search to locate the claim for Al Neviaser.

7. Click the Edit icon in the Action column and confirm the auto-populated details. Seven tabs appear within the claim: Patient Info, Provider Info, Payer Info, Encounter Notes, Claim Info, Charge Capture, and Submission. Certain patient demographic and encounter information is auto-populated in the claim.
8. Within the Patient Info tab, review the auto-populated information and document any additional information needed. Click the Save button.
9. Click the Provider Info tab.
10. Review the auto-populated information and document any additional information needed. Click the Save button.
11. Click the Payer Info tab.
12. Review the auto-populated information and document any additional information needed. Click the Save button.
13. Click the Encounter Notes tab.
14. Review the auto-populated information. Select the Yes radio button to indicate that the HIPAA form is on file for Al Neviaser and document the current date in the Dated field.
15. Document any additional information needed. Click the Save button.
16. Click the Claim Info tab.
17. Review the auto-populated information and document any additional information needed. Click the Save button.
18. Click the Charge Capture tab.
19. Document the encounter date in the DOS From and DOS To columns.
20. Document "99396" in the CPT/HCPCS column.
21. Document "11" in the POS column.
22. Document "1" in the DX column.
23. Document "105.00" in the Fee column.
24. In the next row, document the encounter date in the DOS From and DOS To columns.
25. Document "90658" in the CPT/HCPCS column.
26. Document "11" in the POS column.
27. Document "1" in DX column.
28. Document "24.00" in the Fee column.
29. In the next row, document the encounter date in the DOS From and DOS To columns.
30. Document "90471" in the CPT/HCPCS column.
31. Document "11" in the POS column.
32. Document "1" in the DX column.
33. Document "10.00" in the Fee column.
34. Click the Save button.
35. Click the Submission tab. Click in the I am ready to submit the Claim box. Click the Yes radio button to indicate that there a signature on file and enter today's date in the Date field (Figure 4-68).

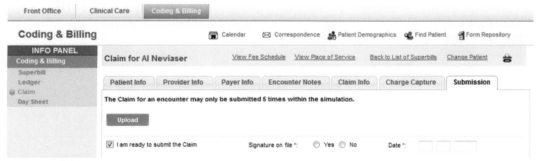

Figure 4-68 Submitting a Claim.

36. Click on the Submit Claim button.
37. Select Ledger from the left Info Panel.
38. Search for Al Neviaser using the Patient Search fields.
39. Select the radio button for Al Neviaser and click the Select button.

40. Click the arrow to the right of Al Neviaser's name to expand his patient ledger.
41. All charges submitted on the claim will auto-populate on the ledger. Click Add Row to enter the payment made by Al Neviaser.
42. Document the current date in the Transaction Date column using the calendar picker.
43. Document the date of service in the DOS column using the calendar picker.
44. Select James A. Martin, MD in the Provider dropdown.
45. Select PTPYMTCK in the Service dropdown.
46. Document "25.00" in the Payment column.
47. Click the Save button. The balance will auto-populate in the Balance column and the total will auto-populate in the Total Ledger Balance field below the table.

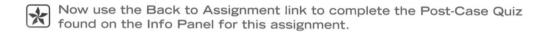 Now use the Back to Assignment link to complete the Post-Case Quiz found on the Info Panel for this assignment.

75. Update Ledger and Prepare Patient Statement for Charles Johnson

■ Objectives

- Search for a patient record.
- Post an insurance payment.
- Post a patient payment.
- Prepare a patient statement.

■ Overview

Charles Johnson received notification from his insurance that they would not be paying for his HBa1C so he sent payment of the $32.00 (with a check) to the Walden-Martin office. In the meantime, the insurance claim had been resubmitted and a reimbursement of $22.00 was issued. Post both payments to Charles Johnson's ledger and prepare a patient statement to send to Charles Johnson.

■ Competencies

- Display sensitivity when requesting payment for services rendered, CAAHEP VII.A-2, ABHES 5-c, 5-h, 7-c
- Describe types of adjustments made to patient accounts, CAAHEP VII.C-4, ABHES 7-c
- Inform a patient of financial obligations for services rendered, CAAHEP VII.P-4, ABHES 5-c, 5-h, 7-c
- Perform accounts receivable procedures to patient accounts including posting charges, payments, and adjustments, CAAHEP VII.P-1, ABHES 7-c
- Utilize an EMR, CAAHEP VI.P-6, ABHES 7-b

Estimated completion time: 25 minutes

Measurable Steps

1. Within the Coding & Billing tab, select Ledger from the left Info Panel (Figure 4-69).

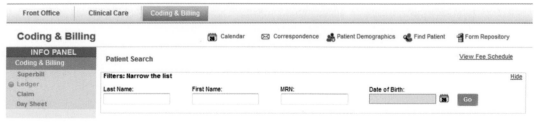

Figure 4-69 Ledger in the left Info Panel.

2. Search for Charles Johnson using the Patient Search fields.
3. Select the radio button for Charles Johnson and click the Select button.
4. Confirm the auto-populated details in the header (Figure 4-70).
5. Click the arrow to the right of Charles Johnson's name to expand his patient ledger.
6. All charges submitted on the claim will auto-populate on the ledger. Click Add Row to enter the payment made by Charles Johnson.
7. Document the current date in the Transaction Date column using the calendar picker.
8. Document the date of service in the DOS column using the calendar picker.
9. Document PTPYMTCK in the Service column.

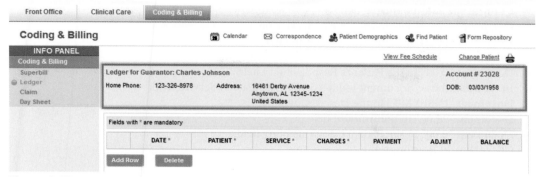

Figure 4-70 Confirm the auto-populated details in the header.

10. Document "32.00" in the Payment column.
11. Click the Add Row button.
12. Document the current date in the Transaction Date column using the calendar picker.
13. Document the date of service in the DOS column using the calendar picker.
14. Document INSPYMT in the Service column.
15. Document "22.00" in the Payment column.
16. Click the Add Row button.
17. Document the current date in the Transaction Date column using the calendar picker.
18. Document the date of service in the DOS column using the calendar picker.
19. Document PTREFUND in the Service column.
20. Document "0.00" in the Charges column.
21. Document "22.00" in the Adjustment column. The balance will auto-populate in the Balance column.
22. Click the Save button.
23. Click on the Form Repository icon.
24. Select Patient Statement from the Patient Forms section of the left Info Panel.
25. Click the Patient Search button (Figure 4-71) to perform a patient search and assign the form to Charles Johnson.

HELPFUL HINT

Performing a patient search before completing a form helps to ensure accurate documentation.

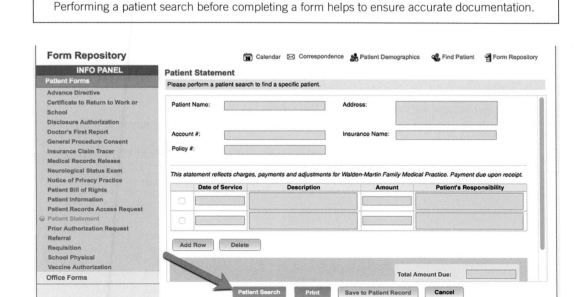

Figure 4-71 Click the Patient Search button to perform a patient search and assign the form to Charles Johnson.

26. Confirm the auto-populated details.
27. Document today's date in the Date of Service field.
28. Document "PTPYMT" in the Description field.
29. Document "32.00" in the Amount field.
30. Document "0.00" in the Patient's Responsibility field.
31. In the second row, document today's date in the Date of Service field.
32. Document "INSPYMT" in the Description field.
33. Document "22.00" in the Amount field.
34. Document "0.00" in the Patient's Responsibility field.
35. Click the Add Row button.
36. Document today's date in the Date of Service field.
37. Document "Pt Refund" in the Description field.
38. Document "22.00" in the Amount field.
39. Document "0.00" in the Patient's Responsibility field.
40. Document "0.00" in the Total Amount Due field (Figure 4-72).

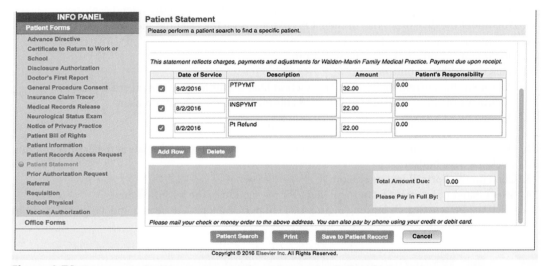

Figure 4-72 Document all of the necessary information on the Patient Statement.

41. Click the Save to Patient Record button. Confirm the date and click the OK button.
42. Click the Find Patient icon.
43. Using the Patient Search fields, search for Charles Johnson's patient record. Once you locate him in the List of Patients, confirm his date of birth.
44. Select the radio button for Charles Johnson and click the Select button. Confirm the auto-populated details.
45. Scroll down to view the Forms section of the Patient Dashboard.
46. Select the form you prepared. The form will open in a new window, allowing you to print.

Now use the Back to Assignment link to complete the Post-Case Quiz found on the Info Panel for this assignment.

Coding & Billing

76. Post Payment to Ledger for Walter Biller and Update Day Sheet

Objectives

- Search for a patient record.
- Update a patient ledger.
- Update the day sheet.

Overview

Walter Biller stopped by the medical office to have Dr. Martin complete a section of his life insurance application form and mail it back to him. The medical assistant informs Walter Biller that there is a $15.00 fee for report preparation and Walter Biller pays the fee with a check. Document this payment in Walter Biller's ledger and on the day sheet.

Competencies

- Identify types of third party plans, information required to file a third party claim and the steps for filing a third party claim, CAAHEP VIII.C-1, ABHES 7-d
- Perform diagnostic coding, CAAHEP IX.P-2, ABHES 7-d
- Utilize an EMR, CAAHEP VI.P-6, ABHES 7-b

Estimated completion time: 20 minutes

Measurable Steps

1. Within the Coding & Billing tab, select Ledger from the left Info Panel (Figure 4-73).

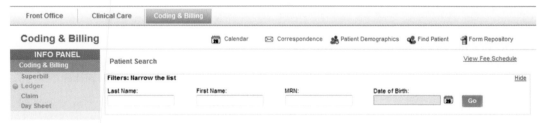

Figure 4-73 Ledger in the left Info Panel.

2. Search for Walter Biller using the Patient Search fields.
3. Select the radio button for Walter Biller and click the Select button.
4. Confirm the auto-populated details in the header.
5. Click the arrow to the right of Walter Biller's name to expand his patient ledger.
6. Document the current date in the Transaction Date column using the calendar picker.
7. Document the date of service in the DOS column using the calendar picker.
8. Select James A. Martin, MD from the Provider dropdown.
9. Place your cursor in the Service column and select the TC button to access the encoder.
10. Enter "report preparation" in the Search field and select CPT Tabular from the dropdown menu.
11. Click the Search button.
12. Click the link in the Search Results pane to show all 16 results and click the 99080 code to expand this code and confirm that it is the most specific code available (Figure 4-74).
13. Click the 99080 code for "Special Reports such as insurance forms" that appears in the tree. This code will auto-populate in the ledger (Figure 4-75).

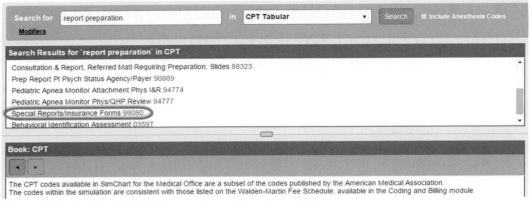

Figure 4-74 Confirm 99080 is the most specific code available.

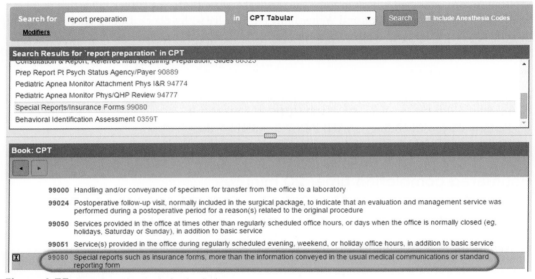

Figure 4-75 Populate the code in the ledger.

14. Document "15.00" in the Charges column.
15. Click Add Row.
16. Document the current date in the Transaction Date column using the calendar picker.
17. Document the date of service in the DOS column using the calendar picker.
18. Select James A. Martin, MD using the dropdown in the Provider field.
19. Document PTPYMTCK in the Service column.
20. Document "15.00" in the Payment column.
21. The balance will auto-populate in the Balance column.
22. Click the Save button.
23. Select Day Sheet from the left Info Panel.
24. Document the current date in the Date column using the calendar picker.
25. Document "Walter Biller" in the Patient Name field.
26. Select James A. Martin, MD using the dropdown in the Provider field.
27. Document "99080" in the Service column.
28. Document "15.00" in the Charges column.
29. Document "15.00" in the Payment column.
30. Document "0.00" in the New Balance column.
31. Click the Save button.

 Now use the Back to Assignment link to complete the Post-Case Quiz found on the Info Panel for this assignment.

77. Complete Superbill, Post Payment to Ledger, and Update Day Sheet for Norma Washington

■ Objectives

- Search for a patient record.
- Complete a superbill.
- Complete a claim.
- Update a patient ledger.
- Update the day sheet.

■ Overview

Norma Washington has degenerative joint disease in her right knee and had blood drawn for a sedimentation rate during an expanded problem-focused office visit with Dr. Walden. Norma Washington made her $25.00 copay (with a credit card) while she was in the office. Document the patient's chief complaint, complete the superbill and claim, update the patient ledger, and update the daysheet.

■ Competencies

- Define basic bookkeeping terms, CAAHEP VII.C-1, ABHES 7-c
- Describe types of adjustments made to patient accounts, CAAHEP VII.C-4, ABHES 7-c
- Identify types of third party plans, information required to file a third party claim and the steps for filing a third party claim, CAAHEP VIII.C-1, ABHES 7-d
- Identify precautions for accepting cash, checks, and credit cards, CAAHEP VII.C-3, ABHES 7-c
- Perform diagnostic coding, CAAHEP IX.P-2, ABHES 7-d
- Perform procedural coding, CAAHEP IX.P-1, ABHES 7-d
- Utilize an EMR, CAAHEP VI.P-6, ABHES 7-b
- Identify types of information contained in the patient's billing record, CAAHEP VII.C-5
- Obtain accurate patient billing information, CAAHEP VII.P-3

Estimated completion time: 30 minutes

Measurable Steps

1. Click on the Find Patient icon.
2. Using the Patient Search field, search for Norma Washington's patient record.
3. Select the radio button for Norma Washington and click the select button.
4. Confirm the auto-populated details in the patient header.

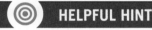
HELPFUL HINT

Confirming patient demographics helps to ensure you have located the correct patient record.

5. Create a new encounter by clicking Office Visit in the left Info Panel (Figure 4-76). If the Create New Encounter window does not appear, click the Add New button to create the new encounter.
6. In the Create New Encounter window, select Follow-Up/Established Visit from the Visit Type dropdown.
7. Select Julie Walden, MD in the Provider dropdown.
8. Click Save.
9. Select Chief Complaint from the dropdown menu.
10. Enter "Follow up on DJD, right knee" in the Chief Complaint box.

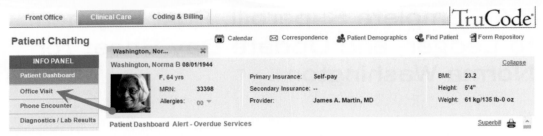

Figure 4-76 Office Visit in the Info Panel.

11. Click the Save button.
12. Select Patient dashboard from the Info Panel.
13. Click the Superbill link below the patient header (Figure 4-77) in the Patient Dashboard.

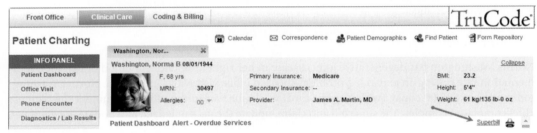

Figure 4-77 Superbill link below the patient header.

14. Select the correct encounter from the Encounters Not Coded table and confirm the auto-populated details.
15. On page one of the superbill, select the ICD-10 radio button.
16. In the Rank 1 row of the Diagnoses box, place the cursor in the text field to access the encoder.
17. Enter "Degenerative Joint Disease" in the Search field and select Diagnosis ICD-10-CM from the dropdown menu.
18. Click the Search button.
19. Click Osteoarthritis and then M17.9 to expand this code and confirm that it is the most specific code available (Figure 4-78).

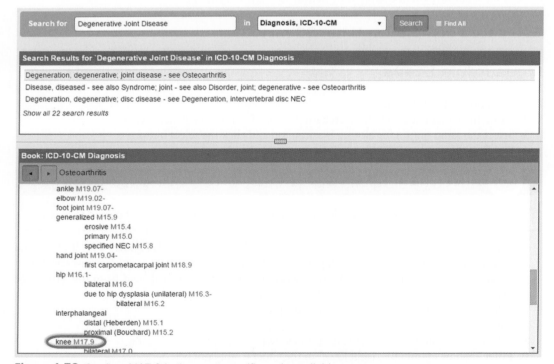

Figure 4-78 Confirm M17.9 is the most specific code available.

Coding & Billing

20. Click the code M17.11 for "Unilateral primary osteoarthritis, right knee" that appears in the tree. This code will auto-populate in the Rank 1 row of the Diagnoses box (Figure 4-79).
21. Document "1" in the Rank column for expanded problem-focused office visit.

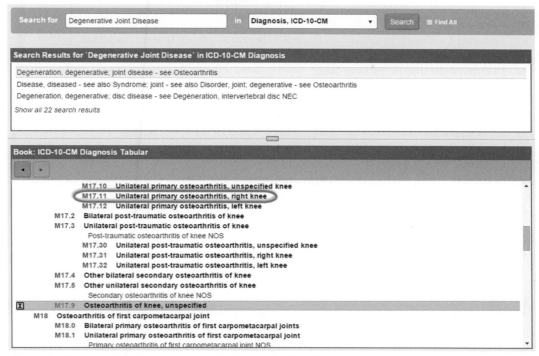

Figure 4-79 Populating the code in the Rank 1 row of the Diagnoses box.

22. Select the View Fee Schedule link to obtain the charges and code for the expanded office visit.
23. Enter "43.00" in the Fee column and "99213" in the Est column for the expanded problem-focused office visit.
24. Click the Save button.
25. Go to page three of the superbill.
26. Document "2" in the Rank column for Venipuncture.
27. Select the View Fee Schedule link to obtain the charges and code for Venipuncture.
28. Enter "10.00" in the Fee column and "36415" in the code column for Venipuncture (Figure 4-80).

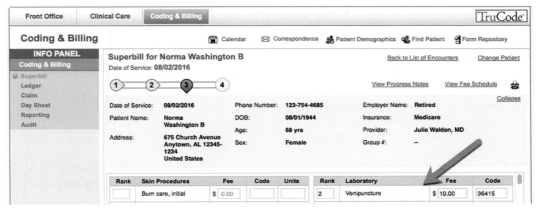

Figure 4-80 Enter "10.00" in the Fee column and "36415" in the code column for Venipuncture.

29. Document "3" in the Rank column for Sedimentation rate.
30. Select the View Fee Schedule link to obtain the charges and code for Sedimentation rate.
31. Enter "16.00" in the Fee column and "85652" in the code column for Sedimentation rate.
32. Click the Save button.

33. Go to page four of the superbill.
34. On page four, document "25.00" in the Copay field.
35. Confirm that the total in the Today's Charges field has populated correctly.
36. Document "44.00" in the Balance Due field.
37. Document any additional information needed.
38. Click the Save button.
39. Select the I am ready to submit the Superbill checkbox at the bottom of the screen.
40. Select the Yes radio button to indicate that the signature is on file.
41. Document the date in the Date field.
42. Click the Submit Superbill button. A confirmation message will appear.
43. Select Claim from the left Info Panel.
44. Search for Norma Washington using the Patient Search fields.
45. Select the radio button for Norma Washington and click the Select button.
46. Select the correct encounter and click the Edit icon in the Action column. Confirm the auto-populated details. Seven tabs appear within the claim: Patient Info, Provider Info, Payer Info, Encounter Notes, Claim Info, Charge Capture, and Submission. Certain patient demographic and encounter information is auto-populated in the claim.
47. Within the Patient Info tab, review the auto-populated information and document any additional information needed. Click the Save button.
48. Click the Provider Info tab.
49. Review the auto-populated information and document any additional information needed. Click the Save button.
50. Click the Payer Info tab.
51. Review the auto-populated information and document any additional information needed. Click the Save button.
52. Click the Encounter Notes tab.
53. Review the auto-populated information. Select the Yes radio button to indicate that the HIPAA form is on file for Norma Washington and document the current date in the Dated field. Click the Save button.
54. Click the Claim Info tab.
55. Review the auto-populated information and document any additional information needed. Click the Save button.
56. Click the Charge Capture tab.
57. Document the encounter date in the DOS From and DOS To columns.
58. Document "99213" in the CPT/HCPCS column.
59. Document "11" in the POS column.
60. Document "1" in the DX column.
61. Document "43.00" in the Fee column.
62. In the next row, document the Encounter date of service in the DOS From and DOS To columns.
63. Document "36415" in the CPT/HCPCS column.
64. Document "11" in the POS column.
65. Document "1" in the DX column.
66. Document "10.00" in the Fee column.
67. In the next row, document the Encounter date of service in the DOS From and DOS To columns.
68. Document "85652" in the CPT/HCPCS column.
69. Document "11" in the POS column.
70. Document "1" in the DX column.
71. Document "16.00" in the Fee column.
72. Click the Save button.
73. Click the Submission tab. Click the I am ready to submit the Claim box (Figure 4-81). Click the Yes radio button to indicate that there is a signature on file and enter today's date in the Date field.
74. Click on the Submit Claim button.
75. Select Ledger from the left Info Panel.
76. Search for Norma Washington using the Patient Search fields.
77. Select the radio button for Norma Washington and click the Select button.
78. Confirm the auto-populated details in the header.
79. Click the arrow to the right of Norma Washington's name to expand her patient ledger.

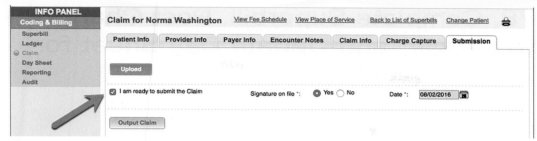

Figure 4-81 Click the "I am ready to submit the Claim" box.

80. All charges submitted on the claim will auto-populate on the ledger. Click Add Row to enter the payment made by Norma Washington.
81. Document the current date in the Transaction Date column using the calendar picker.
82. Document the date of service in the DOS column using the calendar picker.
83. Select Julie Walden, MD using the dropdown in the Provider field.
84. Document PTPYMTCC in the Service column.
85. Document "25.00" in the Payment column. The balance will auto-populate in the Balance column.
86. Click the Save button.
87. Select Day Sheet from the left Info Panel.
88. Document the current date in the Date column using the calendar picker.
89. Document "Norma Washington" in the Patient column.
90. Select the correct provider in the Provider column.
91. Document "99213" in the Service column.
92. Document "43.00" in the Charges column.
93. Document "25.00" in the Payment column.
94. Document "0.00" in the Adjustment column.
95. Document "18.00" in the New Balance column.
96. Document "0.00" in the Old Balance column.
97. Click Add Row button.
98. Document the current date in the Date column using the calendar picker.
99. Document "Norma Washington" in the Patient column.
100. Select the correct provider in the Provider column.
101. Document "36415" in the Service column.
102. Document "10.00" in the Charges column.
103. Document "0.00" in the Payment column.
104. Document "0.00" in the Adjustment column.
105. Document "28.00" in the New Balance column.
105. Document "18.00" in the Old Balance column.
106. Click Add Row button.
107. Document the current date in the Date column using the calendar picker.
108. Document "Norma Washington" in the Patient column.
109. Select the correct provider in the Provider column.
110. Document "85652" in the Service column.
111. Document "16.00" in the Charges column.
112. Document "0.00" in the Payment column.
113. Document "0.00" in the Adjustment column.
114. Document "44.00" in the New Balance column.
115. Document "28.00" in the Old Balance column.
116. Click the Save button.

★ Now use the Back to Assignment link to complete the Post-Case Quiz found on the Info Panel for this assignment.

78. Complete Superbill, Post Charges to Ledger, and Update Day Sheet for Robert Caudill

■ Objectives

- Search for a patient record.
- Document a patient's chief complaint.
- Complete a superbill.
- Complete a claim.
- Update a patient ledger.
- Update the day sheet.

■ Overview

Jean Burke, NP saw Robert Caudill for a partial nail removal for an ingrowing nail that is billed at $115.00 and Robert Caudill made his $25.00 copay with a check. Document the patient's chief complaint, complete a superbill and claim, update the patient ledger, and update the day sheet.

■ Competencies

- Define basic bookkeeping terms, CAAHEP VII.C-1, ABHES 7-c
- Describe types of adjustments made to patient accounts, CAAHEP VII.C-4, ABHES 7-c
- Explain patient financial obligations for services rendered, CAAHEP VII.C-6, ABHES 5-c, 7-c
- Identify types of information contained in the patient's billing record, CAAHEP VII.C-5, ABHES 7-b, 7-c
- Perform accounts receivable procedure to patient accounts including posting charges, payments, and adjustments, CAAHEP VII.P-1, ABHES 7-c
- Perform diagnostic coding, CAAHEP IX.P-2, ABHES 7-d
- Perform procedural coding, CAAHEP IX.P-1, ABHES 7-d
- Define medical necessity as it applies to procedural and diagnostic coding, CAAHEP IX.C-5

Estimated completion time: 30 minutes

Measurable Steps

1. Click on the Find Patient icon.
2. Using the Patient Search field, search for Robert Caudill's patient record.
3. Select the radio button for Robert Caudill and click the Select button.
4. Confirm the auto-populated details in the patient header.

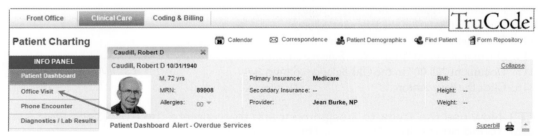

Figure 4-82 Office Visit in the Info Panel.

5. Create a new encounter by clicking Office Visit in the left Info Panel (Figure 4-82).
6. Click Add New to add today's encounter.

7. In the Create New Encounter window, select Follow-Up/Established Visit from the Visit Type dropdown.
8. Select Jean Burke, NP from the Provider dropdown.
9. Click the Save button.
10. Select Chief Complaint from the dropdown menu.
11. Insert "partial nail removal for an ingrowing nail" in the Chief Complaint box.
12. Click the Save button.
13. Select Patient Dashboard from the left Info Panel.
14. Select the Superbill link below the patient header.
15. Select the correct encounter from the Encounters Not Coded table.
16. On page one of the superbill, click the ICD-10 radio button.
17. In the Rank 1 row of the Diagnoses box, place the cursor in the text field to access the encoder.
18. Enter "Ingrowing nail" in the Search field and select Diagnosis ICD-10-CM from the dropdown menu.
19. Click the Search button.
20. Click the code L60.0 to expand this code and confirm that it is the most specific code available (Figure 4-83).

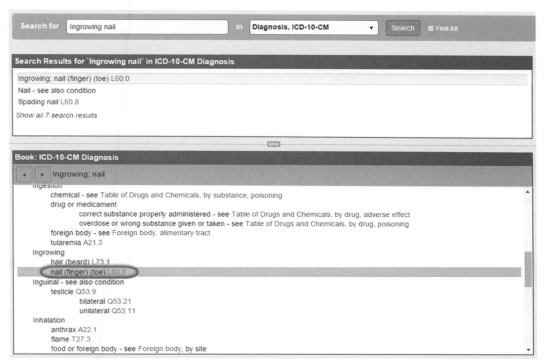

Figure 4-83 Confirm L60.0 is the most specific code available.

21. Click the code L60.0 for "Ingrowing nail" that appears in the tree. This code will auto-populate in the Rank 1 row of the Diagnoses box (Figure 4-84).
22. Click Save.
23. Go to page three of the superbill.
24. Document Rank "1" for Nail Removal, partial in Skin Procedures.
25. Select the View Fee Schedule link to obtain the charges and code for Nail Removal, partial.
26. Enter "115.00" in the Fee column and "11730" in the code column for Nail Removal, partial.
27. Click Save and then go to page four of the superbill.
28. On page four, document "25.00" in the Copay field.
29. Confirm that the total in the Today's Charges field has populated correctly.
30. Document "90.00" in the Balance Due field.
31. Document any additional information needed.
32. Select the I am ready to submit the Superbill checkbox at the bottom of the screen.
33. Select the Yes radio button to indicate that the signature is on file.

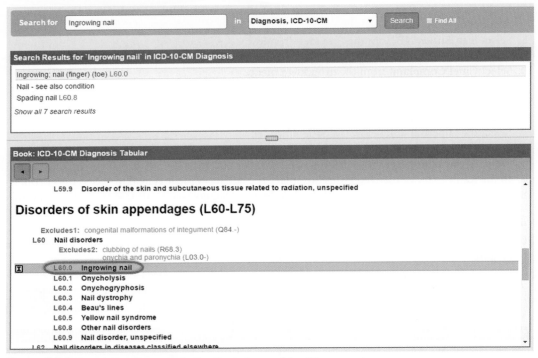

Figure 4-84 Populating the code in the Rank 1 row of the Diagnoses box.

34. Document the date in the Date field.
35. Click the Submit Superbill button. A confirmation message will appear.
36. Select Claim from the left Info Panel.
37. Search for Robert Caudill using the Patient Search fields.
38. Select the radio button for Robert Caudill and click the Select button.
39. Select the correct encounter and click the Edit icon in the Action column. Confirm the auto-populated details. Seven tabs appear within the claim: Patient Info, Provider Info, Payer Info, Encounter Notes, Claim Info, Charge Capture, and Submission. Certain patient demographic and encounter information is auto-populated in the claim.
40. Within the Patient Info tab, review the auto-populated information and document any additional information needed. Click the Save button.
41. Click the Provider Info tab.
42. Review the auto-populated information and document any additional information needed. Click the Save button.
43. Click the Payer Info tab.
44. Review the auto-populated information and document any additional information needed. Click the Save button.
45. Click the Encounter Notes tab.
46. Review the auto-populated information. Select the Yes radio button to indicate that the HIPAA form is on file for Robert Caudill and document the current date in the Dated field. Click the Save button.
47. Click the Claim Info tab.
48. Review the auto-populated information and document any additional information needed. Click the Save button.
49. Click the Charge Capture tab.
50. Document the encounter date in the DOS From and DOS To columns.
51. Document "11730" in the CPT/HCPCS column.
52. Document "11" in the POS column.
53. Document "1" in the DX column.
54. Document "115.00" in the Fee column (Figure 4-85).

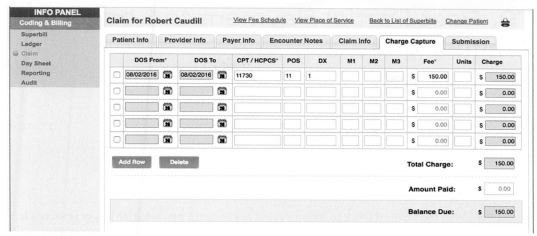

Figure 4-85 Document the necessary information in the Charge Capture tab of the claim.

55. Click the Save button.
56. Click the Submission tab. Click in the I am ready to submit the Claim box. Click the Yes radio button to indicate that there a signature on file and enter today's date in the Date field.
57. Click on the Submit Claim button.
58. Select Ledger from the left Info Panel.
59. Search for Robert Caudill using the Patient Search fields.
60. Select the radio button for Robert Caudill and click the Select button.
61. Confirm the auto-populated details in the header.
62. Click the arrow to the right of Robert Caudill's name to expand his patient ledger.
63. All charges submitted on the claim will auto-populate on the ledger. Click Add Row to enter the payment made by Robert Caudill.
64. Document the current date in the Transaction Date column using the calendar picker.
65. Document the date of service in the DOS column using the calendar picker.
66. Select Jean Burke, NP using the dropdown in the Provider field.
67. Document PTPYMTCK in the Service column.
68. Document "25.00" in the Payment column. The balance will auto-populate in the Balance column.
69. Click the Save button.
70. Select the Day Sheet from the left Info Panel.
71. Document the current date in the Date column using the calendar picker.
72. Document "Robert Caudill" in the Patient Name column.
73. Select Jean Burke, NP using the dropdown in the Provider field.
74. Document "11730" in the Service column.
75. Document "115.00" in the Charges column.
76. Document "25.00" in the Payment column.
77. Document "0.00" in the Adjustment column.
78. Document "90.00" in the New Balance column.
79. Document "0.00" in the Old Balance column.
80. Click the Save button.

✦ Now use the Back to Assignment link to complete the Post-Case Quiz found on the Info Panel for this assignment.

79. Post Partial Payment to Ledger for Amma Patel

■ Objectives

- Search for a patient record.
- Update a patient ledger.

■ Overview

Amma Patel calls the medical office to inquire about her account balance. Her ledger reflects a balance of $204.00. Amma Patel pays $50.00 over the phone with a credit card. Post the payment to the patient ledger and print a copy to send to Amma Patel.

■ Competencies

- Define basic bookkeeping terms, CAAHEP VII.C-1, ABHES 7-c
- Define Uniform Anatomical Gift Act, CAAHEP X.C-7e, ABHES 4-f
- Display professionalism through written and verbal communications, ABHES 7-g
- Display sensitivity when requesting payment for services rendered, CAAHEP VII.A-2, ABHES 5-c, 5-h, 7-c
- Explain patient financial obligations for services rendered, CAAHEP VII.C-6, ABHES 5-c, 7-c
- Identify types of information contained in the patient's billing record, CAAHEP VII.C-5, ABHES 7-b, 7-c
- Perform accounts receivable procedure to patient accounts including posting charges, payments, and adjustments, CAAHEP VII.P-1, ABHES 7-c
- Perform billing and collection procedures including accounts payable and receivable, ABHES 7-c

Estimated completion time: 15 minutes

Measurable Steps

1. Within the Coding & Billing tab, select Ledger from the left Info Panel (Figure 4-86).

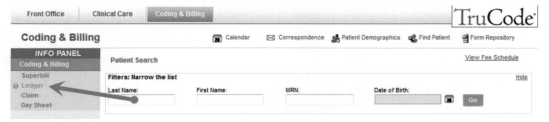

Figure 4-86 Ledger in the Info Panel.

2. Search for Amma Patel using the Patient Search fields.
3. Select the radio button for Amma Patel and click the Select button.
4. Confirm the auto-populated details in the header (Figure 4-87).
5. Click the arrow to the right of Amma Patel's name to expand her patient ledger.
6. All charges submitted on the claim will auto-populate on the ledger. Click Add Row to enter the payment made by Amma Patel.
7. Document the current date in the Transaction Date column using the calendar picker.
8. Document the date of service in the DOS column using the calendar picker.
9. Document PTPYMTCC in the Service column.
10. Document "50.00" in the Payment column.

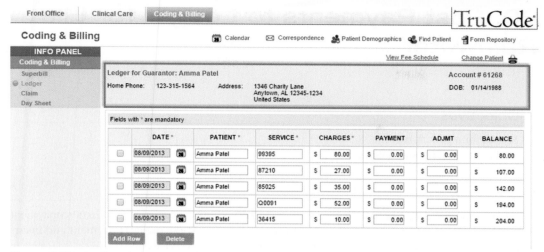

Figure 4-87 Confirm the auto-populated details in the header.

11. Click the Save button.
12. Click the Print icon in the top right corner (Figure 4-88).

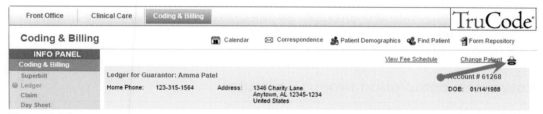

Figure 4-88 Print icon.

Now use the Back to Assignment link to complete the Post-Case Quiz found on the Info Panel for this assignment.

80. Post Payments to Ledger for Ella Rainwater

■ Objectives

- Search for a patient record.
- Post an insurance adjustment.

■ Overview

The claim submitted for Ella Rainwater was for $133.00. Ella Rainwater paid a $25.00 copayment with a check and the insurance reimbursement was $100.00. Post the patient's payment and insurance reimbursement to the patient ledger using INSPYMT as the service code.

■ Competencies

- Identify types of third party claims, information required to file a third party claim, and the steps for filing a third party claim, CAAHEP VIII.C-1, ABHES 7-d
- Perform accounts receivable procedures to patient accounts including posting charges, payments, and adjustments, CAAHEP VII.P-1, ABHES 7-c
- Perform procedural coding, CAAHEP IX.P-1, ABHES 7-d

Estimated completion time: 15 minutes

Measurable Steps

1. Within the Coding & Billing tab, select Ledger from the left Info Panel (Figure 4-89).

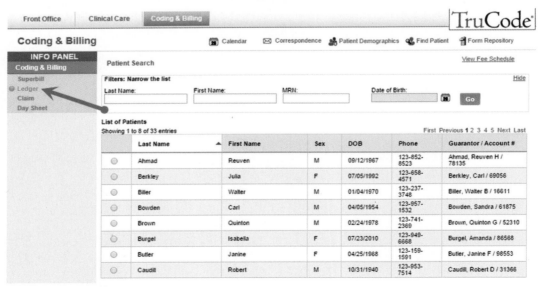

	Last Name	First Name	Sex	DOB	Phone	Guarantor / Account #
○	Ahmad	Reuven	M	09/12/1967	123-852-8523	Ahmad, Reuven H / 78135
○	Berkley	Julia	F	07/05/1992	123-658-4571	Berkley, Carl / 69056
○	Biller	Walter	M	01/04/1970	123-237-3748	Biller, Walter B / 16611
○	Bowden	Carl	M	04/05/1954	123-957-1532	Bowden, Sandra / 61875
○	Brown	Quinton	M	02/24/1978	123-741-2369	Brown, Quinton G / 52310
○	Burgel	Isabella	F	07/23/2010	123-949-6668	Burgel, Amanda / 86568
○	Butler	Janine	F	04/25/1968	123-159-1591	Butler, Janine F / 98553
○	Caudill	Robert	M	10/31/1940	123-953-7514	Caudill, Robert D / 31366

Figure 4-89 Ledger in the Info Panel.

2. Search for Ella Rainwater using the Patient Search fields.
3. Select the radio button for Ella Rainwater and click the Select button.
4. Confirm the auto-populated details in the header. Click the arrow to the right of Ella Rainwater's name to expand her patient ledger (Figure 4-90).

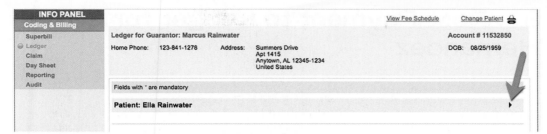

Figure 4-90 Click the arrow to the right of Ella Rainwater's name to expand her patient ledger.

5. All charges submitted on the claim will auto-populate on the ledger. Click Add Row to enter the payment made by Ella Rainwater and the reimbursement from the insurance company.
6. Document the current date in the Transaction Date column using the calendar picker.
7. Document the date of service in the DOS column using the calendar picker.
8. Select James A. Martin, MD from the Provider dropdown.
9. Document PTPYMTCK in the Service column.
10. Document "25.00" in the Payment column.
11. Click Add Row.
12. Document the current date in the Transaction Date column using the calendar picker.
13. Document the date of service in the DOS column using the calendar picker.
14. Select James A. Martin, MD from the Provider dropdown.
15. Document INSPYMT in the Service column.
16. Document "-100.00" in the Adjustment column. The balance will auto-populate in the Balance column.
17. Click the Save button.

Now use the Back to Assignment link to complete the Post-Case Quiz found on the Info Panel for this assignment.

Coding & Billing

81. Post Payment to Ledger for Casey Hernandez

Objectives

- Search for a patient record.
- Post an insurance payment.
- Post a payment.

Overview

Casey Hernandez's mother, Sofia, paid a $25.00 copayment at the time of Casey's comprehensive visit. Walden-Martin just received the $30.00 insurance payment for the service. Post the insurance payment (INSPYMT) to the ledger.

Competencies

- Discuss developmental stages of life, ABHES 5-d, 8-k
- Identify types of third party plans, information required to file a third party claim, and the steps for filing a third party claim, CAAHEP VIII.C-1, ABHES 7-d
- Perform accounts receivable procedures to patient accounts including posting charges, payments, and adjustments, CAAHEP VII.P-1, ABHES 7-c
- Post adjustments, ABHES 7-c
- Recognize barriers to communication, CAAHEP V.C-3, ABHES 5-h, 7-g, 8-j
- Utilize an EMR, CAAHEP VI.P-6, ABHES 7-b

Estimated completion time: 15 minutes

Measurable Steps

1. Within the Coding & Billing tab, select Ledger from the left Info Panel.
2. Search for Casey Hernandez using the Patient Search fields.
3. Select the radio button for Casey Hernandez and click the Select button.
4. Confirm the auto-populated details in the header (Figure 4-91).

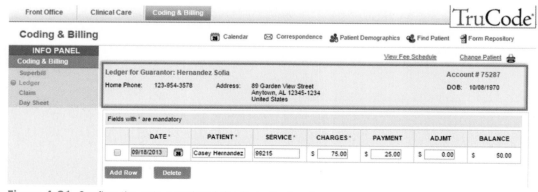

Figure 4-91 Confirm the auto-populated details in the header.

5. Click the arrow to the right of Casey Hernandez's name to expand her patient ledger.
6. All charges submitted on the claim will auto-populate on the ledger. Click Add Row to enter the payment made by the insurance company.
7. Document the current date in the Transaction Date column using the calendar picker.

8. Document the date of service in the DOS column using the calendar picker.
9. Document INSPYMT in the Service field.
10. Document "30.00" in the Payment column.
11. The balance will auto-populate in the Balance column.
12. Click the Save button.

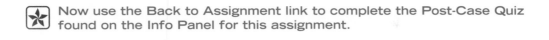 Now use the Back to Assignment link to complete the Post-Case Quiz found on the Info Panel for this assignment.

82. Post Insurance Payment and Adjustment to Ledger for Casey Hernandez

◾ Objectives

- Search for a patient record.
- Post an insurance adjustment to a ledger.
- Post an insurance payment to a ledger.

◾ Overview

Casey Hernandez's insurance company has agreed to pay $60.00 as payment for her spirometry procedure. Document an adjustment of $18.00 for the procedure. Post the insurance payment, using INSPYMT as the service code, and post the adjustment to the patient ledger.

◾ Competencies

- Identify types of third party plans, information required to file a third party claim, and the steps for filing a third party claim, CAAHEP VIII.C-1, ABHES 7-d
- Properly utilize PDR, drug handbook, and other drug reference to identify a drug's classification, usual dosage, usual side effects, and contraindications, ABHES 6-d
- Respond appropriately to patients with abnormal behavior patterns, ABHES 5-a
- Explain patient financial obligations for services rendered, CAAHEP VII.C-6
- Interpret information on an insurance card, CAAHEP VIII.P-1

Estimated completion time: 20 minutes

Measurable Steps

1. Within the Coding & Billing tab, select Ledger from the left Info Panel (Figure 4-92).

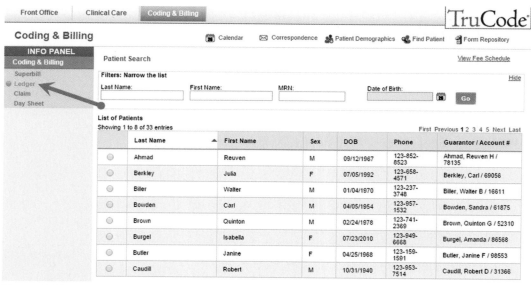

Figure 4-92 Ledger in the Info Panel.

2. Search for Casey Hernandez using the Patient Search fields.
3. Select the radio button for Casey Hernandez and click the Select button.
4. Confirm the auto-populated details in the header (Figure 4-93).

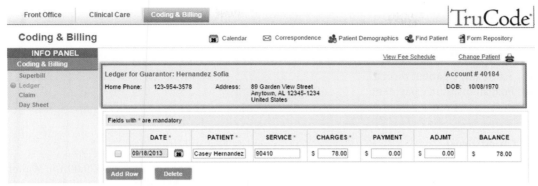

Figure 4-93 Confirm the auto-populated details in the header.

5. Click the arrow to the right of Casey Hernandez's name to expand her patient ledger.
6. All charges submitted on the claim will auto-populate on the ledger. Click Add Row to enter the payment made by the insurance company and the adjustment.
7. Select the Add Row button.
8. Document the current date in the Transaction Date column using the calendar picker.
9. Document the date of service in the DOS column using the calendar picker.
10. Document INSPYMT in the Service column.
11. Document "60.00" in the Payment column.
12. Document "-18.00" in the Adjustment column. The balance will auto-populate in the Balance column.
13. Click the Save button.

⬛ Now use the Back to Assignment link to complete the Post-Case Quiz found on the Info Panel for this assignment.

Coding & Billing

83. Post Insurance Payment and Adjustment to Ledger for Walter Biller

■ Objectives

- Search for a patient record.
- Post an insurance payment.
- Post an insurance adjustment.

■ Overview

Walter Biller's insurance company has agreed to pay $65.00 of the total fee of $79.00 for Walter Biller's visit, which included a glucometer procedure. Using INSPYMT as the service code, post the insurance payment and adjustment to the patient ledger for Walter Biller.

■ Competencies

- Define scope of practice for the medical assistant within the state that the medical assistant is employed, ABHES 4-f
- Identify types of third party plans, information required to file a third party claim, and the steps for filing a third party claim, CAAHEP VIII.C-1, ABHES 7-d
- Perform accounts receivable procedures to patient accounts including posting charges, payments, and adjustments, CAAHEP VII.P-1, ABHES 7-c
- Post adjustments, ABHES 7-c

Estimated completion time: 20 minutes

Measurable Steps

1. Within the Coding & Billing tab, select Ledger from the left Info Panel (Figure 4-94).

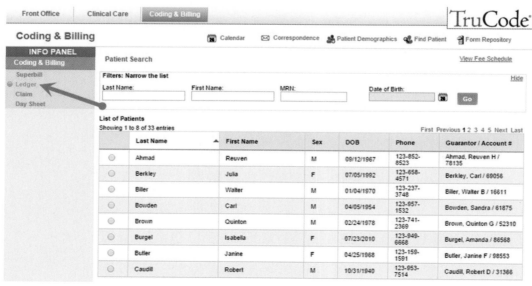

Figure 4-94 Ledger in the Info Panel.

2. Search for Walter Biller using the Patient Search fields.
3. Select the radio button for Walter Biller and click the Select button.

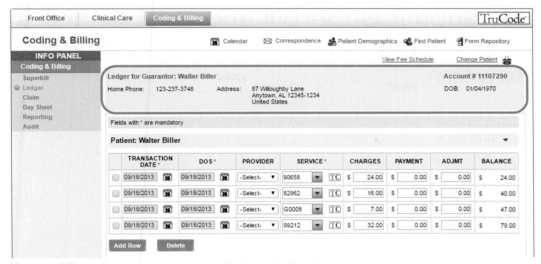

Figure 4-95 Confirm the auto-populated details in the header.

4. Confirm the auto-populated details in the header (Figure 4-95).
5. Click the arrow to the right of Walter Biller's name to expand his patient ledger.
6. All charges submitted on the claim will auto-populate on the ledger. Click Add Row to enter the payment made by the insurance company and the adjustment.
7. Document the current date in the Transaction Date column using the calendar picker.
8. Document the date of service in the DOS column using the calendar picker.
9. Document INSPYMT in the Service column.
10. Document "65.00" in the Payment column.
11. Document "-14.00" in the Adjustment column. The balance will auto-populate in the Balance column and the total will auto-populate in the Total field below the table.
12. Click the Save button.

> ★ Now use the Back to Assignment link to complete the Post-Case Quiz found on the Info Panel for this assignment.

84. Submit Superbill and Post Charges and Payments to Ledger for Carl Bowden

■ Objectives

- Search for a patient record.
- Document a patient's chief complaint.
- Complete a superbill.
- Complete a claim.
- Update a patient ledger.

■ Overview

Carl Bowden had a recent detailed visit with Dr. Walden because he was experiencing chest pain, shortness of breath, palpitations, and fatigue after his recent myocardial infarction. An ECG and lab work (CBC, CMP, and lipid panel) were obtained in the office. The ECG showed no new changes and Carl Bowden was diagnosed with unstable angina. Dr. Walden prescribed Nitroglycerin SL and referred Carl Bowden to Cardiac Rehab, with the diagnoses of unstable angina and shortness of breath. Carl Bowden received the following services: EP Detailed OV, ECG w/interpretation, CBC w/auto differential, metabolic panel comprehensive, and lipid panel. Carl Bowden paid a $25.00 copayment with a credit card at the time of the visit. Document the patient's chief complaint, complete and submit the superbill and claim, and post payments to the ledger for Carl Bowden.

■ Competencies

- Define basic bookkeeping terms, CAAHEP VII.C-1, ABHES 7-c
- Explain patient financial obligations for services rendered, CAAHEP VII.C-6, ABHES 5-c, 7-c
- Identify types of information contained in the patient's billing record, CAAHEP VII.C-5, ABHES 7-b, 7-c
- Obtain specimens and perform CLIA-waived immunology test, CAAHEP I.P-11d, ABHES 9-b
- Perform diagnostic coding, CAAHEP IX.P-2, ABHES 7-d

Estimated completion time: 50 minutes

Measurable Steps

1. Click on the Find Patient icon.
2. Using the Patient Search field, search for Carl Bowden's patient record.

 HELPFUL HINT

Confirming patient demographics helps to ensure you have located the correct patient record.

3. Verify Carl Bowden's date of birth, select the radio button for Carl Bowden, and click the select button.
4. Confirm the auto-populated details in the patient header.
5. Create a new encounter by clicking Office Visit in the left Info Panel (Figure 4-96).
6. In the Create New Encounter window, select Follow-Up/Established Visit from the Visit Type dropdown.
7. Select Julie Walden, MD from the Provider dropdown.
8. Click Save.

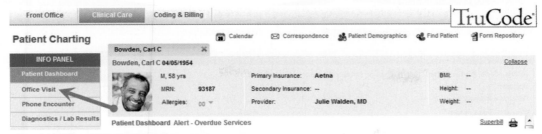

Figure 4-96 Office Visit in the Info Panel.

9. Select Chief Complaint from the dropdown menu.
10. Enter "chest pain, shortness of breath, palpitations, and fatigue" in the Chief Complaint box.
11. Click the Save button.
12. Select Patient Dashboard in the left Info Panel.
13. Click the Superbill link below the patient header.
14. Select the correct encounter from the Encounters Not Coded table and confirm the auto-populated details.
15. On page one of the superbill, select the ICD-10 radio button.
16. In the Rank 1 row of the Diagnoses box, place the cursor in the text field to access the encoder.
17. Enter "Unstable angina" in the Search field and select Diagnosis ICD-10-CM from the dropdown menu.
18. Click the Search button.
19. Click the code I20.0 to expand this code and confirm that it is the most specific code available (Figure 4-97).

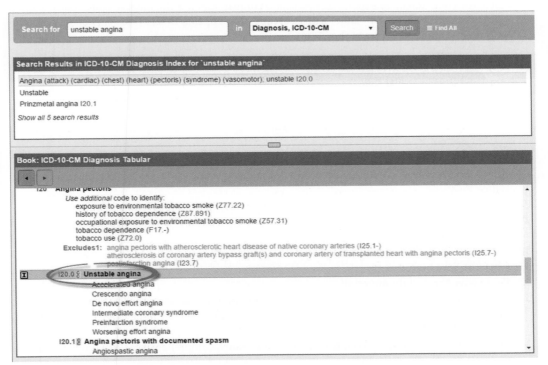

Figure 4-97 Confirm I20.0 is the most specific code available.

20. Click the code I20.0 for "Unstable angina" that appears in the tree. This code will auto-populate in the Rank 1 row of the Diagnoses box (Figure 4-98).
21. In the Rank 2 row of the Diagnoses box, place the cursor in the text field to access the encoder.
22. Enter "Shortness of breath" in the Search field and select Diagnosis ICD-10-CM from the dropdown menu.
23. Click the Search button.

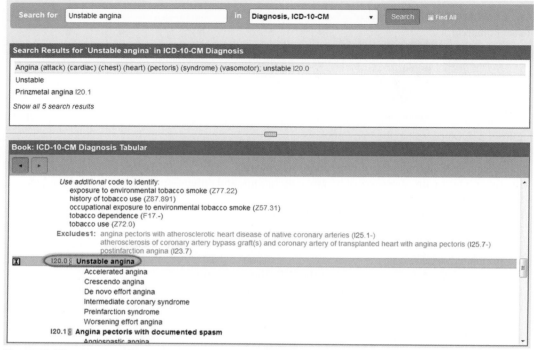

Figure 4-98 Populating the code in the Rank 1 row of the Diagnoses box.

24. Click the code R06.02 to expand this code and confirm that it is the most specific code available.
25. Click the code R06.02 for "Shortness of breath" that appears in the tree. This code will auto-populate in the Rank 2 row of the Diagnoses box.

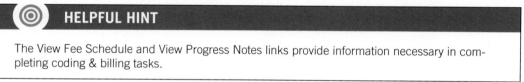

HELPFUL HINT

The View Fee Schedule and View Progress Notes links provide information necessary in completing coding & billing tasks.

26. Document "1" in the Rank column for Detailed Office Visit.
27. Select the View Fee Schedule link to obtain the charges and code for the Established Detailed Office Visit.
28. Enter "65.00" in the Fee column and "99214" in the Est column for Detailed Office Visit.
29. Document "2" in the Rank column for ECG w/ interpretation. View the Fee Schedule to obtain the charges and code.
30. Enter "89.00" in the Fee column and "93000" in the Code column for ECG, w/interpretation.
31. Click the Save button.
32. Go to page three of the superbill.
33. Document "3" in the Rank column for CBC w/ auto differential. View the Fee Schedule to obtain the charges and code. Enter "35.00" in the Fee column and "85025" in the Code column for CBC w/auto differential.
34. Document "4" in the Rank column for Metabolic panel, comprehensive. View the Fee Schedule to obtain the charge and code.
35. Enter "55.00" in the Fee column "80053" in the Code column for Metabolic panel, comprehensive.
36. Document "5" in the Rank column for Lipid panel. View the Fee Schedule to obtain the charge and code.
37. Enter "47.00" in the Fee column and "80061" in the Code column for Lipid panel.
38. Document "6" in the Rank column for Venipuncture. View the Fee Schedule to obtain the charge and code.
39. Enter "10.00" in the Fee column and "36415" in the Code column for Venipuncture.

40. Click the Save button.
41. Go to page four of the superbill.
42. Document "25.00" in the Copay field.
43. Confirm that the total in the Today's Charges field has populated correctly.
44. Document "276.00" in the Balance Due field (Figure 4-99).

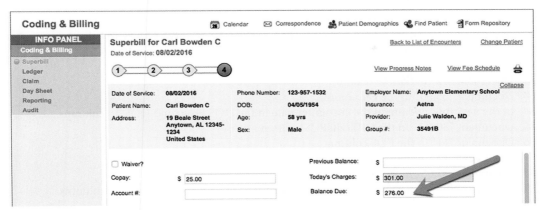

Figure 4-99 Document "276.00" in the Balance Due field.

45. Fill out any additional fields as needed.
46. Click the Save button.
47. Select the I am ready to submit the Superbill checkbox at the bottom of the screen.
48. Document the date in the Date field.
49. Click the Submit Superbill button. A confirmation message will appear.
50. Select Claim from the left Info Panel.
51. Search for Carl Bowden using the Patient Search fields.
52. Select the radio button for Carl Bowden and click the Select button.
53. Select the correct encounter and click the Edit icon in the Action column. Confirm the auto-populated details. Seven tabs appear within the claim: Patient Info, Provider Info, Payer Info, Encounter Notes, Claim Info, Charge Capture, and Submission. Certain patient demographic and encounter information is auto-populated in the claim.
54. Within the Patient Info tab, review the auto-populated information and document any additional information needed. Click the Save button.
55. Click the Provider Info tab.
56. Review the auto-populated information and document any additional information needed. Click the Save button.
57. Click the Payer Info tab.
58. Review the auto-populated information and document any additional information needed. Click the Save button.
59. Click the Encounter Notes tab.
60. Review the auto-populated information. Select the Yes radio button to indicate that the HIPAA form is on file for Carl Bowden and document the current date in the Dated field. Click the Save button.
61. Click the Claim Info tab.
62. Review the auto-populated information and document any additional information needed. Click the Save button.
63. Click the Charge Capture tab.
64. Document the encounter date in the DOS From and DOS To columns.
65. Document "99214" in the CPT/HCPCS column.
66. Document "11" in the POS column.
67. Document "12" in the DX column.
68. Document "65.00" in the Fee column.
69. In the next row, document the encounter date in the DOS From and DOS To columns.
70. Document "93000" in the CPT/HCPCS column.
71. Document "11" in the POS column.

72. Document "12" in the DX column.
73. Document "89.00" in the Fee column.
74. In the next row, document the encounter date in the DOS From and DOS To columns.
75. Document "85025" in the CPT/HCPCS column.
76. Document "11" in the POS column.
77. Document "12" in the DX column.
78. Document "35.00" in the Fee column.
79. In the next row, document the encounter date in the DOS From and DOS To columns.
80. Document "80053" in the CPT/HCPCS column.
81. Document "11" in the POS column.
82. Document "12" in the DX column.
83. Document "55.00" in the Fee column.
84. In the next row, document the encounter date in the DOS From and DOS To columns.
85. Document "80061" in the CPT/HCPCS column.
86. Document "11" in the POS column.
87. Document "12" in the DX column.
88. Document "47.00" in the Fee column.
89. In the next row, document the encounter date in the DOS From and DOS To columns.
90. Document "36415" in the CPT/HCPCS column.
91. Document "11" in the POS column.
92. Document "12" in the DX column.
93. Document "10.00" in the Fee column.
94. Click the Save button (Figure 4-100).

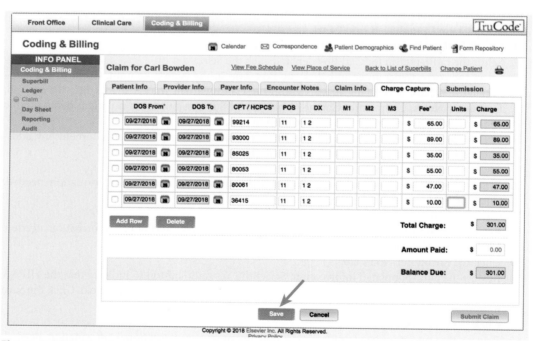

Figure 4-100 After documenting all the necessary information in the Charge Capture tab of the claim, click the Save button.

95. Click the Submission tab. Click in the I am ready to submit the Claim box. Click the Yes radio button to indicate that there a signature on file and enter today's date in the Date field.
96. Click on the Submit Claim button.

97. Select Ledger from the left Info Panel.
98. Search for Carl Bowden using the Patient Search fields.
99. Select the radio button for Carl Bowden and click the Select button.
100. Click the arrow to the right of Carl Bowden's name to expand his patient ledger.
101. All charges submitted on the claim will auto-populate on the ledger. Click Add Row to enter the payment made by Carl.
102. Document the date in the Transaction Date column using the calendar picker.
103. Document the date of service in the DOS column using the calendar picker.
104. Select Julie Walden, MD from the Provider dropdown.
105. Document PTPYMTCC in the Service column.
106. Document "25.00" in the Payment column. The balance will auto-populate in the Balance column.
107. Click the Save button.

 Now use the Back to Assignment link to complete the Post-Case Quiz found on the Info Panel for this assignment.

85. Document Progress Note, Complete Superbill, Update Ledger, and Post Payment to Day Sheet for Casey Hernandez

■ Objectives

- Search for a patient record.
- Document in the progress note.
- Complete a superbill.
- Complete a claim.
- Update a patient ledger.
- Update the day sheet.

■ Overview

Casey Hernandez is experiencing asthma symptoms, having difficulty breathing and wheezing. Her albuterol inhaler has been providing little relief. Her vital signs are T: 99.8°F, P: 96 reg, thready, R: 26, labored, O2 Sat of 91%, post nebulizer treatment O2 Sat 95%, BP 136/86 left arm, sitting. After seeing Casey (problem-focused office visit), Jean Burke, NP orders the medical assistant to administer a nebulizer treatment, which helps, and instructs Casey to return to the office as needed. Casey's mom pays a $25.00 copayment with a check. Document in the progress note, submit a superbill and claim, update the ledger, and post the charges and payment to the day sheet.

■ Competencies

- Demonstrate the principles of self-boundaries, CAAHEP V.A-2, ABHES 5-f, 10-b
- Display professionalism through written and verbal communications, ABHES 7-g
- Document patient care accurately in the medical record, CAAHEP X.P-3, ABHES 4-a
- Identify body systems, CAAHEP I.C-2, ABHES 2-a
- Perform accounts receivable procedures to patient accounts including posting charges, payments, and adjustments, CAAHEP VII.P-1, ABHES 7-c
- Perform diagnostic coding, CAAHEP IX.P-2, ABHES 7-d

Estimated completion time: 50 minutes

Measurable Steps

1. Click on the Find Patient icon.
2. Using the Patient Search fields, search for Casey's patient record. Once you locate Casey's patient record in the List of Patients, confirm her date of birth.

HELPFUL HINT

Confirming date of birth helps to ensure that you have located the correct patient record.

3. Select the radio button for Casey Hernandez and click the Select button.
4. Create a new encounter by clicking Office Visit in the left Info Panel.
5. In the Create New Encounter window, select Urgent Visit from the Visit Type dropdown.
6. Select Jean Burke, NP from the Provider dropdown.

Coding & Billing

7. Click the Save button.
8. Select Progress Notes from the Record dropdown menu.
9. Document the date using the calendar picker.
10. Document "Experiencing asthma symptoms, dyspnea, and wheezing." in the Subjective field.
11. Document "T: 99.8°F, P: 96 reg, thready, R: 26, labored, O2 Sat 91%. post nebulizer treatment O2 Sat 95%, BP: 136/86 left arm, sitting" in the Objective field.
12. Document "Asthma" in the Assessment field.
13. Document "Patient to return to office as needed" in the Plan field.
14. Click the Save button.

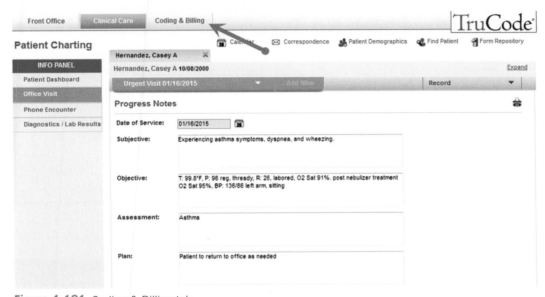

Figure 4-101 Coding & Billing tab.

15. Click the Coding & Billing tab (Figure 4-101) and select Superbill from the left Info Panel.
16. Using the Patient Search field, search for Casey's patient record.
17. Select the radio button for Casey Hernandez and click the select button.
18. Confirm the auto-populated details.
19. Select the correct encounter from the Encounters Not Coded table and confirm auto-populated details.
20. On page one of the superbill, select the ICD-10 radio button.
21. In the Rank 1 row of the Diagnoses box, place the cursor in the text field to access the encoder.
22. Enter "Asthma" in the Search field and select Diagnosis ICD-10-CM from the dropdown menu.
23. Click the Search button.
24. Click the code J45.909 to expand this code and confirm that it is the most specific code available (Figure 4-102).
25. Click the code J45.909 for "Unspecified asthma, uncomplicated" that appears in the tree. This code will auto-populate in the Rank 1 row of the Diagnoses box (Figure 4-103).

> ◎ **HELPFUL HINT**
>
> The View Fee Schedule and View Progress Notes links provide information necessary in completing coding & billing tasks.

26. Document "1" in the Rank column for problem-focused office visit.
27. Select the View Fee Schedule link to obtain the charges and code for the Established Problem-Focused Office Visit (Figure 4-104).
28. Enter "32.00" in the Fee column and "99212" in the Est column for Problem-Focused Office Visit.
29. Document "2" in the Rank column for Nebulizer. View the fee schedule to obtain the fee and code.

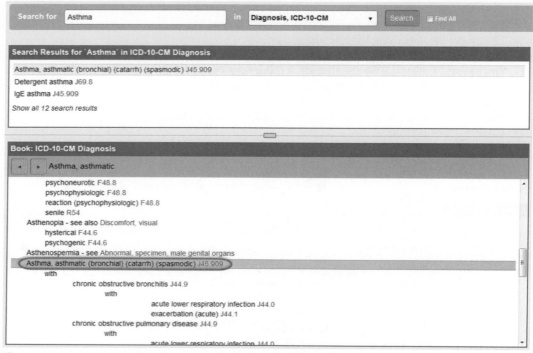

Figure 4-102 Confirm J45.909 is the most specific code available.

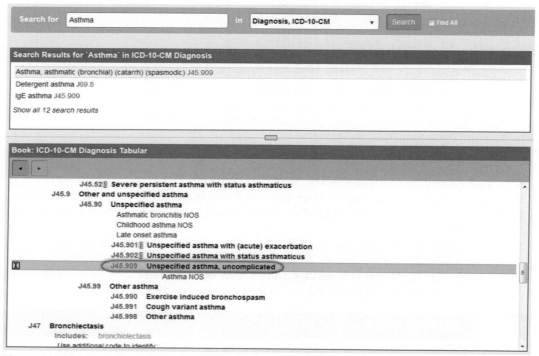

Figure 4-103 Populating the code in the Rank 1 row of the Diagnoses box.

30. Enter "49.22" in the Fee column and "94640" in the Code column for Nebulizer.
31. Click the Save button.
32. Go to page four of the superbill.
33. On page four, document "25.00" in the Copay field.
34. Confirm that the total in the Today's Charges field has populated correctly.
35. Document "56.22" in the Balance Due field.

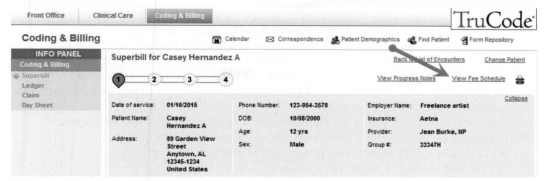

Figure 4-104 View Fee Schedule link.

36. Fill out additional fields as needed.
37. Click the Save button.
38. Select the I am ready to submit the Superbill checkbox at the bottom of the screen.
39. Select the Yes radio button to indicate that the signature is on file.
40. Document the date in the Date field.
41. Click the Submit Superbill button. A confirmation message will appear.
42. Select Claim from the left Info Panel.
43. Search for Casey Hernandez using the Patient Search fields.
44. Select the radio button for Casey Hernandez and click the Select button.
45. Select the correct encounter and click the Edit icon in the Action column. Confirm the auto-populated details. Seven tabs appear within the claim: Patient Info, Provider Info, Payer Info, Encounter Notes, Claim Info, Charge Capture, and Submission. Certain patient demographic and encounter information is auto-populated in the claim.
46. Within the Patient Info tab, review the auto-populated information and document any additional information needed. Click the Save button.
47. Click the Provider Info tab.
48. Review the auto-populated information and document any additional information needed. Click the Save button.
49. Click the Payer Info tab.
50. Review the auto-populated information and document any additional information needed. Click the Save button.
51. Click the Encounter Notes tab.
52. Review the auto-populated information. Select the Yes radio button to indicate that the HIPAA form is on file for Casey Hernandez and document the current date in the Dated field. Click the Save button.
53. Click the Claim Info tab.
54. Review the auto-populated information and document any additional information needed. Click the Save button.
55. Click the Charge Capture tab.
56. Document the encounter date in the DOS From and DOS To columns.
57. Document "99212" in the CPT/HCPCS column.
58. Document "11" in the POS column.
59. Document "1" in the DX column.
60. Document "32.00" in the Fee column.
61. In the next row, document the encounter date in the DOS From and DOS To columns.
62. Document "94640" in the CPT/HCPCS column.
63. Document "11" in the POS column.
64. Document "1" in the DX column.
65. Document "49.22" in the Fee column.
66. Click the Save button.
67. Click the Submission tab. Click in the I am ready to submit the Claim box. Click the Yes radio button to indicate that there is a signature on file and enter today's date in the Date field.
68. Click on the Submit Claim button.

69. Select Ledger from the left Info Panel.
70. Search for Casey Hernandez using the Patient Search fields.
71. Select the radio button for Casey Hernandez and click the Select button.
72. Confirm the auto-populated details in the header.
73. Click the arrow to the right of Casey Hernandez's name to expand her patient ledger.
74. All charges submitted on the claim will auto-populate on the ledger. Click Add Row to enter the payment made by Casey Hernandez.
75. Document the current date in the Transaction Date column using the calendar picker.
76. Document the date of service in the DOS column using the calendar picker.
77. Select Jean Burke, NP using the dropdown in the Provider field.
78. Document PTPYMTCK in the Service column.
79. Document "25.00" in the Payment column.
80. The balance will auto-populate in the Balance column and the total will auto-populate in the Total Ledger Balance field below the grid.
81. Click the Save button.
82. Select Day Sheet from the left Info Panel.
83. Document the current date in the Date column using the calendar picker.
84. Document "Casey Hernandez" in the Patient column.
85. Select Jean Burke, NP using the dropdown in the Provider field.
86. Document "99212" in the Service column.
87. Document "32.00" in the Charges column.
88. Document "25.00" in the Payment column.
89. Document "0.00" in the Adjustment column.
90. Document "7.00" in the New Balance column.

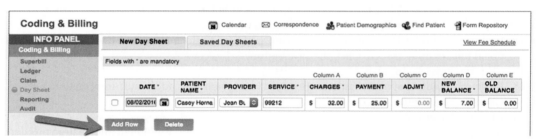

Figure 4-105 After you enter the necessary information in the first row of the Day Sheet, click the Add Row button to add another row.

91. Document "0.00" in the Old Balance column.
92. Click the Add Row button (Figure 4-105).
93. Document the current date in the Date column using the calendar picker.
94. Document "Casey Hernandez" in the Patient column.
95. Select Jean Burke, NP using the dropdown in the Provider field.
96. Document "94640" in the Service column.
97. Document "49.22" in the Charges column.
98. Document "0.00" in the Payment column.
99. Document "0.00" in the Adjustment column.
100. Document "56.22" in the New Balance column.
101. Document "7.00" in the Old Balance column.
102. Click the Save button.

Now use the Back to Assignment link to complete the Post-Case Quiz found on the Info Panel for this assignment.

86. Complete Superbill and Post Payment to Ledger for Janine Butler

■ **Objectives**

- Search for a patient record.
- Complete a superbill.
- Complete a claim.

■ **Overview**

During a routine review of medical records, the medical assistant discovers that services performed on April 2 (expanded problem-focused office visit and a rapid strep test, that was positive for strepto-coccal pharyngitis), were not billed to Janine Butler. Correct this mistake by completing and submit-ting the superbill and claim for Janine Butler.

■ **Competencies**

- Collect, label, and process specimens: Perform wound collection procedures, ABHES 9-d
- Define the principles of standard precautions, CAAHEP III.C-5, ABHES 8-a
- Identify CLIA-waived tests associated with common diseases, CAAHEP I.C-10, ABHES 9-b
- Obtain specimens and perform CLIA-waived microbiologic test, CAAHEP I.P-11e, ABHES 9-b
- Perform diagnostic coding, CAAHEP IX.P-2, ABHES 7-d
- Perform selected CLIA-waived tests that assist with diagnosis and treatment: kit testing-quick strep, ABHES 9-b
- Recognize the implications for failure to comply with Center for Disease Control (CDC) regula-tions in healthcare settings, CAAHEP III.A-1

Estimated completion time: 30 minutes

Measurable Steps

1. Click on the Find Patient icon.
2. Using the Patient Search field, search for Janine Butler's patient record.
3. Select the radio button for Janine Butler and click the select button.
4. Confirm the auto-populated details in the patient header.
5. After reviewing the encounter, click the Superbill link below the patient header (Figure 4-106).

> **HELPFUL HINT**
>
> Confirming patient demographics helps to ensure you have located the correct patient record.

6. Select the correct encounter from the Encounters Not Coded table and confirm the auto-popu-lated details.
7. On page one of the superbill, select the ICD-10 radio button.
8. In the Rank 1 row of the Diagnoses box, place the cursor in the text field to access the encoder.
9. Enter "Streptococcal pharyngitis" in the Search field and select Diagnosis ICD-10-CM from the dropdown menu.
10. Click the Search button.
11. Click the code J02.0 to expand this code and confirm that it is the most specific code available (Figure 4-107).
12. Click the code J02.0 for "Streptococcal pharyngitis" that appears in the tree. This code will auto-populate in the Rank 1 row of the Diagnoses box (Figure 4-108).

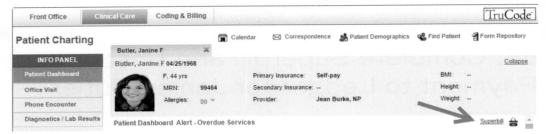

Figure 4-106 Superbill link below the patient header.

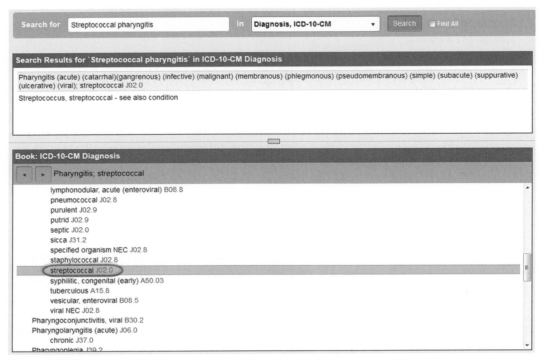

Figure 4-107 Confirm J02.0 is the most specific code available.

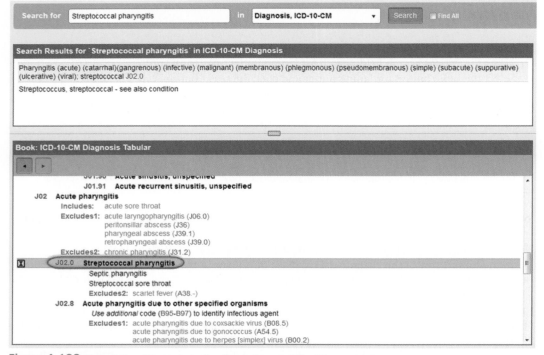

Figure 4-108 Populating the code in the Rank 1 row of the Diagnoses box.

13. Document "1" in the Rank column for the expanded problem-focused office visit.
14. Select the View Fee Schedule link to obtain the charges and code for the Established Expanded Office Visit.

◎ **HELPFUL HINT**

The View Fee Schedule and View Progress Notes links provide information necessary in completing coding & billing tasks.

15. Enter "43.00" in the Fee column and "99213" in the Est column for Expanded Problem-Focused Office Visit.
16. Click the Save button.
17. Go to page three of the superbill.
18. Document "2" in the Rank column for the Strep, rapid. View the Fee Schedule to obtain the charges and code. Enter "21.00" in the Fee column and "87880"in the Code column for Strep, rapid (Figure 4-109).

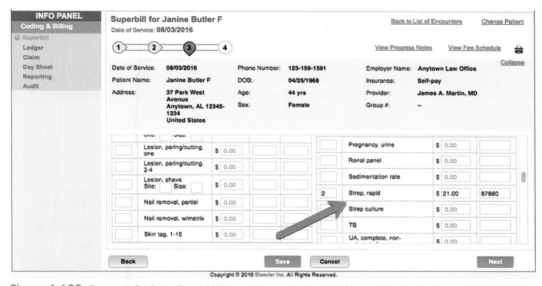

Figure 4-109 On page 3 of the Superbill, input the correct rank, fee, and code for the rapid strep test.

19. Click the Save button.
20. Go to page four of the superbill.
21. On page four, document "0.00" in the Copay field.
22. Confirm that the total in the Today's Charges field has populated correctly.
23. Document "64.00" in the Balance Due field.
24. Fill out additional fields as needed.
25. Click the Save button.
26. Select the I am ready to submit the Superbill checkbox at the bottom of the screen.
27. Select the Yes radio button to indicate that the signature is on file.
28. Document the date in the Date field.
29. Click the Submit Superbill button. A confirmation message will appear.
30. Select Claim from the left Info Panel.
31. Search for Janine Butler using the Patient Search fields.

◎ **HELPFUL HINT**

Performing a patient search before completing a form helps to ensure accurate documentation.

32. Select the radio button for Janine Butler and click the Select button.
33. Select the correct encounter and click the Edit icon in the Action column. Confirm the auto-populated details. Seven tabs appear within the claim: Patient Info, Provider Info, Payer Info,

Encounter Notes, Claim Info, Charge Capture, and Submission. Certain patient demographic and encounter information is auto-populated in the claim.

34. Within the Patient Info tab, review the auto-populated information and document any additional information needed. Click the Save button.
35. Click the Provider Info tab.
36. Review the auto-populated information and document any additional information needed. Click the Save button.
37. Click the Payer Info tab.
38. Review the auto-populated information and document any additional information needed. Click the Save button.
39. Click the Encounter Notes tab.
40. Review the auto-populated information. Select the Yes radio button to indicate that the HIPAA form is on file for Janine Butler and document the current date in the Dated field. Click the Save button.
41. Click the Claim Info tab.
42. Review the auto-populated information and document any additional information needed. Click the Save button.
43. Click the Charge Capture tab.
44. Document the encounter date in the DOS From and DOS To columns.
45. Document "99213" in the CPT/HCPCS column.
46. Document "11" in the POS column.
47. Document "1" in the DX column.
48. Document "43.00" in the Fee column.
49. In the next row, document the encounter date in the DOS From and DOS To columns.
50. Document "87880" in the CPT/HCPCS column.
51. Document "11" in the POS column.
52. Document "1" in the DX column.
53. Document "21.00" in the Fee column.
54. Click the Save button (Figure 4-110).

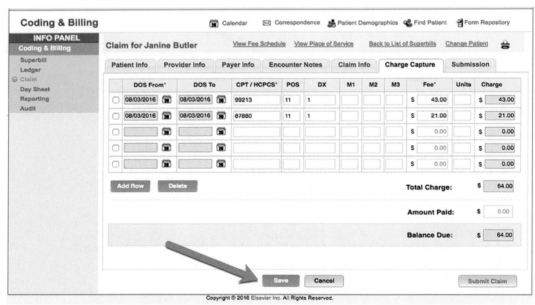

Figure 4-110 After all the necessary information is filled out in the Charge Capture tab of the claim, click the Save button.

55. Click the Submission tab. Click in the I am ready to submit the Claim box. Click the Yes radio button to indicate that there is a signature on file and enter today's date in the Date field.
56. Click on the Submit Claim button.

[*] Now use the Back to Assignment link to complete the Post-Case Quiz found on the Info Panel for this assignment.

Coding & Billing

87. Complete Claim for Diego Lupez

■ Objectives

- Search for a patient record.
- Analyze the content of a patient ledger.
- Complete a claim.

■ Overview

Diego Lupez calls Walden-Martin after hours and leaves a voicemail message stating he would like to know the balance of his anemia follow-up appointment after his deductible payment has been applied to the balance. While viewing the ledger, the medical assistant notices that Diego Lupez's total balance is greater than the charge for the anemia follow-up. Workers' Compensation paid $0.00 on Diego Lupez's visit for stepping on a nail and no claim was submitted to the health insurance carrier. Submit a claim for this visit so the health insurance carrier can consider the charges.

■ Competencies

- File patient medical records, CAAHEP VI.P-5, ABHES 7-a, 7-b

Estimated completion time: 30 minutes

Measurable Steps

1. Within the Coding & Billing tab, select Claim from the left Info Panel (Figure 4-111).

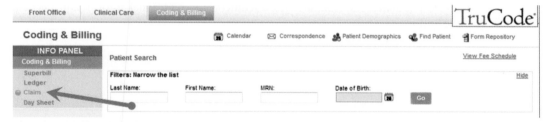

Figure 4-111 Claim in the Info Panel.

2. Perform a patient search to locate the claim for Diego Lupez.
3. Select the correct encounter and click the Edit icon in the Action column. Confirm the auto-populated details. Seven tabs appear within the claim: Patient Info, Provider Info, Payer Info, Encounter Notes, Claim Info, Charge Capture, and Submission. Certain patient demographic and encounter information is auto-populated in the claim.
4. Within the Patient Info tab, review the auto-populated information and document any additional information needed. Click the Save button.
5. Click the Provider Info tab.
6. Review the auto-populated information and document any additional information needed. Click the Save button.
7. Click the Payer Info tab.
8. Review the auto-populated information and indicate that this claim is now going to be submitted to the health insurance carrier. Click the Save button.
9. Click the Encounter Notes tab.
10. Select the Yes radio button to indicate that the HIPAA form is on file for Diego Lupez and document the current date in the Dated field (Figure 4-112).
11. Document any additional information needed and click the Save button.

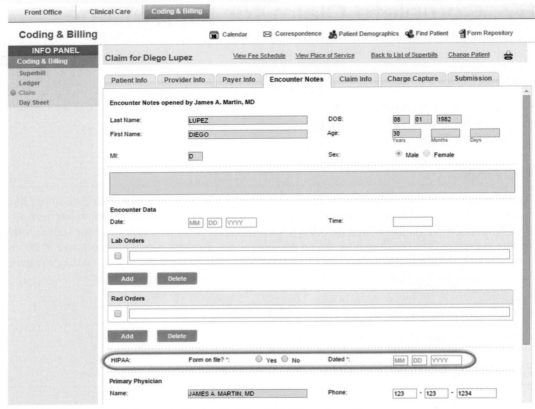

Figure 4-112 Yes radio button indicates that the HIPAA form is on file.

12. Click the Claim Info tab.
13. Review the auto-populated information and document any additional information needed. Click the Save button.
14. Click the Charge Capture tab and review all information.
15. Click the Submission Tab.
16. Select the I am ready to submit the Claim checkbox (Figure 4-113).

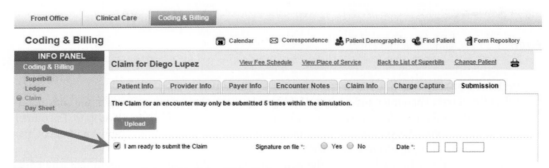

Figure 4-113 "I am ready to submit the Claim" checkbox.

17. Select the Yes radio button and document the date.
18. Click the Save button.

⭐ Now use the Back to Assignment link to complete the Post-Case Quiz found on the Info Panel for this assignment.

Coding & Billing

88. Complete Superbill, Ledger, and Claim, then Prepare Patient Statement for Ella Rainwater

■ Objectives

- Search for a patient record.
- Complete a superbill.
- Complete a claim.
- Update a patient ledger.
- Prepare a patient statement.

■ Overview

Ella Rainwater's annual wellness visit included a routine pap smear that was not billed to her or her insurance company. Ella paid her $25.00 copay with a check during the visit. Complete and submit the superbill and claim, update the ledger, and then prepare a patient statement for the missed charge.

■ Competencies

- Identify types of third party plans, information required to file a third party claim, and the steps for filing a third party claim, CAAHEP VIII.C-1, ABHES 7-d
- Inform a patient of financial obligations for services rendered, CAAHEP VII.P-4, ABHES 5-c, 5-h, 7-c
- Report relevant information concisely and accurately, CAAHEP V.P-11, ABHES 5-f, 7-g
- Perform diagnostic coding, CAAHEP IX.P-2, ABHES 7-d

Estimated completion time: 50 minutes

Measurable Steps

1. Click on the Find Patient icon.
2. Using the Patient Search field, search for Ella Rainwater's patient record.
3. Select the radio button for Ella Rainwater and click the select button.
4. Confirm the auto-populated details in the patient header.

 HELPFUL HINT

Confirming patient demographics helps to ensure you have located the correct patient record.

5. Click the Superbill link below the patient header.
6. Select the correct encounter from the Encounters Not Coded table and confirm the auto-popu-lated details.
7. On page one of the superbill, select the ICD-10 radio button.
8. In the Rank 1 row of the Diagnoses box, place the cursor in the text field to access the encoder.
9. Enter "Routine pap smear" in the Search field and select Diagnosis ICD-10-CM from the drop-down menu.
10. Click the Search button.
11. Click the code Z01.419 to expand this code and confirm that it is the most specific code available (Figure 4-114).

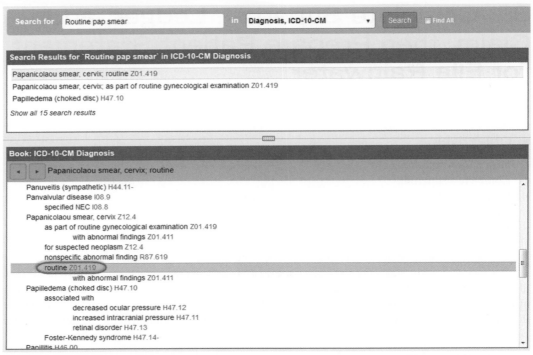

Figure 4-114 Confirm Z01.419 is the most specific code available.

12. Click the code Z01.419 for "Encounter for gynecological examination (general) (routine) without abnormal findings" that appears in the tree. This code will auto-populate in the Rank 1 row of the Diagnosis box (Figure 4-115).

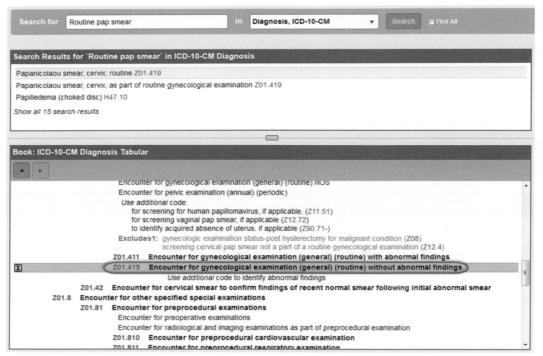

Figure 4-115 Populating the code in the Rank 1 row of the Diagnoses box.

13. Document "1" in the Rank column for Well Visit 40-64y.
14. Select the View Fee Schedule link to obtain the charges and code for the Well Visit.

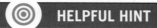
The View Fee Schedule and View Progress Notes links provide information necessary in completing coding & billing tasks.

15. Enter "105.00" in the Fee column and "99396" in the Est column for the Well Visit 40-64y.
16. Click the Save button and go to page two of the superbill.
17. Document "2" in the Rank column for Pap in Preventive Services. View the Fee Schedule to obtain the charges. Enter "52.00" in the Fee column and "Q0091" in the Code column for Pap.
18. Click the Save button.
19. Go to page four of the superbill.
20. On page four, document "25.00" in the Copay field.
21. Confirm that the total in the Today's Charges field has populated correctly.
22. Document "132.00" in the Balance Due field. Fill out additional fields as needed.
23. Click the Save button.
24. Select the I am ready to submit the Superbill checkbox at the bottom of the screen.
25. Select the Yes radio button to indicate that the signature is on file.
26. Document the date in the Date field.
27. Click the Submit Superbill button. A confirmation message will appear (Figure 4-116).

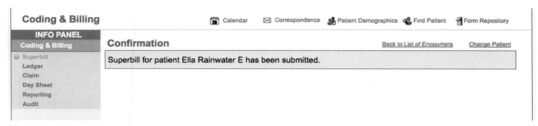

Figure 4-116 A confirmation message will appear after the Submit Superbill button is clicked.

28. Select Claim from the left Info Panel and perform a patient search to locate the claim for Ella Rainwater.
29. Select the correct encounter and click the Edit icon in the Action column. Confirm the auto-populated details. Seven tabs appear within the claim: Patient Info, Provider Info, Payer Info, Encounter Notes, Claim Info, Charge Capture, and Submission. Certain patient demographic and encounter information is auto-populated in the claim.
30. Within the Patient Info tab, review the auto-populated information and document any additional information needed. Click the Save button.
31. Click the Provider Info tab.
32. Review the auto-populated information and document any additional information needed. Click the Save button.
33. Click the Payer Info tab.
34. Review the auto-populated information and document any additional information needed. Click the Save button.
35. Click the Encounter Notes tab.
36. Review the auto-populated information and Document "Pap smear" in the Lab Orders table.
37. Select the Yes radio button to indicate that the HIPAA form is on file for Ella Rainwater and document the current date in the Dated field.
38. Document any additional information needed and click the Save button.
39. Click the Claim Info tab.
40. Review the auto-populated information and document any additional information needed. Click the Save button.
41. Click the Charge Capture tab.
42. Document the encounter date in the DOS From and DOS To columns.
43. Document "99396" in the CPT/HCPCS column.

44. Document "11" in the POS column.
45. Document "1" in the DX column.
46. Document "105.00" in the Fee column.
47. In the next row, document the encounter date in the DOS From and DOS To columns.
48. Document "Q0091" in the CPT/HCPCS column.
49. Document "11" in the POS column.
50. Document "1" in the DX column.
51. Document "52.00" in the Fee column.
52. Click the Save button.
53. Click the Submission tab. Click in the I am ready to submit the Claim box. Click on the Yes radio button to indicate that there is a signature on file and enter today's date in the Date field.
54. Click the Save button. Click the Submit Claim button.
55. Select Ledger from the left Info Panel.
56. Search for Ella Rainwater using the Patient Search fields.
57. Select the radio button for Ella Rainwater and click the Select button.
58. Confirm the auto-populated details in the header.
59. Click the arrow to the right of Ella Rainwater's name to expand her patient ledger (Figure 4-117).

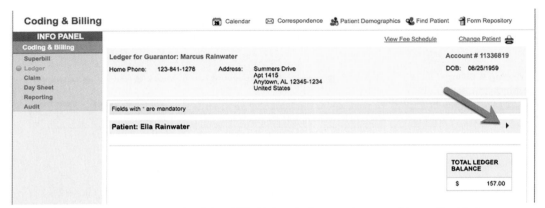

Figure 4-117 Click the arrow to the right of Ella Rainwater's name to expand her patient ledger.

60. All charges submitted on the claim will auto-populate on the ledger. Click Add Row to enter the payment made by Ella Rainwater.
61. Document the current date in the Transaction Date column using the calendar picker.
62. Document the date of service in the DOS column using the calendar picker.
63. Select James A. Martin, MD using the dropdown in the Provider field.
64. Select PTPYMTCK in the Service column.
65. Document "25.00" in the Payment column. The balance will auto-populate in the Balance column.
66. Click the Save button.
67. Click on the Form Repository icon.
68. Select Patient Statement from the Patient Forms section of the left Info Panel.
69. Click the Patient Search button to perform a patient search and assign the form to Ella Rainwater.

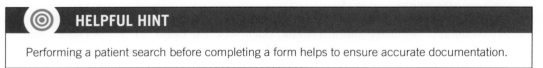

HELPFUL HINT

Performing a patient search before completing a form helps to ensure accurate documentation.

70. Document the date of service in the Date of Service field.
71. Document Routine Pap Smear in the Description field.
72. Document 157.00 in the Amount field.
73. In the next row, document the date of service in the Date of Service field.
74. Document "Patient Payment" in the description field.
75. Document "-25.00" in the Amount field.

Coding & Billing

76. Document "0.00" in the Patient's Responsibility field.
77. Document "0.00" in the Total Amount Due field.
78. Document "0.00" in the Please Pay in Full by field.
79. Click the Save to Patient Record button.
80. Select the date and click OK.
81. Click the Clinical Care tab at the top. Using the Patient Search fields, search for Ella Rainwater's patient record. Once you locate her in the List of Patients, confirm her date of birth.
82. Select the form you prepared from the Patient Dashboard. The form will open in a new window, allowing you to print.

 Now use the Back to Assignment link to complete the Post-Case Quiz found on the Info Panel for this assignment.

89. Post Insurance Payments to Ledger for Al Neviaser

■ Objectives

- Search for a patient record.
- Document insurance reimbursement.

■ Overview

The medical assistant just received Al Neviaser's explanation of benefits. The insurance reimbursement is the following:

Preventative Visit: $80.00
Influenza Vaccine: $20.00
Administration: $10.00

Post the insurance reimbursements to the ledger. The actual charges billed totaled $139.00. Therefore, document a $29.00 insurance adjustment.

■ Competencies

- Identify types of third party plans, information required to file a third party claim, and the steps for filing a third party claim, CAAHEP VIII.C-1, ABHES 7-d

Estimated completion time: 25 minutes

Measurable Steps

1. Within the Coding & Billing tab, select Ledger from the left Info Panel (Figure 4-118).

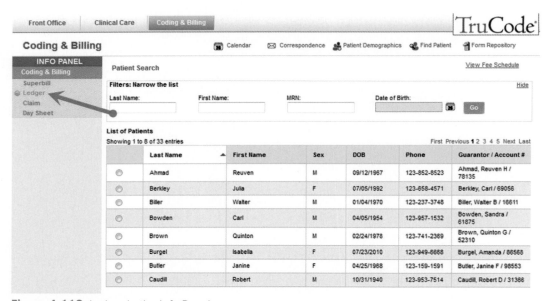

Figure 4-118 Ledger in the Info Panel.

2. Using the Patient Search fields, search for Al Neviaser's patient record.
3. Select the radio button for Al Neviaser and click the Select button.

4. Confirm the auto-populated details in the header (Figure 4-95).
5. Click the arrow to the right of Al Neviaser's name to expand his patient ledger.
6. Click the Add Row button.
7. Document the current date in the Transaction Date column using the calendar picker. Document the Date of Service in the DOS field.
8. Document "INSPYMT" in the Service column.
9. Document "110.00" in the Payment column.
10. Document "-29.00" in the Adjustment column. The balance will auto-populate in the Balance column.
11. Click the Save button (Figure 4-119).

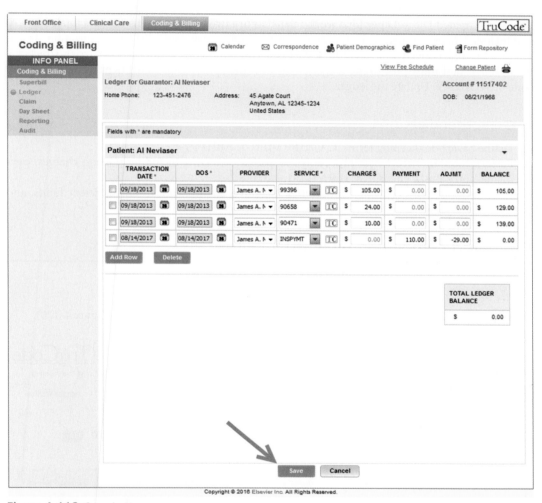

Figure 4-119 Save button.

⊕ Now use the Back to Assignment link to complete the Post-Case Quiz found on the Info Panel for this assignment.

90. Update Ledger for Diego Lupez

■ Objectives

- Search for a patient record.
- Update a patient ledger.

■ Overview

Dr. Martin treated Diego Lupez for a work-related injury two weeks ago. His services totaled $91.70 and included an established patient, problem-focused office visit, and a DTP immunization. Today, Walden-Martin received a payment of $80.00 from the Workers' Compensation carrier, which the medical assistant must post to the ledger along with the appropriate adjustment using the service code of WCPYMT. Update the ledger.

■ Competencies

- Define basic bookkeeping terms, CAAHEP VII.C-1, ABHES 7-c
- Perform accounts receivable procedures to patient accounts including posting charges, payments, and adjustments, CAAHEP VII.P-1, ABHES 7-c
- Perform billing and collection procedures including credit balance, non-sufficient funds, and refunds, ABHES 7-c

Estimated completion time: 30 minutes

Measurable Steps

1. Within the Coding & Billing module, select Ledger from the left Info Panel (Figure 4-120).

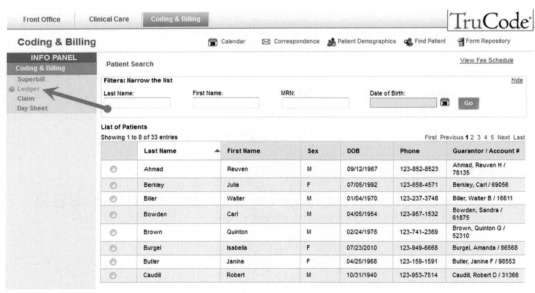

Figure 4-120 Ledger in the Info Panel.

2. Using the Patient Search field, search for Diego Lupez's patient record.
3. Select the radio button for Diego Lupez and click the Select button.
4. Confirm the auto-populated details in the header (Figure 4-121).
5. Click the arrow to the right of Diego Lupez's name to expand his patient ledger.

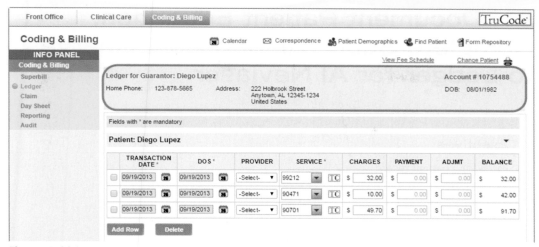

Figure 4-121 Confirm the auto-populated details in the header.

6. Select the Add Row button.
7. Document the current date in the Transaction Date column using the calendar picker.
8. Document the date of service in the DOS column using the calendar picker.
9. Select James A. Martin, MD from the Provider dropdown.
10. Document WCPYMT in the Service column.
11. Document "80.00" in the Payment column.
12. Document "-11.70" in the Adjustment column. The balance will auto-populate in the Balance column.
13. Click the Save button (Figure 4-122).

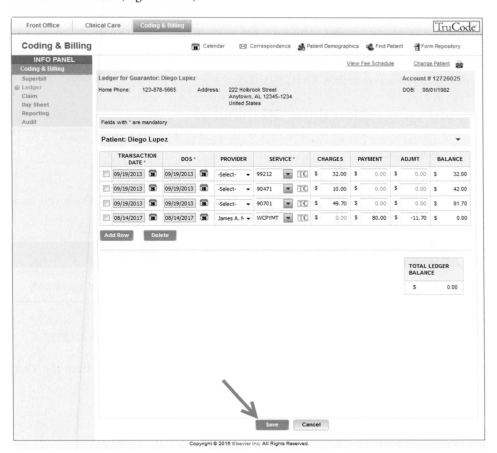

Figure 4-122 Save button.

⭐ Now use the Back to Assignment link to complete the Post-Case Quiz found on the Info Panel for this assignment.

91. Document Patient Education, Complete Superbill, and Post Charges to Ledger for Al Neviaser

■ Objectives

- Search for a patient record.
- Print a patient education handout.
- Complete a superbill.
- Complete a claim.
- Update a patient ledger.

■ Overview

Al Neviaser's recent test results show hyperlipidemia. Dr. Martin discusses Al Neviaser's risk for coronary artery disease and asks the medical assistant to print a patient education form. Al Neviaser supplies his copay of $25.00 with a check. Document the patient education, complete and submit the superbill and claim for the expanded problem-focused office visit, and post the payment to the ledger.

■ Competencies

- Explain the purpose of routine maintenance of administrative and clinical equipment, CAAHEP VI.C-9, ABHES 7-f
- Instruct and prepare a patient for a procedure or a treatment, CAAHEP I.P-8, ABHES 2-c, 8-h
- Perform diagnostic coding, CAAHEP IX.P-2, ABHES 7-d
- Use language/verbal skills that enable patients' understanding, CAAHEP V.P- 5, ABHES 5-h, 7-g
- Identify special dietary needs, CAAHEP IV.C-3

Estimated completion time: 35 minutes

Measurable Steps

1. Click on the Find Patient icon.
2. Using the Patient Search fields, search for Al Neviaser's patient record. Once you locate his patient record in the List of Patients, confirm his date of birth.

> ◎ **HELPFUL HINT**
>
> Confirming date of birth will help to ensure that you have located the correct patient record.

3. Select the radio button for Al Neviaser and click the Select button.
4. Create a new encounter by clicking Office Visit in the left Info Panel (Figure 4-123).
5. Click Add New to create a new encounter.
6. In the Create New Encounter window, select Follow-Up/Established Visit from the Visit Type dropdown.
7. Select James A. Martin, MD from the Provider dropdown.
8. Click the Save button.
9. Select Patient Education from the Record dropdown menu (Figure 4-124).
10. Select Diagnosis from the Category dropdown menu.
11. Select Cardiovascular System from the Subcategory dropdown menu.
12. Select the Coronary Artery Disease checkbox in the Teaching Topics field.

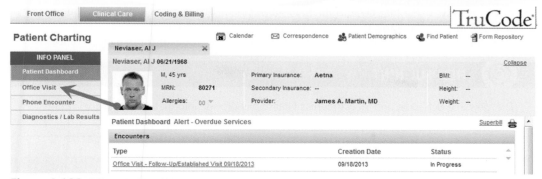

Figure 4-123 Office Visit in the Info Panel.

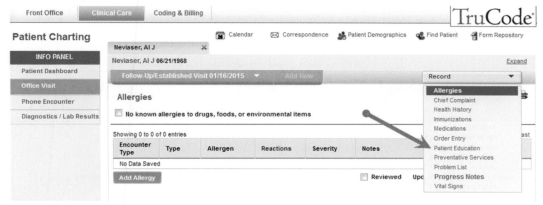

Figure 4-124 Patient Education in the Record dropdown menu.

13. Click the Save button. This teaching topic will move from the New tab to the Saved tab.
14. Expand the accordion of the saved patient education category to view and print the handout.
15. Select Patient Dashboard from the Info Panel.
16. Click the Superbill link below the patient header (Figure 4-125).

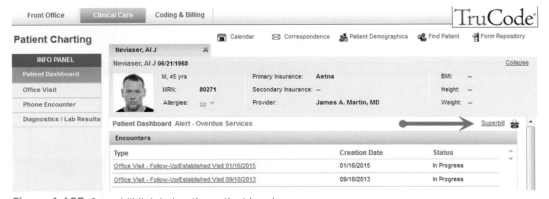

Figure 4-125 Superbill link below the patient header.

17. Select the correct encounter from the Encounters Not Coded table and confirm the auto-populated details.
18. On page one of the superbill, select the ICD-10 radio button.
19. In the Rank 1 row of the Diagnoses box, place the cursor in the text field to access the encoder.
20. Enter "Hyperlipidemia" in the Search field and select Diagnosis ICD-10-CM from the dropdown menu.
21. Click the Search button.
22. Click the code E78.5 to expand this code and confirm that it is the most specific code available (Figure 4-126).

Coding & Billing

23. Click the code E78.5 for "Hyperlipidemia, unspecified" that appears in the tree. This code will auto-populate in the Rank 1 row of the Diagnoses box (Figure 4-127).
24. Click the View Fee Schedule link to obtain the charges and code for the expanded office visit.

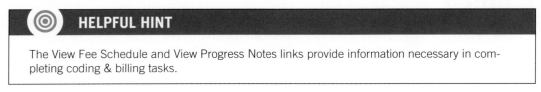

HELPFUL HINT

The View Fee Schedule and View Progress Notes links provide information necessary in completing coding & billing tasks.

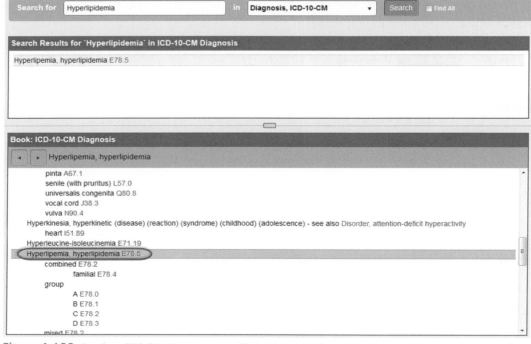

Figure 4-126 Confirm E78.5 is the most specific code available.

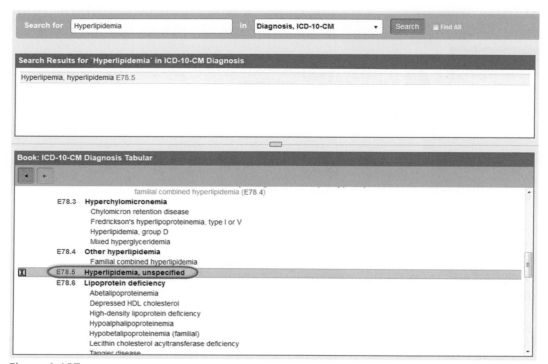

Figure 4-127 Populating the code in the Rank 1 row of the Diagnoses box.

25. Document "1" in the Rank column for Expanded problem focused office visit with the corresponding fee of "43.00" and CPT code of "99213" in the Est column.
26. Click the Save button.
27. Go to page four of the superbill.
28. On page four, document "25.00" in the Copay field.
29. Confirm that the total in the Today's Charges field has populated correctly.
30. Document "18.00" in the Balance Due field (Figure 4-128).

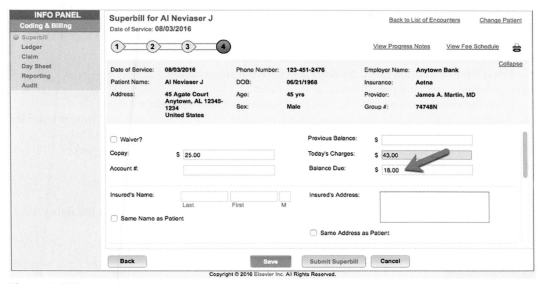

Figure 4-128 Document the Balance Due.

31. Fill out other fields as needed.
32. Click the Save button.
33. Select the I am ready to submit the Superbill checkbox at the bottom of the screen.
34. Select the Yes radio button to indicate that the signature is on file.
35. Document the date in the Date field.
36. Click the Submit Superbill button. A confirmation message will appear.
37. Select Claim from the left Info Panel and perform a patient search to locate the claim for Al Neviaser.
38. Select the correct encounter and click the Edit icon in the Action column. Confirm the auto-populated details. Seven tabs appear within the claim: Patient Info, Provider Info, Payer Info, Encounter Notes, Claim Info, Charge Capture, and Submission. Certain patient demographic and encounter information is auto-populated in the claim.
39. Within the Patient Info tab, review the auto-populated information and document any additional information needed. Click the Save button.
40. Click the Provider Info tab.
41. Review the auto-populated information and document any additional information needed. Click the Save button.
42. Click the Payer Info tab.
43. Review the auto-populated information and document any additional information needed. Click the Save button.
44. Click the Encounter Notes tab.
45. Review the auto-populated information.
46. Select the Yes radio button to indicate that the HIPAA form is on file for Al Neviaser and document the current date in the Dated field.
47. Document any additional information needed and click the Save button.
48. Click the Claim Info tab.
49. Review the auto-populated information and document any additional information needed. Click the Save button.

50. Click the Charge Capture tab.
51. Document the encounter date in the DOS From and DOS To columns.
52. Document "99213" in the CPT/HCPCS column.
53. Document "11" in the POS column.
54. Document "1" in the DX column.
55. Document "43.00" in the Fee column.
56. Click the Save button.
57. Click the Submission tab. Click in the I am ready to submit the Claim box. Click on the Yes radio button to indicate that there is a signature on file and enter today's date in the Date field.
58. Click the Save button. Click the Submit Claim button.
59. Within the Coding & Billing tab, select Ledger from the left Info Panel.
60. Search for Al Neviaser using the Patient Search fields.
61. Select the radio button for Al Neviaser and click the Select button.
62. Confirm the auto-populated details in the header.
63. Click the arrow to the right of Al Neviaser's name to expand his patient ledger.
64. All charges submitted on the claim will auto-populate on the ledger. Click Add Row to enter the payment made by Al Neviaser.
65. Document the current date in the Transaction Date column using the calendar picker.
66. Document the date of service in the DOS column using the calendar picker.
67. Select James A. Martin, MD using the dropdown in the Provider field.
68. Select PTPYMTCK using the dropdown in the Service column.
69. Document "25.00" in the Payment column. The balance will auto-populate in the Balance column (Figure 4-129).
70. Click the Save button.

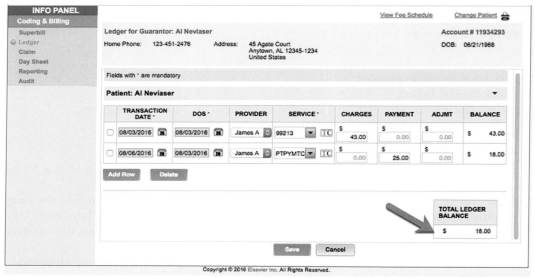

Figure 4-129 The balance will auto-populate in the Balance column.

Now use the Back to Assignment link to complete the Post-Case Quiz found on the Info Panel for this assignment.

92. Prepare Patient Statement for Janine Butler

■ Objectives

- Search for a patient record.
- Create a patient statement.

■ Overview

During a routine review of medical records, the medical assistant discovers charges that were not billed to Janine Butler for a visit (established problem-focused office visit - $32.00) addressing strep throat (strep, rapid - $21.00) on December 16. Correct this error and prepare a patient statement to send to Janine Butler.

■ Competencies

- Define basic bookkeeping terms, CAAHEP VII.C-1, ABHES 7-c
- Explain patient financial obligations for services rendered, CAAHEP VII.C-6, ABHES 5-c, 7-c
- Inform a patient of financial obligations for services rendered, CAAHEP VII.P-4, ABHES 5-c, 5-h, 7-c

Estimated completion time: 30 minutes

Measurable Steps

1. Click on the Form Repository icon.
2. Select Patient Statement from the Patient Forms section of the left Info Panel.
3. Click the Patient Search button to perform a patient search and assign the form to Janine Butler.

 HELPFUL HINT

Performing a patient search before completing a form helps to ensure accurate documentation.

4. Select the radio button for Janine Butler and click the Select button. Confirm the auto-populated details.
5. Document the date of service in the Date of Service field.
6. Document "Office Visit" in the Description field.
7. Document "32.00" in the Amount field.
8. Document "32.00" in the Patient's Responsibility field.
9. Document the date of service in the Date of Service column.
10. Document "Rapid strep test" in the Description column.
11. Document "21.00" in the Amount column.
12. Document "21.00" in the Patient's Responsibility column.
13. Document "53.00" in the Total Amount Due field.
14. Click the Save to Patient Record button.
15. Confirm the date and click OK.
16. Click on the Find Patient icon.
17. Using the Patient Search fields, search for Janine Butler's patient record. Once you locate her in the List of Patients, confirm her date of birth.
18. Select the form you prepared from the Forms section of the Patient Dashboard. The form will open in a new window, allowing you to print (Figure 4-130).

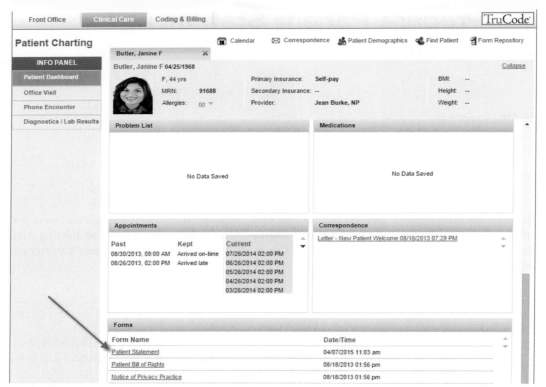

Figure 4-130 Select the form you prepared.

⬚ Now use the Back to Assignment link to complete the Post-Case Quiz found on the Info Panel for this assignment.

93. Document Progress Note and Submit Superbill for Diego Lupez

■ Objectives

- Search for a patient record.
- Document in the progress note.
- Complete a superbill.

■ Overview

Diego Lupez is seeing Dr. Martin for a follow-up for his anemia. He is feeling better since starting B12 injections and monitoring his diet. His vitals are T: 97.4°F (Tym), P: 66 reg, thready, R: 12 reg, shallow, BP: 126/72 sitting, left arm. His hemoglobin is 11.6 g/dL, hematocrit 34.8%, RBC 4.7 million/mm3, WBC 7,200/mm3, Platelets 346,000/mm3. Dr. Martin's diagnosis is pernicious anemia and the plan is to continue current therapy and return to the clinic in six months. Diego Lupez pays a $25.00 copayment with a credit card. Document in the progress note and submit a superbill for the problem-focused office visit and CBC with auto differential.

■ Competencies

- Define basic bookkeeping terms, CAAHEP VII.C-1, ABHES 7-c
- Define the principles of standard precautions, CAAHEP III.C-5, ABHES 8-a
- Perform diagnostic coding, CAAHEP IX.P-2, ABHES 7-d
- Perform venipuncture, CAAHEP I.P-2b, ABHES 9-d

Estimated completion time: 35 minutes

Measurable Steps

1. Click on the Find Patient icon.
2. Using the Patient Search fields, search for Diego Lupez's patient record. Once you locate his patient record in the List of Patients, confirm his date of birth.

 HELPFUL HINT

Confirming date of birth will help to ensure that you have located the correct patient record.

3. Select the radio button for Diego Lupez and click the Select button.
4. Create a new encounter by clicking Office Visit in the left Info Panel.
5. In the Create New Encounter window, select Follow-Up/Established Visit from the Visit Type dropdown.
6. Select James A. Martin, MD in the Provider dropdown.
7. Click the Save button.
8. Select Progress Notes from the Record dropdown menu.
9. Document the date using the calendar picker.
10. Document "Anemia follow-up, patient feeling better taking B12 injections and following prescribed diet" in the Subjective field.
11. Document "T:97.4°F (Tym), P: 66 reg, thready, R: 12 reg, shallow, BP: 126/72 sitting, left arm, Hematocrit 34.8%, RBC 4.7 T/L, WBC 7,200/mm3, Platelets 346,000/mm3" in the Objective field.
12. Document "Pernicious anemia" in the Assessment field.

13. Document "Continue current therapy and return to clinic in six months" in the Plan field.
14. Click the Save button (Figure 4-131).
15. After reviewing the encounter, select Patient Dashboard in the Info Panel and then click the Superbill link below the patient header.

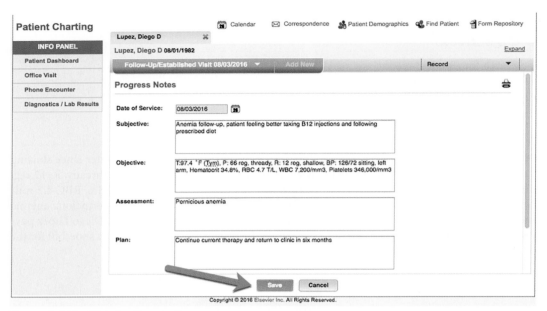

Patient Charting

Calendar   Correspondence   Patient Demographics   Find Patient   Form Repository

Lupez, Diego D

INFO PANEL

Lupez, Diego D 08/01/1982   Expand

Patient Dashboard

Office Visit   Follow-Up/Established Visit 08/03/2016 ▼   Add New   Record   ▼

Phone Encounter   **Progress Notes**

Diagnostics / Lab Results

Date of Service: 08/03/2016

Subjective: Anemia follow-up, patient feeling better taking B12 injections and following prescribed diet

Objective: T:97.4 °F (Tym), P: 66 reg, thready, R: 12 reg, shallow, BP: 126/72 sitting, left arm, Hematocrit 34.8%, RBC 4.7 T/L, WBC 7,200/mm3, Platelets 346,000/mm3

Assessment: Pernicious anemia

Plan: Continue current therapy and return to clinic in six months

Save   Cancel

Copyright © 2016 Elsevier Inc. All Rights Reserved.

Figure 4-131 Click the Save button.

16. Select the correct encounter from the Encounters Not Coded table and confirm the auto-populated details.
17. On page one of the superbill, select the ICD-10 radio button.
18. In the Rank 1 row of the Diagnoses box, place the cursor in the text field to access the encoder.
19. Enter "Pernicious Anemia" in the Search field and select Diagnosis ICD-10-CM from the drop-down menu.
20. Click the Search button.
21. Click the code D51.0 to expand this code and confirm that it is the most specific code available (Figure 4-132).
22. Click the code D51.0 for "Vitamin B12 deficiency anemia due to intrinsic factor deficiency" that appears in the tree. This code will auto-populate in the Rank 1 row of the Diagnoses box (Figure 4-133).
23. Click the View Fee Schedule link to obtain the charges for the Problem-Focused office visit.

◎ **HELPFUL HINT**

The View Fee Schedule and View Progress Notes links provide information necessary in completing coding & billing tasks.

24. Document "1" in the Rank column for Problem-focused Office Visit with the corresponding fee of "32.00" and the CPT code "99212" in the Est column.
25. Click the Save button.
26. Go to page three of the superbill.
27. On page three of the superbill, document "2" in the Rank column for Venipuncture. View the Fee Schedule to obtain the charges and code.
28. Enter "10.00" in the Fee column and "36415" in the Code column for Venipuncture.
29. Document "3" in the Rank column for CBC, w/o auto differential. View the Fee Schedule to obtain the charges and code.
30. Enter "25.00" in the Fee column and "85027" in the Code column for CBC, w/o auto differential.

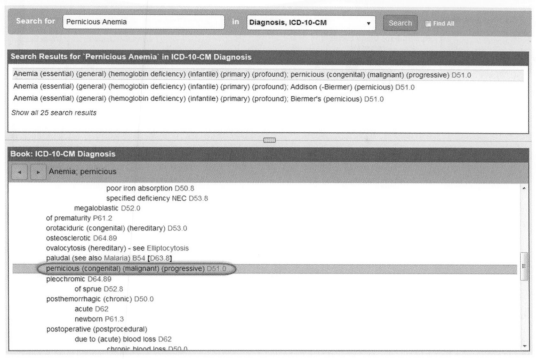

Figure 4-132 Confirm D51.0 is the most specific code available.

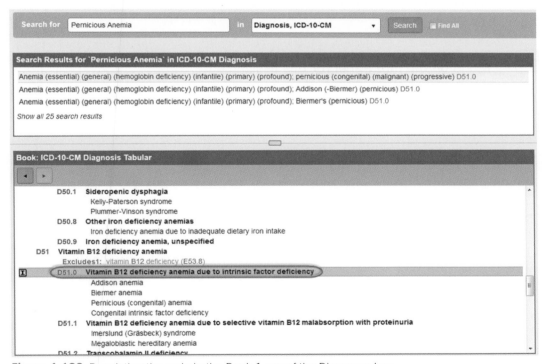

Figure 4-133 Populating the code in the Rank 1 row of the Diagnoses box.

31. Click the Save button and then go to page four of the superbill (Figure 4-134).
32. On page four, document "25.00" in the Copay field.

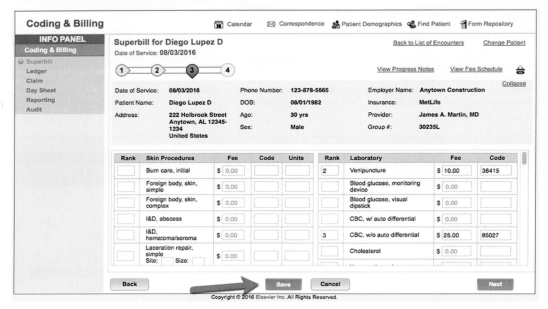

Figure 4-134 Click the Save button and then go to page four of the superbill.

33. Confirm that the total in the Today's Charges field has populated correctly.
34. Document "42.00" in the Balance Due field.
35. Fill out additional fields as needed.
36. Click the Save button.
37. Select the I am ready to submit the Superbill checkbox at the bottom of the screen.
38. Select the Yes radio button to indicate that the signature is on file.
39. Document the date in the Date field.
40. Click the Submit Superbill button. A confirmation message will appear.

 Now use the Back to Assignment link to complete the Post-Case Quiz found on the Info Panel for this assignment.

Coding & Billing

94. Document Progress Note, Complete Superbill and Ledger for Ella Rainwater, then Post Services on Day Sheet

■ Objectives

- Search for a patient record.
- Document in the patient progress note.
- Complete a superbill.
- Complete a claim.
- Update a patient ledger.
- Update the day sheet.

■ Overview

Ella Rainwater has a history of hypertension and is seeing Dr. Martin for a blood pressure check and states that she has been feeling "just fine" since her last visit. Her vitals are T: 98.2°F (Tym), P: 94 reg, strong, R: 24 reg, normal, BP: 146/92 sitting, left arm. Dr. Martin prescribes Norvasc 5 mg PO qd for Ella Rainwater and orders her to return in two weeks to recheck her blood pressure. Ella submitted her copayment of $25.00 with a credit card during the visit. Document this visit in the progress note, complete and submit the superbill and claim, and post visit charges to the ledger and day sheet for a problem-focused office visit for this established patient.

■ Competencies

- Define and use medical abbreviations when appropriate and acceptable, ABHES 3-d
- Describe types of adjustments made to patient accounts, CAAHEP VII.C-4, ABHES 7-c
- Perform diagnostic coding, CAAHEP IX.P-2, ABHES 7-d
- Properly utilize PDR, drug handbook, and other drug reference to identify a drug's classification, usual dosage, usual side effects, and contraindications, ABHES 6-d

Estimated completion time: 35 minutes

Measurable Steps

1. Click on the Find Patient icon.
2. Using the Patient Search fields, search for Ella Rainwater's patient record. Once you locate her patient record in the List of Patients, confirm her date of birth.

 HELPFUL HINT

Confirming date of birth helps to ensure that you have located the correct patient record.

3. Select the radio button for Ella Rainwater and click the Select button.
4. Create a new encounter by clicking Office Visit in the left Info Panel (Figure 4-135).
5. In the Create New Encounter window, select Follow-Up/Established Visit from the Visit Type dropdown.
6. Select James A. Martin, MD from the Provider dropdown.
7. Click the Save button.
8. Select Progress Notes from the Record dropdown menu.

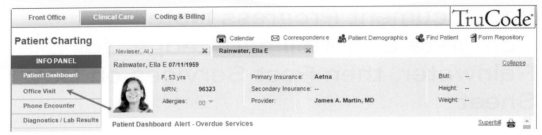

Figure 4-135 Office Visit in the Info Panel.

9. Document the date using the calendar picker.
10. Document "Patient states that she has been feeling "just fine" since her last visit" in the Subjective field.
11. Document "VS: T: 98.2°F, P: 94, reg, strong R: 24, reg, normal BP:146/92 left arm" in the Objective field.
12. Document "Benign hypertension" in the Assessment field.
13. Document "Norvasc 5 mg PO qd. Patient to return in 2 weeks for recheck of BP" in the Plan field.
14. Click the Save button.
15. After reviewing the encounter, select Patient Dashboard from the Info Panel.
16. Click the Superbill link below the patient header.
17. Select the correct encounter from the Encounters Not Coded table and confirm the auto-populated details.

> ◎ **HELPFUL HINT**
>
> The View Fee Schedule and View Progress Notes links provide information necessary in completing coding & billing tasks.

18. On page one of the superbill, select the ICD-10 radio button.
19. In the Rank 1 row of the Diagnoses box, place the cursor in the text field to access the encoder.
20. Enter "Hypertension" in the Search field and select Diagnosis ICD-10-CM from the dropdown menu.
21. Click the Search button.
22. Click the code I10 to expand this code and confirm that it is the most specific code available (Figure 4-136).
23. Click the code I10 for "Essential (primary) hypertension" that appears in the tree. This code will auto-populate in the Rank 1 row of the Diagnoses box (Figure 4-137).
24. Document "1" in the Rank column for problem focused office visit. Click the View Fee Schedule link to obtain the charges and code for the Problem focused office visit.
25. Enter "32.00" in the Fee column and "99212" in the Est column for Problem focused office visit.
26. Click the Save button (Figure 4-138).
27. Go to page four of the superbill.
28. On page four, document "25.00" in the Copay field.
29. Confirm that the total in the Today's Charges field has populated correctly.
30. Document "7.00" in the Balance Due field.
31. Fill out additional fields as needed.
32. Click the Save button.
33. Select the I am ready to submit the Superbill checkbox at the bottom of the screen.
34. Select the Yes radio button to indicate that the signature is on file.
35. Document the date in the Date field.
36. Click the Submit Superbill button. A confirmation message will appear.
37. Select Claim from the left Info Panel and perform a patient search to locate the claim for Ella Rainwater.
38. Select the correct encounter and click the Edit icon in the Action column. Confirm the auto-populated details. Seven tabs appear within the claim: Patient Info, Provider Info, Payer Info, Encounter Notes, Claim Info, Charge Capture, and Submission. Certain patient demographic and encounter information is auto-populated in the claim.

Coding & Billing

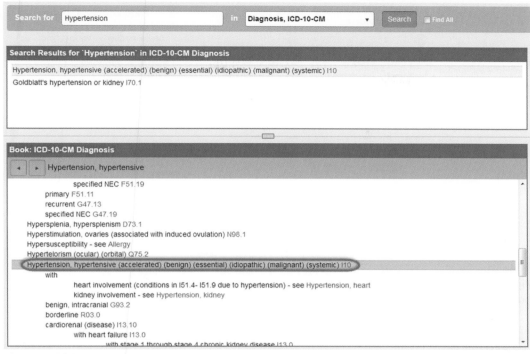

Figure 4-136 Confirm I10 is the most specific code available.

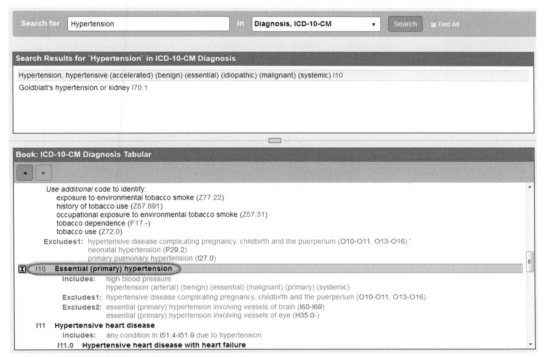

Figure 4-137 Populating the code in the Rank 1 row of the Diagnoses box.

39. Within the Patient Info tab, review the auto-populated information and document any additional information needed. Click the Save button.
40. Click the Provider Info tab.
41. Review the auto-populated information and document any additional information needed. Click the Save button.
42. Click the Payer Info tab.

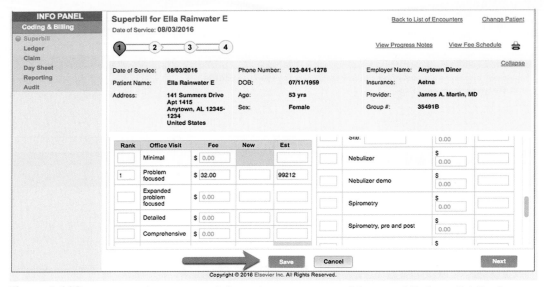

Figure 4-138 Document the necessary information on page one of the superbill, then click the Save button.

43. Review the auto-populated information and document any additional information needed. Click the Save button.
44. Click the Encounter Notes tab.
45. Review the auto-populated information.
46. Select the Yes radio button to indicate that the HIPAA form is on file for Ella Rainwater and document the current date in the Dated field (Figure 4-139).

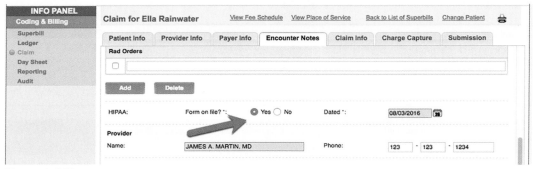

Figure 4-139 Select the Yes radio button and document the current date in the Dated field.

47. Document any additional information needed and click the Save button.
48. Click the Claim Info tab.
49. Review the auto-populated information and document any additional information needed. Click the Save button.
50. Click the Charge Capture tab.
51. Document the encounter date in the DOS From and DOS To columns.
52. Document "99212" in the CPT/HCPCS column.
53. Document "11" in the POS column.
54. Document "1" in the DX column.
55. Document "32.00" in the Fee column.
56. Click the Save button.
57. Click the Submission tab. Click in the I am ready to submit the Claim box. Click the Yes radio button to indicate that there is a signature on file and enter today's date in the Date field.
58. Click the Save button. Click the Submit Claim button.
59. Within the Coding & Billing tab, select Ledger from the left Info Panel.
60. Search for Ella Rainwater using the Patient Search fields.

61. Select the radio button for Ella Rainwater and click the Select button.
62. Confirm the auto-populated details in the header.
63. Click the arrow to the right of Ella Rainwater's name to expand her patient ledger.
64. All charges submitted on the claim will auto-populate on the ledger. Click Add Row to enter the payment made by Ella Rainwater.
65. Document the current date in the Transaction Date column using the calendar picker.
66. Document the date of service in the DOS column using the calendar picker.
67. Select James A. Martin, MD using the dropdown in the Provider field.
68. Select PTPYMTCC using the dropdown in the Service column.
69. Document "25.00" in the Payment column. The balance will auto-populate in the Balance column.
70. Click the Save button.
71. Select Day Sheet from the left Info Panel.
72. Document the current date in the Date column using the calendar picker.
73. Document "Ella Rainwater" in the Patient column.
74. Select James A. Martin, MD from the Provider dropdown.
75. Document "99212" in the Service column.
76. Document "32.00" in the Charges column.
77. Document "25.00" in the Payment column.
78. Document "0.00" in the Adjustment column.
79. Document "7.00" in the New Balance column.
80. Document "0.00" in the Old Balance column.
81. Click the Save button.

Now use the Back to Assignment link to complete the Post-Case Quiz found on the Info Panel for this assignment.

95. Document Progress Note, Submit Superbill, and Post Charges to Ledger for Robert Caudill

■ Objectives

- Search for a patient record.
- Document in the progress note.
- Use a fee schedule.
- Complete a superbill.
- Complete a claim.
- Update a patient ledger.

■ Overview

Robert Caudill has a history of diabetes mellitus type 2 and complains of dizziness, blurred vision, and mild confusion. Jean Burke, NP notices that Robert Caudill's skin is cool and clammy during the acute care visit. Robert Caudill's pulse is 116 and his BP is 90/58. Jean Burke, NP orders a blood glucose finger stick and the results are 42. Jean Burke, NP diagnoses Robert Caudill with hypoglycemia and gives him a glucose tablet with a glass of orange juice. She then performs a repeat blood glucose finger stick and the results are 90. She lowers the dosage of Robert Caudill's glimepiride from 4 mg per day to 2 mg per day. She also instructs Robert Caudill to track his morning blood sugars for two weeks and call Walden-Martin at the end of each week to report his readings. Robert Caudill pays his $25.00 copay with a credit card during the visit. Document in the progress note, complete and submit the superbill and claim for the expanded problem-focused office, and two blood glucose levels, and post payment to the ledger for Robert Caudill.

■ Competencies

- Assist provider with a patient exam, CAAHEP I.P-9, ABHES 8-c, 8-d
- Describe how to use the most current procedural coding system, CAAHEP IX.C-1, ABHES 7-d
- Measure and record vital signs, CAAHEP I.P-1, ABHES 4-a, 8-b
- Perform diagnostic coding, CAAHEP IX.P-2, ABHES 7-d

Estimated completion time: 35 minutes

Measurable Steps

1. Click on the Find Patient icon.
2. Using the Patient Search fields, search for Robert Caudill's patient record. Once you locate his patient record in the List of Patients, confirm his date of birth.

 HELPFUL HINT

Confirming date of birth will help to ensure that you have located the correct patient record.

3. Select the radio button for Robert Caudill and click the Select button.
4. Create a new encounter by clicking Office Visit in the left Info Panel (Figure 4-140).
5. In the Create New Encounter window, select Follow-Up/Established Visit from the Visit Type dropdown.
6. Select Jean Burke, NP from the Provider dropdown.

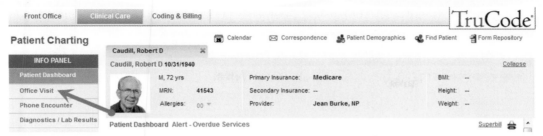

Figure 4-140 Office Visit in the Info Panel.

7. Click the Save button.
8. Select Progress Notes from the Record dropdown menu (Figure 4-141).

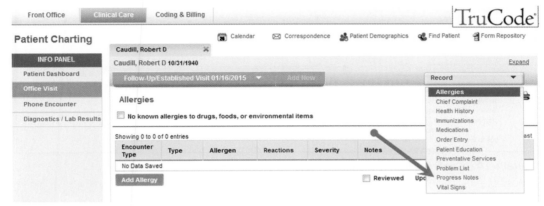

Figure 4-141 Progress Notes from the Record dropdown menu.

9. Document the date using the calendar picker.
10. Document "Patient complains of dizziness, blurred vision, and mild confusion" in the Subjective field.
11. Document "Skin is cool and clammy, P 116, BP 90/58, blood glucose 42 mg/dL" in the Objective field.
12. Document "Hypoglycemia" in the Assessment field.
13. Document "Patient to decrease glimepiride to 2 mg per day, track morning blood sugars for two weeks and report the results after the first week and again after the second week, refer to diabetic education classes" in the Plan field.
14. Click the Save button.
15. After reviewing the encounter, select Patient Dashboard from the Info Panel.
16. Click the Superbill link below the patient header.
17. Select the correct encounter from the Encounters Not Coded table and confirm the auto-populated details.

◎ **HELPFUL HINT**

The View Fee Schedule and View Progress Notes links provide information necessary in completing coding & billing tasks.

---

18. On page one of the superbill, select the ICD-10 radio button.
19. In the Rank 1 row of the Diagnoses box, place the cursor in the text field to access the encoder.
20. Enter "Hypoglycemia" in the Search field and select Diagnosis ICD-10-CM from the dropdown menu.
21. Click the Search button.
22. Click the code E16.2 to expand this code and confirm that it is the most specific code available (Figure 4-142).
23. Click the code E16.2 for "hypoglycemia, unspecified" that appears in the tree. This code will auto-populate in the Rank 1 row of the Diagnoses box (Figure 4-143).

Coding & Billing

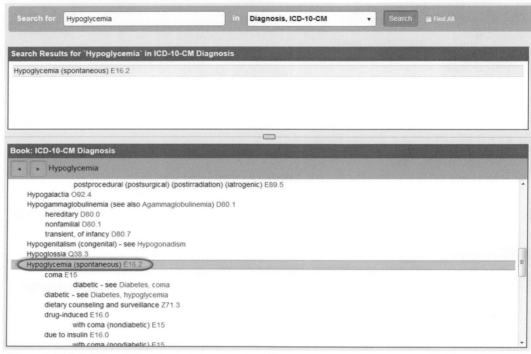

Figure 4-142 Confirm E16.2 is the most specific code available.

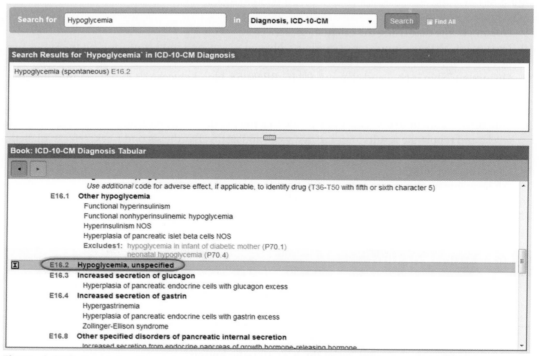

Figure 4-143 Populating the code in the Rank 1 row of the Diagnoses box.

24. Click the View Fee Schedule link to obtain the charges for the Expanded Office Visit.
25. Document "1" in the Rank column for Expanded Problem-Focused Office Visit with the corresponding fee of 43.00 and CPT code of 99213.
26. Click the Save button.
27. Go to page three of the superbill.

28. Document "2" in the Rank column for Blood glucose, monitoring device. View the Fee Schedule to obtain the charges and code.
29. Enter "32.00" in the Fee column and "82962" in the Code column for Blood glucose, monitoring device.
30. Click the Save button.
31. Go to page four of the superbill.
32. On page four, document "25.00" in the Copay field.
33. Confirm that the total in the Today's Charges field has populated correctly.
34. Document "50.00" in the Balance Due field.
35. Fill out additional fields as needed.
36. Click the Save button.
37. Select the I am ready to submit the Superbill checkbox at the bottom of the screen.
38. Select the Yes radio button to indicate that the signature is on file.
39. Document the date in the Date field.
40. Click the Submit Superbill button. A confirmation message will appear.
41. Select Claim from the left Info Panel and perform a patient search to locate the claim for Robert Caudill.
42. Select the correct encounter and click the Edit icon in the Action column. Confirm the auto-populated details. Seven tabs appear within the claim: Patient Info, Provider Info, Payer Info, Encounter Notes, Claim Info, Charge Capture, and Submission. Certain patient demographic and encounter information is auto-populated in the claim.
43. Within the Patient Info tab, review the auto-populated information and document any additional information needed. Click the Save button.
44. Click the Provider Info tab.
45. Review the auto-populated information and document any additional information needed. Click the Save button.
46. Click the Payer Info tab.
47. Review the auto-populated information and document any additional information needed. Click the Save button.
48. Click the Encounter Notes tab.
49. Review the auto-populated information.
50. Select the Yes radio button to indicate that the HIPAA form is on file for Robert Caudill and document the current date in the Dated field.
51. Document any additional information needed and click the Save button.
52. Click the Claim Info tab.
53. Review the auto-populated information and document any additional information needed. Click the Save button.
54. Click the Charge Capture tab.
55. Document the encounter date in the DOS From and DOS To columns.
56. Document "99213" in the CPT/HCPCS column.
57. Document "11" in the POS column.
58. Document "1" in the DX column.
59. Document "43.00" in the Fee column.
60. Click the Save button.
61. In the next row, document the encounter date in the DOS From and DOS To columns.
62. Document "82962" in the CPT/HCPCS column.
63. Document "11" in the POS column.
64. Document "1" in the DX column.
65. Document "16.00" in the Fee column.
66. Document "2" in the Units column.
67. Click the Save button (Figure 4-144).
68. Click the Submission tab. Click in the I am ready to submit the Claim box. Click on the Yes radio button to indicate that there is a signature on file and enter today's date in the Date field.
69. Click the Save button. Click the Submit Claim button.
70. Within the Coding & Billing tab, select Ledger from the left Info Panel.
71. Search for Robert Caudill using the Patient Search fields.
72. Select the radio button for Robert Caudill and click the Select button.

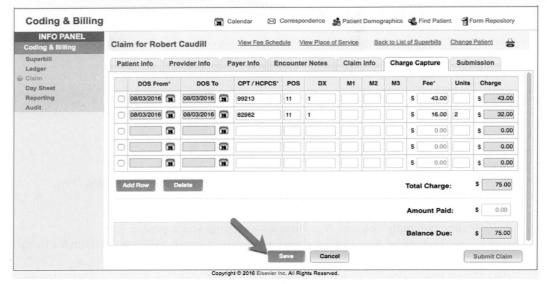

Figure 4-144 Insert the necessary information into the Charge Capture tab of the claim, and then click the Save button.

73. Confirm the auto-populated details in the header.
74. Click the arrow to the right of Robert Caudill's name to expand his patient ledger.
75. All charges submitted on the claim will auto-populate on the ledger. Click Add Row to enter the payment made by Robert Caudill.
76. Document the current date in the Transaction Date column using the calendar picker.
77. Document the date of service in the DOS column using the calendar picker.
78. Select Jean Burke, NP using the dropdown in the Provider field.
79. Select PTPYMTCC using the dropdown in the Service column.
80. Document "25.00" in the Payment column. The balance will auto-populate in the Balance column.
81. Click the Save button.

 Now use the Back to Assignment link to complete the Post-Case Quiz found on the Info Panel for this assignment.

96. Document Encounter and Complete Payment Process for Julia Berkley

■ Objectives

- Search for a patient record.
- Document a patient encounter.
- Use a fee schedule.
- Complete a superbill.
- Complete a claim.
- Update a ledger.

■ Overview

Julia Berkley is a senior at Anytown University and a new patient at Walden-Martin. Until now, she has been healthy with no relevant medical history. However, she felt a small mass in her left breast last month during a self-exam. She denies any nipple pain or discharge, and there is no redness or puckering to the breast. Julia Berkley smokes about five cigarettes a day and has been drinking more coffee lately to stay up late studying for final exams. She takes a daily multivitamin and got a flu shot last week at the campus clinic. The shot was administered to her right arm and she had no reaction. Dr. Martin asks Julia Berkley about any past surgeries. Her surgical history includes a tonsillectomy and adenoidectomy when she was 11. She was once pregnant, but the pregnancy resulted in a miscarriage at 10 weeks gestation last year on July 1. Julia Berkley has had yearly pap smears and pelvic exams since she was 17 years old. Although Dr. Martin feels that her mass is due to increased density in the breast, he orders a bilateral screening mammogram as a baseline. Julia paid her $25.00 copay (new patient, problem-focused visit) with a credit card. Document the encounter, complete and submit the superbill and claim, and update the patient ledger for Julia Berkley.

■ Competencies

- Administer parenteral (excluding IV) medications, CAAHEP I.P-7, ABHES 2-c, 8-f
- Define types of information contained in the patient's medical record, CAAHEP VI.C-4, ABHES 7-b
- Identify the abbreviations and symbols used in calculating medication dosages, CAAHEP II.C-5, ABHES 3-d, 6-b, 6-c
- Perform diagnostic coding, CAAHEP IX.P-2, ABHES 7-d
- Perform procedural coding, CAAHEP IX.P-1, ABHES 7-d
- Perform specialty procedures including but not limited to minor surgery, cardiac, respiratory, OB-GYN, neurological, gastroenterology, ABHES 8-e
- Schedule a patient procedure, CAAHEP VI.P-2, ABHES 7-e

Estimated completion time: 1 hour, 30 minutes

Measurable Steps

1. Click on the Find Patient icon.
2. Using the Patient Search fields, search for Julia Berkley's patient record. Once you locate her patient record in the List of Patients, confirm her date of birth.

 HELPFUL HINT

Confirming date of birth will help to ensure that you have located the correct patient record.

3. Select the radio button for Julia Berkley and click the Select button.
4. Create a new encounter by clicking Office Visit in the left Info Panel.
5. In the Create New Encounter window, select New Patient Visit from the Visit Type dropdown.
6. Select James A. Martin, MD from the Provider dropdown.
7. Click the Save button.
8. Select Immunizations from the Record dropdown menu (Figure 4-145).

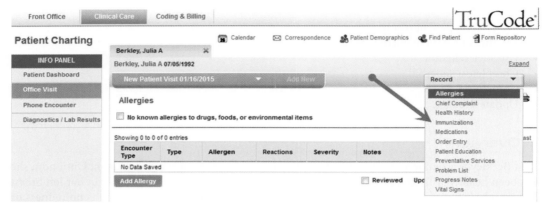

Figure 4-145 Immunizations in the Record dropdown menu.

9. Locate the row for the "Flu" vaccine and click the green plus sign to the far right of that row. That row will become active so you can add an immunization to Julia Berkley's record.
10. Document Unknown in the Type column. Within the Date column, use the calendar picker to select the date administered.
11. Within the Provider column, document "Anytown University Campus Clinic" in the text box.
12. Within the Reaction column, document "Patient has no reaction" in the text box.
13. Click the Save button. The Immunizations table will display the new immunization.
14. Select Health History from the Record dropdown menu.
15. Click on the No previous health history box.
16. Click on the No previous hospitalization box.
17. Click the Add New button beneath the Past Surgeries section.
18. Document the year that the patient would have been 11 years old in the Date field and "Tonsillectomy" in the Type of Surgery field, along with any additional information needed.
19. Click the Save button. The Health History table will display the newly added health history.
20. Click the Add New button beneath the Past Surgeries section.
21. Document the year that the patient would have been 11 years old in the Date field and "Adenoidectomy" in the Type of Surgery field, along with any additional information needed.
22. Click the Save button. The Health History table will display the newly added health history.
23. Click Save, then click the Pregnancy History tab.
24. Document "1" in the Gravida field.
25. Document "0" in the Para field.
26. Document "1" in the Abortions field.
27. Document "Yes" in the Spontaneous field.
28. Document "0" in the Living field.
29. Click the Save button (Figure 4-146). The Pregnancy History table will display the newly added health history.
30. Select Medications from the Record dropdown menu.
31. Within the Over-the-Counter Products tab, click the Add Medication button to add multivitamins to Julia Berkley's medications. An Add Over-the-Counter Product window will appear.
32. Document "Multivitamin" in the Generic Name field.
33. Document "1" in the Dose field.

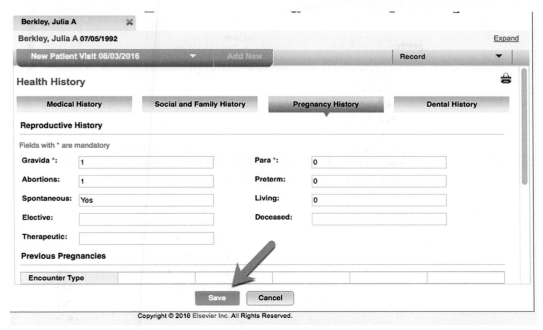

Figure 4-146 Within the Pregnancy History tab, fill out the necessary information, and then click the Save button.

34. Document "once daily" in the Frequency field.
35. Select oral from the Route dropdown menu.
36. Document any additional information needed and select the Active radio button in the Status field.
37. Click the Save button. The Medications table will display the new medication.
38. Select Chief Complaint from the Record dropdown menu.
39. Document "Mass. Julia denies any nipple pain or discharge. No redness or puckering to the breast." in the Chief Complaint field.
40. Document "Left breast" in the Location field.
41. Document "1 month" in the Duration field.
42. Select the No radio button at the top of the column in each section to indicate that Julia Berkley denies having these symptoms.
43. Click the Save button. The chief complaint you just added will move below the Saved tab.
44. Select Order Entry from the Record dropdown menu.
45. Select the TruCode encoder button in the top right corner. The encoder tool will open in a new tab.
46. Enter "Breast mass" in the Search field and select Diagnosis, ICD-10-CM from the corresponding dropdown menu.
47. Click the Search button.
48. Click the code N63 that appears in red to expand this code and confirm that it is the most specific code available (Figure 4-147).
49. Copy the code N63 for "Unspecified lump in breast" that populates in the search results (Figure 4-148).
50. Click the Add button below the Out-of-Office table to add an order.
51. In the Add Order window, select Requisitions from the Order dropdown menu.
52. Select Radiology from the Requisition Type dropdown menu.
53. Paste the diagnosis within the body of the Notes field so that is available for documentation.
54. Document any additional information provided and click the Save button. The Out-of-Office table will display the new order.
55. Click the Form Repository icon.
56. Select the Requisition form from the left Info Panel.
57. Select Radiology from the Requisition Type dropdown menu.

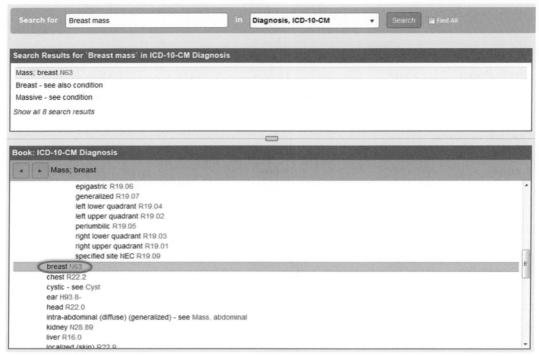

Figure 4-147 Confirm N63 is the most specific code available.

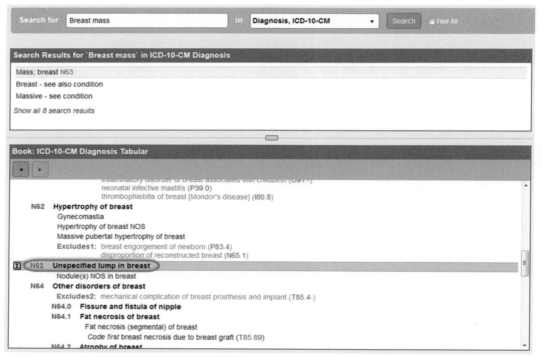

Figure 4-148 Copy the code N63 for "Unspecified lump in breast".

58. Click the Patient Search button to assign the form to Julia Berkley (Figure 4-149). Confirm the auto-populated patient demographics.
59. In the Diagnosis field, document "Screening for Malignant Neoplasms, Mammogram".
60. Place the cursor in the Diagnosis Code field to access the encoder. Accessing the encoder tool this way will auto-populate any selected codes where the cursor is placed.

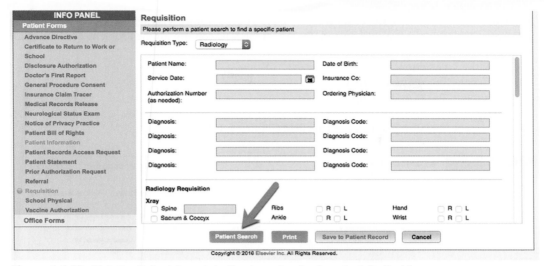

INFO PANEL
Patient Forms
Advance Directive
Certificate to Return to Work or School
Disclosure Authorization
Doctor's First Report
General Procedure Consent
Insurance Claim Tracer
Medical Records Release
Neurological Status Exam
Notice of Privacy Practice
Patient Bill of Rights
Patient Information
Patient Records Access Request
Patient Statement
Prior Authorization Request
Referral
⦿ Requisition
School Physical
Vaccine Authorization
Office Forms

Requisition

Please perform a patient search to find a specific patient

Requisition Type: Radiology

Patient Name:		Date of Birth:	
Service Date:	📅	Insurance Co:	
Authorization Number (as needed):		Ordering Physician:	
Diagnosis:		Diagnosis Code:	
Diagnosis:		Diagnosis Code:	
Diagnosis:		Diagnosis Code:	
Diagnosis:		Diagnosis Code:	

Radiology Requisition

Xray
☐ Spine _____ Ribs ☐ R ☐ L   Hand ☐ R ☐ L
☐ Sacrum & Coccyx Ankle ☐ R ☐ L   Wrist ☐ R ☐ L

[Patient Search] [Print] [Save to Patient Record] [Cancel]

Figure 4-149 Click the Patient Search button to assign the form to Julia Berkley.

61. Enter "Screening for Malignant Neoplasms, Mammogram" in the Search field and select Diagnosis, ICD-10-CM from the dropdown menu.
62. Click the Search button.
63. Click the code Z12.9 to expand this code and confirm that it is the most specific code available.
64. Click the yellow information icon to the left of the code to view the instructional notes, which mention the external cause of the code is also required for this diagnosis.
65. Click the code Z12.31 for "Encounter for screening mammogram for malignant neoplasm of breast" that appears in the tree. This code will auto-populate in the ICD-10 field of the Add Problem window.
66. Document any additional information needed and click the Save to Patient Record button. Confirm the date and click OK.
67. Click the Clinical Care tab.
68. Using the Patient Search fields, search for Julia Berkley's patient record. Once you locate her in the List of Patients, confirm her date of birth.
69. Select the radio button for Julia Berkley and click the Select button. Confirm the auto-populated details.
70. Within the patient dashboard, scroll down to view the saved forms in the Forms section.
71. Select the form you prepared. The form will open in a new window, allowing you to print.
72. After reviewing the encounter, click the Superbill link below the patient header.
73. Select the correct encounter from the Encounters Not Coded table and confirm the auto-populated details.

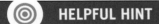 **HELPFUL HINT**

The View Fee Schedule and View Progress Notes links provide information necessary in completing coding & billing tasks.

74. On page one of the superbill, select the ICD-10 radio button.
75. In the Rank 1 row of the Diagnoses box, place the cursor in the text field to access the encoder.
76. Enter "Breast mass" in the Search field and select Diagnosis ICD-10-CM from the dropdown menu.
77. Click the Search button.
78. Click the code N63 to expand this code and confirm that it is the most specific code available.
79. Click the code N63 for "Unspecified lump in breast" that appears in the tree. This code will auto-populate in the Rank 1 row of the Diagnoses box.
80. Click the View Fee Schedule link to obtain the fee and code for the NP Problem-Focused Office Visit.

81. Document "1" in the Rank column for Problem Focused Office Visit.
82. Enter "50.00" in the Fee column and "99202" in the New column for the Problem-Focused office visit.
83. Click the Save button.
84. Go to page four of the superbill.
85. Document "25.00" in the Copay field.
86. Confirm that the total in the Today's Charges field has populated correctly.
87. Document "25.00" in the Balance Due field (Figure 4-150).

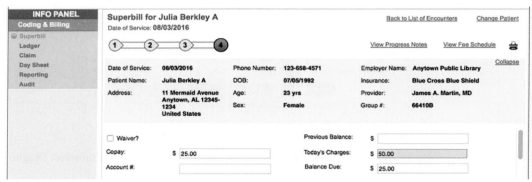

Figure 4-150 Document the copay and the balance due.

88. Fill out additional fields as needed.
89. Click the Save button.
90. Select the I am ready to submit the Superbill checkbox at the bottom of the screen.
91. Select the Yes radio button to indicate that the signature is on file.
92. Document the date in the Date field.
93. Click the Submit Superbill button. A confirmation message will appear.
94. Select Claim from the left Info Panel and perform a patient search to locate the claim for Julia Berkley.
95. Select the correct encounter and click the Edit icon in the Action column. Confirm the auto-populated details. Seven tabs appear within the claim: Patient Info, Provider Info, Payer Info, Encounter Notes, Claim Info, Charge Capture, and Submission. Certain patient demographic and encounter information is auto-populated in the claim.
96. Within the Patient Info tab, review the auto-populated information and document any additional information needed. Click the Save button.
97. Click the Provider Info tab.
98. Review the auto-populated information and document any additional information needed. Click the Save button.
99. Click the Payer Info tab.
100. Review the auto-populated information and document any additional information needed. Click the Save button.
101. Click the Encounter Notes tab.
102. Review the auto-populated information.
103. Select the Yes radio button to indicate that the HIPAA form is on file for Julia Berkley and document the current date in the Dated field.
104. Document any additional information needed and click the Save button.
105. Click the Claim Info tab.
106. Review the auto-populated information and document any additional information needed. Click the Save button.
107. Click the Charge Capture tab.
108. Document the encounter date in the DOS From and DOS To columns.
109. Document "99202" in the CPT/HCPCS column.
110. Document "11" in the POS column.
111. Document "1" in the DX column.
112. Document "50.00" in the Fee column.

113. Click the Save button.
114. Click the Submission tab. Click in the I am ready to submit the Claim box. Click on the Yes radio button to indicate that there a signature on file and enter today's date in the Date field.
115. Click the Submit Claim button.
116. Within the Coding & Billing tab, select Ledger from the left Info Panel.
117. Search for Julia Berkley using the Patient Search fields.
118. Select the radio button for Julia Berkley and click the Select button.
119. Confirm the auto-populated details in the header.
120. Click the arrow to the right of Julia Berkley's name to expand her patient ledger.
121. All charges submitted on the claim will auto-populate on the ledger. Click Add Row to enter the payment made by Julia Berkley.
122. Document the current date in the Transaction Date column using the calendar picker.
123. Document the date of service in the DOS column using the calendar picker.
124. Select James A. Martin, MD using the dropdown in the Provider field.
125. Document PTPYMTCC in the Service column.
126. Document "25.00" in the Payment column. The balance will auto-populate in the Balance column and the total will auto-populate in the Total Ledger Balance field below the table (Figure 4-151).
127. Click the Save button.

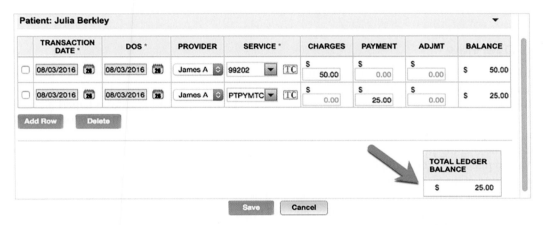

Figure 4-151 The balance will auto-populate in the Balance column and the total will auto-populate in the Total Ledger Balance field below the table.

Now use the Back to Assignment link to complete the Post-Case Quiz found on the Info Panel for this assignment.

97. Complete Referral Form, Document Chief Complaint and Progress Note, and Complete Payment Process for Robert Caudill

■ Objectives

- Search for a patient record.
- Create a referral form.
- Document a chief complaint.
- Document in the progress note.
- Use a fee schedule.
- Complete a superbill.
- Complete a claim.
- Update a patient ledger.
- Update the day sheet.

■ Overview

Robert Caudill is seeing Jean Burke, NP for a follow-up appointment after an episode of hypoglycemia. His blood sugars have been running between 92 and 150 before meals. Dr. Walden reviews Robert Caudill's recent lipid panel results, sees that his LDL is 150, and diagnoses hyperlipidemia. Dr. Walden prescribes one Lipitor 10 mg every day at bedtime. Robert Caudill mentions that he has increasing lower leg discomfort and cramping when walking short distances. He also states that he has some tingling in his feet. Diabetic patients are at an increased risk for vascular disease so Dr. Walden refers Robert Caudill for a vascular consult. Robert Caudill pays a $25.00 copay with a check at the time of his visit. Complete a referral form, document the chief complaint, and document the progress note for Robert Caudill's problem-focused office visit. Then, complete the payment process by completing the superbill, claim, ledger, and day sheet with the charges and payments associated with this encounter.

■ Competencies

- Define types of information contained in the patient's medical record, CAAHEP VI.C-4, ABHES 7-b
- Outline managed care requirements for patient referral, CAAHEP VIII.C-2, ABHES 7-d
- Facilitate referrals to community resources in the role of a patient navigator, CAAHEP V.P-10

Estimated completion time: 1 hour, 30 minutes

Measurable Steps

1. Click on the Find Patient icon.
2. Using the Patient Search fields, search for Robert Caudill's patient record. Once you locate his patient record in the List of Patients, confirm his date of birth.

 HELPFUL HINT

Confirming a patient's date of birth will help to ensure that you have located the correct patient record.

Coding & Billing

3. Select the radio button for Robert Caudill and click the Select button.
4. Create a new encounter by clicking Office Visit in the left Info Panel.
5. In the Create New Encounter window, select Follow-Up/Established Visit from the Visit Type dropdown.
6. Select Jean Burke, NP from the Provider dropdown.
7. Click the Save button.
8. Select Chief Complaint from the Record dropdown menu (Figure 4-152).

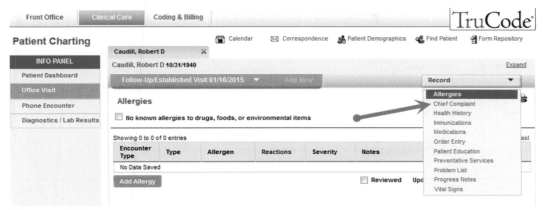

Figure 4-152 Chief Complaint from the Record dropdown menu.

9. Document "Follow-up appointment after episode of Hypoglycemia. Increasing lower leg discomfort and cramping when walking short distances. Tingling in feet." in the Chief Complaint field.
10. Document "Legs and feet" in the Location field.
11. Select the No radio button at the top of the column in each section to indicate that Robert Caudill denies having these symptoms.
12. Select the Yes radio button for Paresthesis in the Neuro section and Myalgia in the MS section.
13. Click the Save button. The chief complaint you just added will move below the Saved tab.
14. Select Progress Notes from the Record dropdown menu.
15. Document the date using the calendar picker.
16. Document "Patient states that he has increasing lower leg discomfort and cramping when walking short distances. He also notes that he has some tingling in his feet." in the Subjective field.
17. Document "Blood sugars have been running between 92 and 150 before meals." in the Objective field.
18. Document "Hyperlipidemia" in the Assessment field.
19. Document "Lipitor 10 mg every day at bedtime and vascular consult" in the Plan field.
20. Click the Save button (Figure 4-153).
21. Click on the Form Repository icon.
22. Select Referral from the Patient Forms section of the left Info Panel.
23. Click the Patient Search button to perform a patient search and assign the form to Robert Caudill.

> ### ◎ HELPFUL HINT
>
> Performing a patient search before completing a form will help to ensure accurate documentation in the patient record.

24. Confirm the auto-populated details and document any additional information needed.
25. Document "DM Type 2, hyperlipidemia" in the Diagnosis field.
26. Document "LDL 150 mg/dL, intermittent claudication and foot paresthesias" in the Significant Clinical Information/Symptoms field.
27. Click the Yes radio button next to Diabetic.

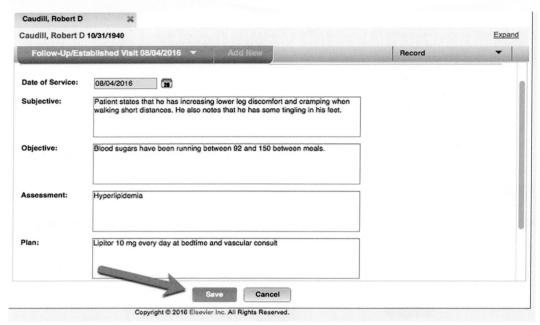

Figure 4-153 Fill in the progress notes and then click the Save button.

28. Document "Lipitor 10 msg daily" in the Medications field.
29. Document any additional information needed.
30. Click the Save to Patient Record button. Confirm the date and click OK.
31. Click on the Find Patient icon.
32. Using the Patient Search fields, search for Robert Caudill's patient record. Once you locate him in the List of Patients, confirm his date of birth.
33. Select the radio button for Robert Caudill and click the Select button. Confirm the auto-populated details.
34. Select the form you prepared from the patient dashboard. The form will open in a new window, allowing you to print.
35. Click the Superbill link below the patient header.
36. Select the correct encounter from the Encounters Not Coded table and confirm the auto-populated details.
37. On page one of the superbill, select the ICD-10 radio button.
38. In the Rank 1 row of the Diagnoses box, place the cursor in the text field to access the encoder.
39. Enter "Type 2 diabetes" in the Search field and select Diagnosis ICD-10-CM from the dropdown menu.
40. Click the Search button.
41. Click the code E11.9 to expand this code and confirm that it is the most specific code available (Figure 4-154).
42. Click the code E11.9 for "Type 2 diabetes mellitus without complications" that appears in the tree. This code will auto-populate in the Rank 1 row of the Diagnoses box (Figure 4-155).
43. In the Rank 2 row of the Diagnoses box, place the cursor in the text field to access the encoder.
44. Enter "Hyperlipidemia" in the Search field and select Diagnosis ICD-10-CM from the dropdown menu.
45. Click the Search button.
46. Click the code E78.5 to expand this code and confirm that it is the most specific code available.
47. Click the code E78.5 for "Hyperlipidemia, unspecified" that appears in the tree. This code will auto-populate in the Rank 2 row of the Diagnoses box.
48. Document "1" in the Rank column for the problem focused office visit. Click the View Fee Schedule link to obtain the fee and code.
49. Enter "32.00" in the Fee column and "99212" in the Est column for the problem-focused office visit.
50. Click the Save button.

Coding & Billing

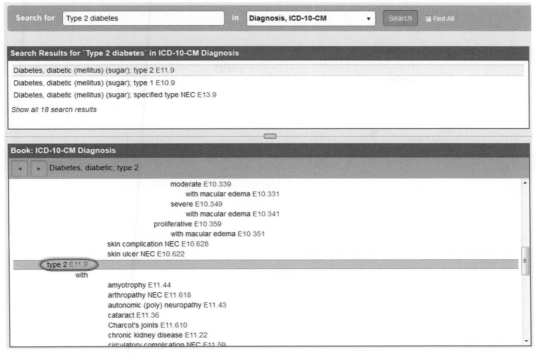

Figure 4-154 Confirm E11.9 is the most specific code available.

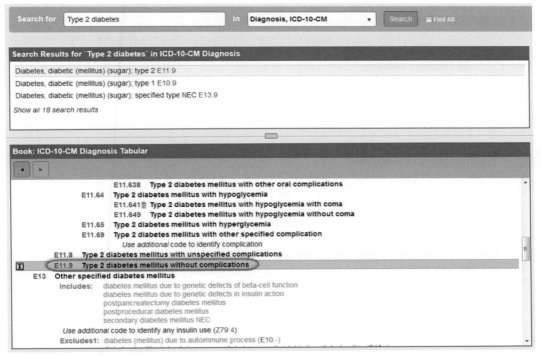

Figure 4-155 Populating the code in the Rank 1 row of the Diagnoses box.

51. Go to page four of the superbill.
52. On page four, document "25.00" in the Copay field.
53. Confirm that the total in the Today's Charges field has populated correctly.
54. Document "7.00" in the Balance Due field (Figure 4-156).
55. Fill out additional fields as needed.
56. Click the Save button.
57. Select the I am ready to submit the Superbill checkbox at the bottom of the screen.

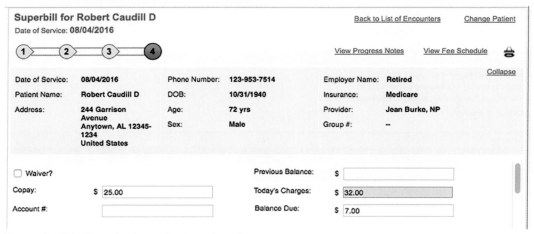

Figure 4-156 Fill in the Copay field, confirm that the total in the Today's Charges field has populated correctly, and document in the Balance Due field.

58. Select the Yes radio button to indicate that the signature is on file.
59. Document the date in the Date field.
60. Click the Submit Superbill button. A confirmation message will appear.
61. Select Claim from the left Info Panel and perform a patient search to locate the claim for Robert Caudill.
62. Select the correct encounter and click the Edit icon in the Action column. Confirm the auto-populated details. Seven tabs appear within the claim: Patient Info, Provider Info, Payer Info, Encounter Notes, Claim Info, Charge Capture, and Submission. Certain patient demographic and encounter information is auto-populated in the claim.
63. Within the Patient Info tab, review the auto-populated information and document any additional information needed. Click the Save button.
64. Click the Provider Info tab.
65. Review the auto-populated information and document any additional information needed. Click the Save button.
66. Click the Payer Info tab.
67. Review the auto-populated information and document any additional information needed. Click the Save button.
68. Click the Encounter Notes tab.
69. Review the auto-populated information.
70. Select the Yes radio button to indicate that the HIPAA form is on file for Robert Caudill and document the current date in the Dated field.
71. Document any additional information needed and click the Save button.
72. Click the Claim Info tab.
73. Review the auto-populated information and document any additional information needed. Click the Save button.
74. Click the Charge Capture tab.
75. Document the encounter date in the DOS From and DOS To columns.
76. Document "99212" in the CPT/HCPCS column.
77. Document "11" in the POS column.
78. Document "12" in the DX column.
79. Document "32.00" in the Fee column.
80. Click the Save button (Figure 4-157).
81. Click the Submission tab. Click in the I am ready to submit the Claim box. Click on the Yes radio button to indicate that there is a signature on file and enter today's date in the Date field.
82. Click the Submit Claim button.
83. Within the Coding & Billing tab, select Ledger from the left Info Panel.
84. Search for Robert Caudill using the Patient Search fields.
85. Select the radio button for Robert Caudill and click the Select button.
86. Confirm the auto-populated details in the header.

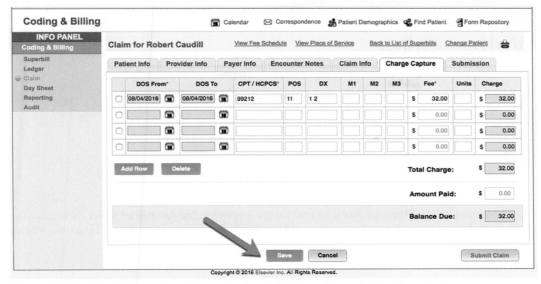

	DOS From*	DOS To	CPT / HCPCS*	POS	DX	M1	M2	M3	Fee*	Units	Charge
☐	08/04/2016	08/04/2016	99212	11	1 2				$ 32.00		$ 32.00
☐									$ 0.00		$ 0.00
☐									$ 0.00		$ 0.00
☐									$ 0.00		$ 0.00

Figure 4-157 After filling out the Charge Capture tab of the claim, click the Save button.

87. Click the arrow to the right of Robert Caudill's name to expand his patient ledger.
88. All charges submitted on the claim will auto-populate on the ledger. Click Add Row to enter the payment made by Robert Caudill.
89. Document the current date in the Transaction Date column using the calendar picker.
90. Document the date of service in the DOS column using the calendar picker.
91. Select Jean Burke, NP using the dropdown in the Provider field.
92. Document PTPYMTCK in the Service column.
93. Document "25.00" in the Payment column. The balance will auto-populate in the Balance column and the total will auto-populate in the Total Ledger Balance field below the grid.
94. Click the Save button.
95. Select Day Sheet from the left Info Panel.
96. Document the current date in the Date column using the calendar picker.
97. Document "Robert Caudill" in the Patient column.
98. Select Jean Burke, NP using the dropdown in the Provider field.
99. Document "99212" in the Service column.
100. Document "32.00" in the Charges column.
101. Document "25.00" in the Payment column.
102. Document "7.00" in the New Balance column.
103. Document "0.00" in the Old Balance column.
104. Click the Save button.

 Now use the Back to Assignment link to complete the Post-Case Quiz found on the Info Panel for this assignment.

Coding & Billing

98. Create Bank Deposit Slip for Walter Biller

■ Objectives

- Search for a patient record.
- Document patient payments on a bank deposit slip.

■ Overview

The first transaction of the day was a $15.00 form completion fee for Walter Biller. Now that the Walden-Martin office is closed, begin a bank deposit slip by documenting this transaction. Walter Biller paid with a check (#3345).

■ Competencies

- Prepare a bank deposit, CAAHEP VII.P-2, ABHES 7-c

Estimated completion time: 10 minutes

Measurable Steps

1. Click on the Form Repository icon.
2. Select Bank Deposit Slip from the Office Forms section of the left Info Panel (Figure 4-158).

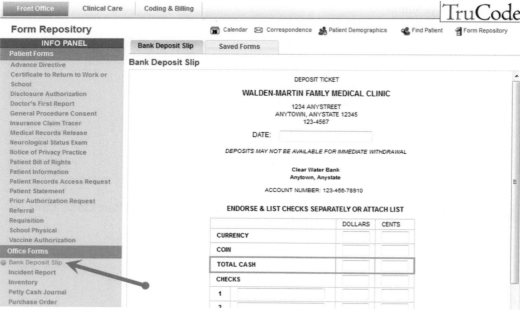

Figure 4-158 Bank Deposit Slip.

3. Document the date in the Date field.
4. Document "Walter Biller" in the first row of the Checks column, followed by "15" in the Dollars column and "00" in the Cents column.
5. Document "15.00" in the Total From Attached List field.
6. Document "1" in the Total Items field.
7. Click the Save button.

8. Select the saved bank deposit from the Select Saved Form dropdown menu.
9. Click the Print button to print (Figure 4-159).

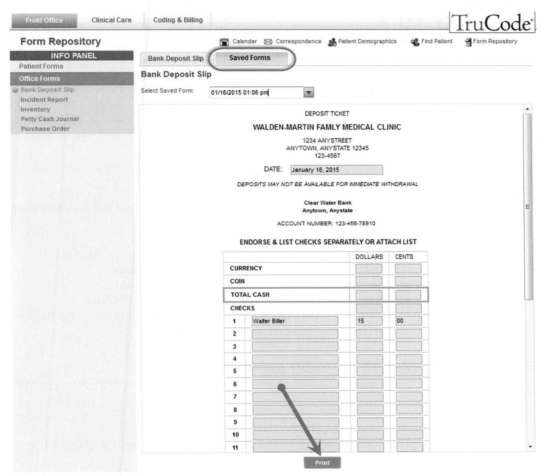

Figure 4-159 Print button.

Now use the Back to Assignment link to complete the Post-Case Quiz found on the Info Panel for this assignment.

99. Document Transactions on Ledger and Day Sheet, then Prepare Bank Deposit Slip

■ Objectives

- Update a patient ledger.
- Document daily transactions on a day sheet.
- Create a bank deposit.

■ Overview

Complete a bank deposit slip and document the daily transactions on the ledger and day sheet using the payments listed below:

- Amma Patel paid $25.00 by check – colposcopy with biopsy – Dr. Martin
- Celia Tapia paid $25.00 by cash – problem-focused 10-minute office visit – Dr. Martin
- Charles Johnson paid $25.00 by check – metabolic panel, basic – Dr. Walden
- Diego Lupez paid $25.00 by check – problem-focused office visit – Dr. Walden
- Ella Rainwater paid $25.00 by check – problem-focused office visit – Dr. Walden
- Janine Butler paid $70.00 by check – new patient detailed office visit (30 minutes) - Dr. Walden
- Quinton Brown paid $24.00 by cash – minimal office visit – Dr. Martin

Estimated completion time: 50 minutes

■ Competencies

- Define basic bookkeeping terms, CAAHEP VII.C-1, ABHES 7-c
- Describe banking procedures as related to the ambulatory care setting, CAAHEP VII.C-2, ABHES 7-c
- Identify precautions for accepting cash, checks, and credit cards, CAAHEP VII.C-3, ABHES 7-c
- Identify types of information contained in the patient's billing record, CAAHEP VII.C-5, ABHES 7-b, 7-c
- Perform accounts receivable procedures to patient accounts including posting charges, payments, and adjustments, CAAHEP VII.P-1, ABHES 7-c
- Obtain accurate patient billing information, CAAHEP VII.P-3

Measurable Steps

1. Within the Coding & Billing tab, select Ledger from the left Info Panel.
2. Search for Amma Patel using the Patient Search fields, then select the radio button for Amma Patel and click the Select button.
3. Click the arrow to the right of Amma Patel's name to expand her patient ledger.
4. Document the current date in the Transaction Date column using the calendar picker.
5. Document the date of service in the DOS column using the calendar picker.
6. Select James A. Martin, MD in the Provider dropdown.
7. In the Service column, select the TC button to access the encoder.
8. Enter "Colposcopy" in the Search field and select CPT Tabular from the dropdown menu.
9. Click the Search button.
10. Click the link to show all 11 search results and click the code 57455 to expand this code and confirm that it is the most specific code available (Figure 4-160).
11. Click the code 57455 for "Colposcopy with biopsy(s) of the cervix" that appears in the tree. This code will auto-populate in the ledger (Figure 4-161).
12. Click the View Fee Schedule link to obtain the charge. Document "178.00" in the Charges field.

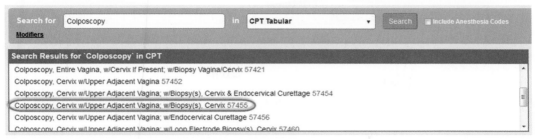

Figure 4-160 Confirm 57455 is the most specific code available.

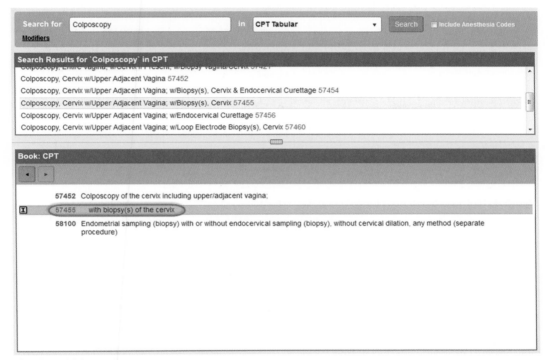

Figure 4-161 Populating the code in the ledger.

13. Document "25.00" in the Payment field.
14. Click the Save button.
15. Select Day Sheet from the left Info Panel (Figure 4-162).
16. Document today's date in the Date field.
17. Document "Amma Patel" in the Patient field.
18. Select James A. Martin, MD using the Provider dropdown.
19. Document "57455" in the Service column.
20. Document "178.00" in the Charges field.
21. Document "25.00" in the Payment field.
22. Document "153.00" in the New Balance field.
23. Document "0.00" in the Old Balance.
24. Click the Save button.
25. Select Ledger from the left Info Panel. Select Change Patient to clear data.
26. Search for Celia Tapia using the Patient Search fields, then select the radio button for Celia Tapia and click the Select button.
27. Click the arrow to the right of Celia Tapia's name to expand her patient ledger.
28. Document the current date in the Transaction Date column using the calendar picker.
29. Document the date of service in the DOS column using the calendar picker.
30. Select James A. Martin, MD in the Provider dropdown.
31. In the Service column, select the TC button to access the encoder. Enter "Problem Focused Office visit" in the Search field and select CPT Tabular from the dropdown menu.

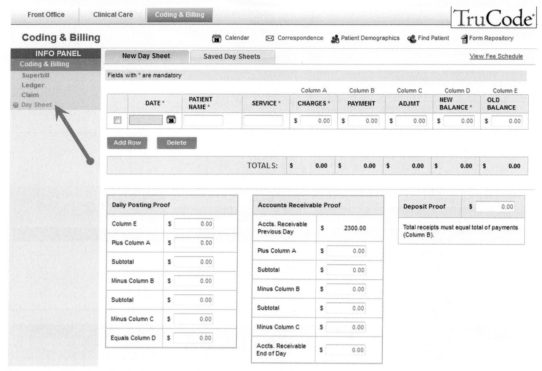

Figure 4-162 Day Sheet from the Info Panel.

32. Click the Search button.
33. Click the code 99212 to expand this code and confirm that it is the most specific code available.
34. Click the code 99212 for "Office or other outpatient visit" that appears in the tree. This code will auto-populate in the ledger.
35. View the Fee Schedule to obtain the charge. Document "32.00" in the Charges field.
36. Document "25.00" in the Payment field.
37. Click the Save button (Figure 4-163).
38. Select Day Sheet from the left Info Panel.
39. Within the Saved Day Sheets tab, select the saved day sheet from the dropdown menu (Figure 4-164).

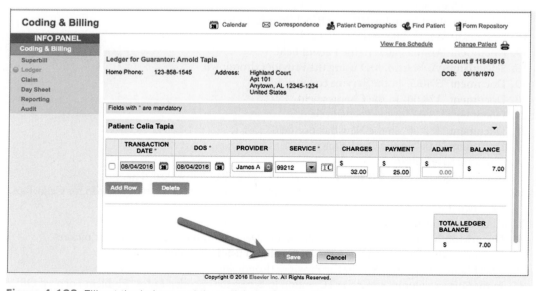

Figure 4-163 Fill out the ledger, and then click the Save button.

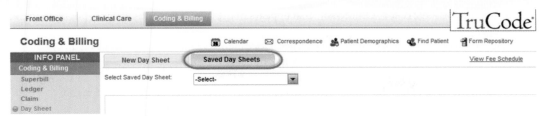

Coding & Billing   📅 Calendar   ✉ Correspondence   👥 Patient Demographics   🔍 Find Patient   📋 Form Repository

INFO PANEL	
Coding & Billing	
Superbill	
Ledger	
Claim	
Day Sheet	

New Day Sheet   **Saved Day Sheets**   View Fee Schedule

Select Saved Day Sheet: -Select-   ▾

Figure 4-164 The saved Day Sheet from the dropdown menu.

40. Click the Add Row button.
41. Document today's date in the Date field.
42. Document "Celia Tapia" in the Patient field.
43. Select James A. Martin, MD using the dropdown in the Provider field.
44. Document "99212" in the Service field.
45. Document "32.00" in the Charges field.
46. Document "25.00" in the Payment field.
47. Document "7.00" in the New Balance field.
48. Click the Save button.
49. Select Ledger from the left Info Panel. Select Change Patient to clear data.
50. Search for Charles Johnson using the Patient Search fields, then select the radio button for Charles Johnson and click the Select button.
51. Click the arrow to the right of Charles Johnson's name to expand his patient ledger.
52. Document the current date in the Transaction Date column using the calendar picker.
53. Document the date of service in the DOS column using the calendar picker.
54. Select Julie Walden, MD in the Provider dropdown.
55. In the Service column, select the TC button to access the encoder. Enter "Metabolic panel" in the Search field and select CPT tabular from the dropdown menu.
56. Click the Search button.
57. Click the code 80048 to expand this code and confirm that it is the most specific code available.
58. Click the code 80048 for "Basic metabolic panel" that appears in the tree. This code will auto-populate in the ledger.
59. View the Fee Schedule to obtain the charges. Document "42.00" in the Charges field.
60. Document "25.00" in the Payment field.
61. Click the Save button.
62. Select Day Sheet from the left Info Panel.
63. Within the Saved Day Sheets tab, select the saved day sheet from the dropdown menu.
64. Click the Add Row button.
65. Document today's date in the Date field.
66. Document "Charles Johnson" in the Patient field.
67. Select Julie Walden, MD using the dropdown in the Provider field.
68. Document "80048" in the Service field.
69. Document "42.00" in the Charges field.
70. Document "25.00" in the Payment field.
71. Document "17.00" in the New Balance field.
72. Document "0.00" in the Old Balance.
73. Click the Save button.
74. Select Ledger from the left Info Panel. Select Change Patient to clear data.
75. Search for Diego Lupez using the Patient Search fields, then select the radio button for Diego Lupez and click the Select button.
76. Click the arrow to the right of Diego Lupez's name to expand his patient ledger.
77. Document the current date in the Transaction Date column using the calendar picker.
78. Document the date of service in the DOS column using the calendar picker.
79. Select Julie Walden, MD in the Provider dropdown.
80. In the Service column, select the TC button to access the encoder. Enter "Problem-Focused Office visit" in the Search field and select CPT tabular from the dropdown menu.
81. Click the Search button.
82. Click the code 99212 to expand this code and confirm that it is the most specific code available.

Coding & Billing

83. Click the code 99212 for "Office visit" that appears in the tree. This code will auto-populate in the ledger.
84. View the Fee Schedule to obtain the charges. Document "32.00" in the Charges field.
85. Document "25.00" in the Payment field. Click the Save button.
86. Select Day Sheet from the left Info Panel.
87. Within the Saved Day Sheets tab, select the saved day sheet from the dropdown menu.
88. Click the Add Row button.
89. Document today's date in the Date field.
90. Document "Diego Lupez" in the Patient field.
91. Select Julie Walden, MD using the dropdown in the Provider field.
92. Document "99212" in the Service field.
93. Document "32.00" in the Charges field.
94. Document "25.00" in the Payment field.
95. Document "7.00" in the New Balance field.
96. Document "0.00" in the Old Balance.
97. Click the Save button.
98. Select Ledger from the left Info Panel. Select Change Patient to clear data.
99. Search for Ella Rainwater using the Patient Search fields, then select the radio button for Ella Rainwater and click the Select button.
100. Click the arrow to the right of Ella Rainwater's name to expand her patient ledger.
101. Document the current date in the Transaction Date column using the calendar picker.
102. Document the date of service in the DOS column using the calendar picker.
103. Select Julie Walden, MD in the Provider dropdown.
104. In the Service column, select the TC button to access the encoder.
105. Enter "Problem Focused Office visit" in the Search field and select CPT Tabular from the dropdown menu.
106. Click the Search button.
107. Click the code 99212 to expand this code and confirm that it is the most specific code available.
108. Click the code 99212 for "Office or other outpatient visit" that appears in the tree. This code will auto-populate in the ledger.
109. View the Fee Schedule to obtain the charges. Document "32.00" in the Charges field.
110. Document "25.00" in the Payment field.
111. Click the Save button.
112. Select Day Sheet from the left Info Panel.
113. Within the Saved Day Sheets tab, select the saved Day Sheet from the dropdown menu.
114. Click the Add Row button.
115. Document today's date in the Date field.
116. Document "Ella Rainwater" in the Patient field.
117. Select Julie Walden, MD using the dropdown in the Provider field.
118. Document "99212" in the Service field.
119. Document "32.00 In the Charges field.
120. Document "25.00" in the Payment field.
121. Document "7.00" in the New Balance field.
122. Document "0.00" in the Old Balance field.
123. Click the Save button.
124. Select Ledger from the left Info Panel. Select Change Patient to clear data.
125. Search for Janine Butler using the Patient Search fields, then select the radio button for Janine Butler and click the Select button.
126. Click the arrow to the right of Janine Butler's name to expand her patient ledger.
127. Document the current date in the Transaction Date column using the calendar picker.
128. Document the date of service in the DOS column using the calendar picker.
129. Select Julie Walden, MD in the Provider dropdown.
130. In the Service column, select the TC button to access the encoder.
131. Enter "Office visit new patient" in the Search field and select CPT Tabular from the dropdown menu.
132. Click the Search button.
133. Click the code 99203 to expand this code and confirm that is the most specific code available.

134. Click the code 99203 for "Office or other outpatient visit" that appears in the tree. This code will auto-populate in the ledger.
135. View the Fee Schedule to obtain the charges. Document "70.00 in the Charges field.
136. Document "70.00" in the Payment field.
137. Click the Save button.
138. Select Day Sheet from the left Info Panel.
139. Within the Saved Day Sheets tab, select the saved day sheet from the dropdown menu.
140. Click the Add Row button.
141. Document today's date in the Date field.
142. Document "Janine Butler" in the Patient field.
143. Select Julie Walden, MD using the dropdown in the Provider field.
144. Document "99203" in the Service field.
145. Document "70.00" in the Charges field.
146. Document "70.00" in the Payment field.
147. Document "0.00" in the Adjustment field.
148. Document "0.00" in the New Balance field.
149. Document "0.00" in the Old Balance field.
150. Click the Save button.
151. Select Ledger from the left Info Panel. Select Change Patient to clear data.
152. Search for Quinton Brown using the Patient Search fields, then select the radio button for Quinton Brown and click the Select button.
153. Click the arrow to the right of Quinton Brown's name to expand his patient ledger.
154. Document the current date in the Transaction Date column using the calendar picker.
155. Document the date of service in the DOS column using the calendar picker.
156. Select James A. Martin, MD in the Provider dropdown.
157. In the Service column, select the TC button to access the encoder.
158. Enter "Minimal Office visit" in the Search field and select CPT Tabular from the dropdown menu.
159. Click the Search button.
160. Click the code 99211 to expand this code and confirm that is the most specific code available.
161. Click the code 99211 for "Office or other outpatient visit" that appears in the tree. This code will auto-populate in the ledger.
162. View the Fee Schedule to obtain the charges. Document "24.00" in the Charges field.
163. Document "24.00" in the Payment field.
164. Click the Save button.
165. Select Day Sheet from the left Info Panel.
166. Within the Saved Day Sheets tab, select the saved day sheet from the dropdown menu.
167. Click the Add Row button.
168. Document today's date in the Date field.
169. Document "Quinton Brown" in the Patient field.
170. Select James A. Martin, MD using the dropdown in the Provider field.
171. Document "99211" in the Service field.
172. Document "24.00" in the Charges field.
173. Document "24.00" in the Payment field.
174. Document "0.00" in the Adjustment field.
175. Document "0.00" in the New Balance field.
176. Document "0.00" in the Old Balance field (Figure 4-165).
177. Click the Save button.
178. Click the Form Repository icon and select Bank Deposit Slip from the Office Forms section.
179. Document today's date in the Date field.
180. In the Currency row, document "49" in the Dollars column and "00" in the Cents column.
181. In the Total Cash row, document "49" in the Dollars column and "00" in the Cents column.
182. In the first row, document "Amma Patel" in the first column, "25" in the Dollars column, and "00" in the Cents column.
183. In the second row, document "Charles Johnson" in the first column, "25" in the Dollars column, and "00" in the Cents column.
184. In the third row, document "Diego Lupez" in the first column, "25" in the Dollars column, and "00" in the Cents column.

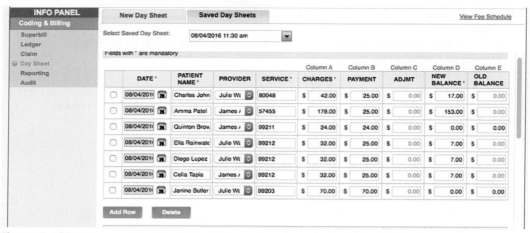

Figure 4-165 The saved day sheet should have all seven patients included.

185. In the fourth row, document "Ella Rainwater" in the first column, "25" in the Dollars column, and "00" in the Cents column.
186. In the fifth row, document "Janine Butler" in the first column, "70" in the Dollars column, and "00" in the Cents column (Figure 4-166).

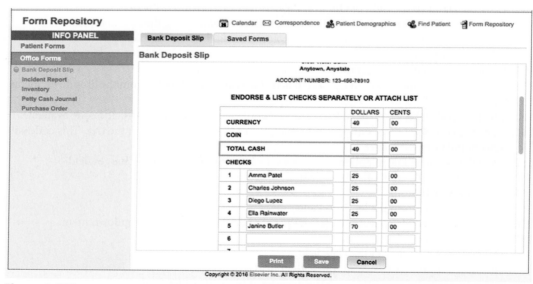

Figure 4-166 Fill out the Bank Deposit with the necessary information.

187. Document "219.00" in the Total From Attached List field.
188. Document "6" in the Total Items field.
189. Click the Save button.

⭐ Now use the Back to Assignment link to complete the Post-Case Quiz found on the Info Panel for this assignment.

Coding & Billing

100. Update Ledger, Create Deposit Slip, and Prepare Patient Statement for Norma Washington

■ Objectives

- Search for a patient record.
- Document patient payments.
- Document patient payments on the deposit slip.
- Prepare a patient statement.

■ Overview

Norma Washington is on a payment plan and sends the agreed-upon payments within the first 10 days of the month. Her first two payments were personal checks as follows: No. 212 for $20.00 and No. 215 for $20.00. Norma Washington's payment is late this month. According to her ledger, she has an outstanding balance of $25.00 on her account. Update the patient ledger to show the two patient payments (PTPYMTCK), create a deposit slip for the payments received, and create a patient statement for the outstanding balance, which is due 2 weeks from today's date.

■ Competencies

- Define basic bookkeeping terms, CAAHEP VII.C-1, ABHES 7-c
- Explain patient financial obligations for services rendered, CAAHEP VII.C-6, ABHES 5-c, 5-h, 7-c
- Identify precautions for accepting cash, checks, and credit cards, CAAHEP VII.C-3, ABHES 7-c
- Identify types of information contained in the patient's billing record, CAAHEP VII.C-5, ABHES 7-b, 7-c
- Inform a patient of financial obligations for services rendered, CAAHEP VII.P-4, ABHES 5-h, 7-c
- Perform accounts receivable procedures to patient accounts including posting charges, payments, and adjustments, CAAHEP VII.P-1, ABHES 7-c

Estimated completion time: 50 minutes

Measurable Steps

1. Within the Coding & Billing tab, select Ledger from the left Info Panel (Figure 4-167).
2. Search for Norma Washington using the Patient Search fields.
3. Select the radio button for Norma Washington and click the Select button.
4. Confirm the auto-populated details in the header (Figure 4-168).
5. Click the arrow to the right of Norma Washington's name to expand her patient ledger.
6. All charges submitted on the claim will auto-populate on the ledger. Click Add Row to enter the payments made by Norma Washington.
7. Document the date in the Transaction Date column using the calendar picker.
8. Document the date of service in the DOS column using the calendar picker.
9. Document PTPYMTCK in the Service column.
10. Document "0.00" in the Charges column.
11. Document "20.00" in the Payment column.
12. Document "0.00" in the Adjustment column. The balance will auto-populate in the Balance column.
13. Click the Add Row button. Document the date in the Transaction Date column using the calendar picker.
14. Document the date of service in the DOS column using the calendar picker.
15. Document PTPYMTCK in the Service column.

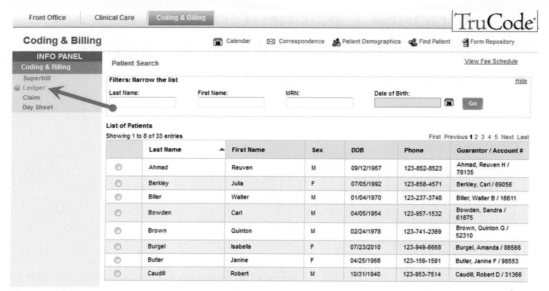

Figure 4-167 Ledger from the Info Panel.

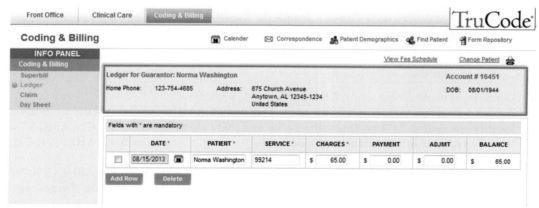

Figure 4-168 Confirm the auto-populated details in the header.

16. Document "0.00" in the Charges column.
17. Document "20.00" in the Payment column. The balance will auto-populate in the Balance column and the total will auto-populate in the Total field below the grid.
18. Click the Save button.
19. Click on the Form Repository icon.
20. Select Bank Deposit Slip from the Office Forms section of the left Info Panel.
21. Document the date in the Date field.
22. Document "Norma Washington" in the first row of the Checks column, followed by "20" in the Dollars column and "00" in the Cents column.
23. Document "Norma Washington" in the second row of the Checks column, followed by "20" in the Dollars column and "00" in the Cents column.
24. Document "40.00" in the Total From Attached List field.
25. Document "2" in the Total Items field.
26. Click the Save button.
27. Select the saved bank deposit from the Select Saved Form dropdown menu.
28. Click the Print button to print (Figure 4-169).
29. Select Patient Statement from the Patient Forms section of the left Info Panel.
30. Search for Norma Washington using the Patient Search fields.
31. Select the radio button for Norma Washington and click the Select button.
32. Confirm the auto-populated details in the header.
33. Document the date that the first payment was received in the first row of the Date of Service column.

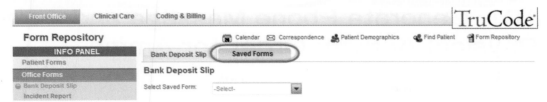

Form Repository   📅 Calendar ✉ Correspondence 👥 Patient Demographics 🔍 Find Patient 📋 Form Repository

INFO PANEL	Bank Deposit Slip Saved Forms
Patient Forms	**Bank Deposit Slip**
Office Forms	
⊙ Bank Deposit Slip	Select Saved Form: -Select- ▼
Incident Report	

Figure 4-169 Saved forms to print.

34. Document Patient Payment in the first row of the Description column.
35. Document "45.00" in the first row of the Patient's Responsibility column.
36. Document the date that the second payment was received in the second row of the Date of Service column.
37. Document Patient Payment in the second row of the Description column.
38. Document "25.00" in the second row of the Patient's Responsibility column.
39. Document "25.00" in the Total Amount Due column.
40. Document two weeks from today's date in the Please Pay in Full by field.
41. Click the Save to Patient Record button. Confirm the date and click OK.

⭐ Now use the Back to Assignment link to complete the Post-Case Quiz found on the Info Panel for this assignment.

101. Generate Phone Message and Physical Activity Order for Amma Patel

- ■ **Objectives**

- Search for a patient record.
- Document a phone encounter.
- Locate an ICD-10 CM code using an encoder.
- Document an order.

- ■ **Overview**

Amma Patel calls the office this morning at 9:15 am to report that she has recently joined a gym. Her health insurance coverage reimburses up to 40% of her membership fee if Dr. Walden writes an order with a diagnosis meeting medical necessity. Amma Patel would like to pick up the prescription today at 3:00 pm. Create a phone encounter for Dr. Walden's review.

After Dr. Walden reviews the phone message, he instructs you to prepare a blank prescription stating "Patient to complete 45 minutes, weight bearing exercise 5-6 days per week". The diagnoses are obesity and primary hypertension. Use the encoder to assign the ICD-10 CM codes in the prescription.

- ■ **Competencies**

- Define scope of practice for the medical assistant within the state that the medical assistant is employed, ABHES 4-f
- Demonstrate professional telephone techniques, CAAHEP V.P-6, ABHES 7-g
- Differentiate between scope of practice and standards of care for medical assistants, CAAHEP X.C-1, ABHES 4-f
- Report relevant information concisely and accurately, CAAHEP V.P-11, ABHES 4-a, 7-d, 7-g
- Perform diagnostic coding, CAAHEP IX.P-2, ABHES 7-d
- Utilize an EMR, CAAHEP VI.P-6, ABHES 7-b
- Document telephone messages accurately, CAAHEP V.P-7

Estimated completion time: 20 minutes

Measurable Steps

1. Click on the Find Patient icon.
2. Using the Patient Search fields, search for Amma Patel's patient record. Once you locate her in the List of Patients, confirm her date of birth.

 HELPFUL HINT

Confirming date of birth will help to ensure that you have located the correct patient record.

3. Select the radio button for Amma Patel and click the Select button. Confirm the auto-populated details in the patient header.
4. Select Phone Encounter from the left Info Panel and confirm or adjust the date and time of the call (Figure 4-170).
5. Document "Amma Patel" in the Caller field.

Coding & Billing

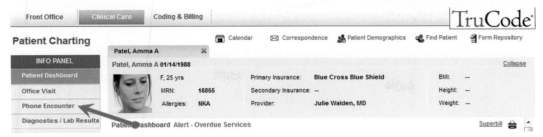

Figure 4-170 Phone Encounter from the Info Panel.

6. Confirm that the correct provider is auto-populated in the Provider field.
7. Document "Patient joined fitness center. Requests prescription with diagnosis for reimbursement of membership dues from insurance carrier. " in the Message field.

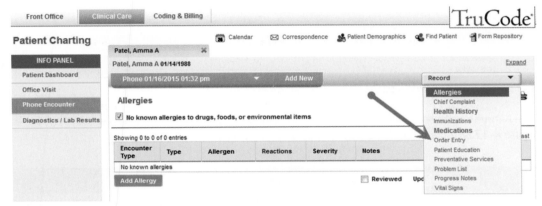

Figure 4-171 Order Entry from the Record dropdown menu.

8. Click the Save button to begin documenting in the new encounter.
9. Select Order Entry from the Record dropdown menu (Figure 4-171).
10. Select the TruCode encoder button in the top right corner. The encoder tool will open in a new tab.
11. Enter "Obesity" in the Search field and select Diagnosis, ICD-10-CM from the corresponding dropdown menu.
12. Click the Search button.
13. Click the code E66.9 that appears in red to expand this code and confirm that it is the most specific code available (Figure 4-172).
14. Copy the E66.9 code for "Obesity, unspecified" that populates in the search results (Figure 4-173).
15. Click the Add button below the Out-of-Office table to add an order.
16. In the Add Order window, select Blank Prescription from the Order dropdown menu (Figure 4-174).
17. Paste the obesity diagnosis within the body of the blank prescription template so that is available for documentation.
18. Return to the TruCode tab, enter "Hypertension" in the Search field and confirm that Diagnosis, ICD-10-CM is still displayed in the corresponding dropdown menu.
19. Click the Search button.
20. Click the code I10 to expand this code and confirm that it is the most specific code available.
21. Copy the I10 code for "Essential (primary) hypertension" that populates in the search results and paste within the body of the blank prescription template so that is available for documentation.
22. Select the checkbox for Julie Walden.
23. Document the details of the fitness order within the body of the blank prescription template, where you pasted the codes: "Patient to complete 45 minutes, weight bearing exercise 5-6 days per week". The diagnoses are obesity (E66.9), hypertension (I10).
24. Complete the Entry By and Date fields using today's date.
25. Document "Patient will pick up prescription today at 3:00 pm." in the Notes field.
26. Click the Save button. The Out-of-Office table will display the new order.

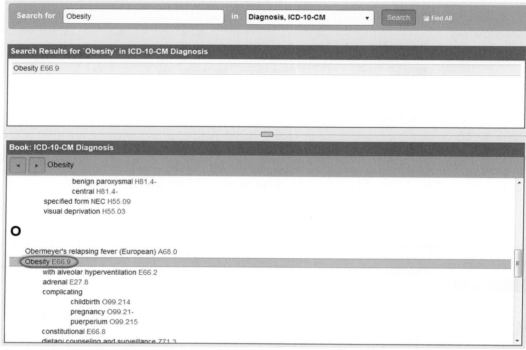

Figure 4-172 Confirm E66.9 is the most specific code available.

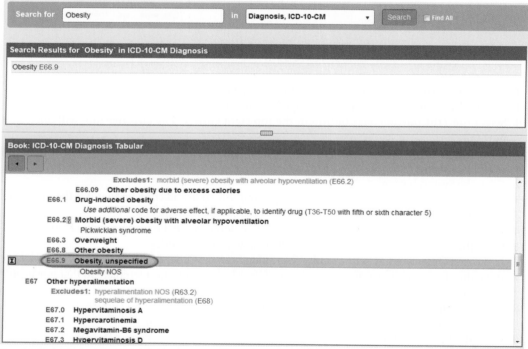

Figure 4-173 Copy the E66.9 code for "Obesity, unspecified."

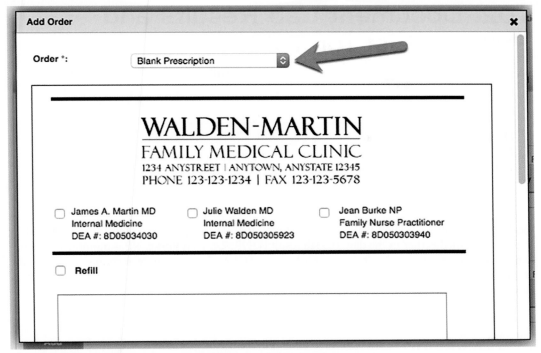

Figure 4-174 Select Blank Prescription from the Order dropdown menu.

> Now use the Back to Assignment link to complete the Post-Case Quiz found on the Info Panel for this assignment.

102. Document Lab Results and Problem List for Tai Yan

■ Objectives

- Document a phone encounter.
- Document lab results.
- Update a problem list using an encoder.

■ Overview

Sarah at University Lab called Walden-Martin today at 4:54 pm regarding a report that Tai Yan's PT/INR was obtained earlier in the day. The lab result is INR: 2.4. Jean Burke, NP is monitoring the patient on long-term anticoagulant therapy for history of CVA. Create a phone encounter to update the problem list using ICD-10 CM codes. The anticoagulant therapy and past stroke were identified on November 19, 2016. Lastly, document the INR results in the Diagnosis Lab Results grid.

■ Competencies

- Apply diagnosis/procedure codes according to current guidelines, AHIMA I.A-1, ABHES 7-d
- Analyze pathology for each body system including diagnostic and treatment measures, CAAHEP I.C-9, ABHES 2-b, 2-c
- Differentiate between normal and abnormal test results, CAAHEP II.P-2, ABHES 2-c
- Perform diagnostic coding, CAAHEP IX.P-2, ABHES 7-d
- Reassure a patient of the accuracy of the test results, CAAHEP II.A-1

Estimated completion time: 20 minutes

Measurable Steps

1. Click on the Find Patient icon.
2. Using the Patient Search fields, search for Tai Yan's patient record. Once you locate her in the List of Patients, confirm her date of birth.

 HELPFUL HINT

Confirming date of birth will help to ensure that you have located the correct patient record.

3. Select the radio button for Tai Yan and click the Select button. Confirm the auto-populated details in the patient header.
4. Select Phone Encounter from the left Info Panel and confirm or adjust the date and time of the call (Figure 4-175).
5. Document "University Lab, Sarah" in the Caller field.
6. Confirm that Jean Burke, NP is auto-populated in the Provider field.
7. Document "INR results are 2.4 for Tai Yan" in the Message field.
8. Click the Save button to begin documenting in the new encounter.
9. Select Problem List from the Record dropdown menu.
10. Click the Add Problem button to add "anticoagulant therapy" as a problem in the Diagnosis field of the Add Problem window.
11. Select the ICD-10 Code radio button and place the cursor in the text box to access the TruCode encoder. Accessing the encoder tool this way will auto-populate any selected codes where the cursor is placed.

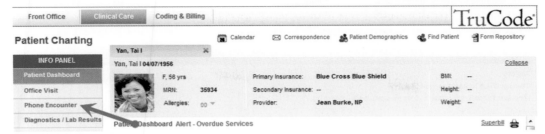

Figure 4-175 Phone Encounter from the Info Panel.

12. Enter "anticoagulant therapy" in the Search field and select Diagnosis, ICD-10-CM from the dropdown menu.
13. Click the Search button.
14. Click the code Z79.01 to expand this code and confirm that it is the most specific code available (Figure 4-176).

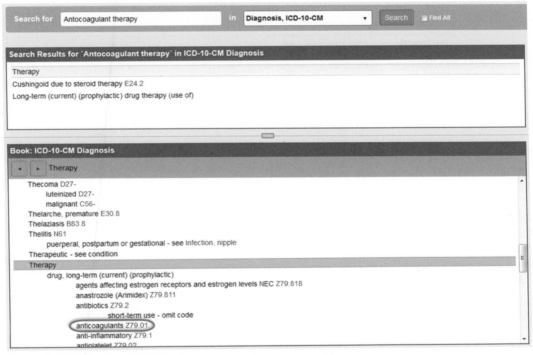

Figure 4-176 Confirm Z79.01 is the most specific code available.

15. Click the code Z79.01 for "Long term (current) use of anticoagulants" that appears in the tree. This code will auto-populate in the ICD-10 field of the Add Problem window (Figure 4-177).
16. Document "November 19, 2016" in the Date Identified field.
17. Select the Active radio button in the Status field.
18. Click the Save button. The Problem List table will display the new problem.
19. Click the Add Problem button to add "personal history of stroke" as a problem in the Diagnosis field of the Add Problem window.
20. Select the ICD-10 Code radio button and place the cursor in the text box to access the encoder. Accessing the encoder tool this way will auto-populate any selected codes where the cursor is placed.
21. Enter "personal history of stroke" in the Search field and select Diagnosis, ICD-10-CM from the dropdown menu.
22. Click the Search button.

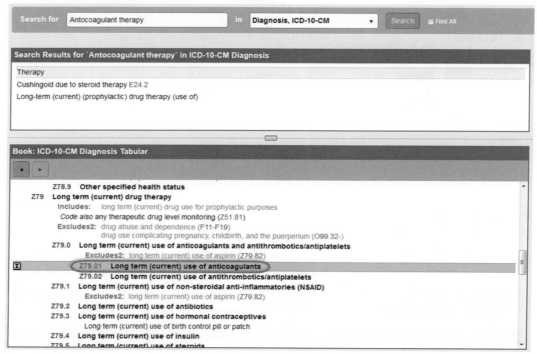

Figure 4-177 Populating the code in the ICD-10 field of the Add Problem window.

23. Click the code Z86.73 to expand this code and confirm that it is the most specific code available.
24. Click the code Z86.73 for "Personal history of transient ischemic attack (TIA), and cerebral infarction without residual deficits" that appears in the tree. This code will auto-populate in the ICD-10 field of the Add Problem window.
25. Select the Active radio button in the Status field.
26. Click the Save button. The Problem List table will display the new problem.
27. Click Diagnostics/Lab Results in the left Info Panel.
28. Click the Add button below the Diagnostics/Lab Results table.
29. Use the calendar picker to document today's date in the Date field.
30. Select Path/Lab from the Type dropdown menu.
31. Document "University Lab; INR: 2.4" in the Notes field.
32. Click the Save button.

 Now use the Back to Assignment link to complete the Post-Case Quiz found on the Info Panel for this assignment.

103. Generate Phone Message and Radiology Order for Ken Thomas

■ **Objectives**

- Complete a phone message.
- Locate an ICD-10 CM code using an encoder.
- Generate a radiology order.

■ **Overview**

Ken Thomas recently visited a chiropractor who recommended that Dr. Martin order an x-ray of the lumbar spine in order to best evaluate the cause of low back pain resulting from a fall down an embankment. Ken Thomas calls the office today at 9:32 am to ask if Dr. Martin would be willing to order this procedure for him. Document this phone message for Dr. Martin using the correspondence repository.

Shortly after the medical assistant finishes the phone message, Dr. Martin approves the lumbar x-ray order. Generate a radiology requisition for Ken Thomas to be performed this Monday. No authorization number is needed and it is a routine study. Use the encoder to generate the ICD-10 CM diagnosis code and the external causes code.

■ **Competencies**

- Analyze pathology for each body system including diagnostic and treatment measures, CAA-HEP I.C-9, ABHES 2-b, 2-c
- Apply diagnosis/procedure codes according to current guidelines, AHIMA I.A-1, ABHES 7-d
- Demonstrate professional telephone techniques, CAAHEP V.P-6, ABHES 7-g
- Identify critical information required for scheduling patient procedures, CAAHEP VI.C-3, ABHES 7-e
- Perform diagnostic coding, CAAHEP IX.P-2, ABHES 7-d
- Relate assertive, aggressive, and passive behaviors to professional communication, CAAHEP V.C-14, ABHES 5-h, 7-g
- Report relevant information concisely and accurately, CAAHEP V.P-11, ABHES 7-g
- Document telephone messages accurately, CAAHEP V.P-7

Estimated completion time: 20 minutes

Measurable Steps

1. Click on the Correspondence icon.
2. Select Phone Messages from the left Info Panel.
3. Use the Patient Search button to perform a patient search and assign the message to Ken Thomas after confirming his date of birth.

HELPFUL HINT

Confirming date of birth will help to ensure that you have located the correct patient record.

4. Document today's date in the Date field.
5. Document "09:32 am" in the Time field.
6. Document "Ken Thomas" in the Caller field.
7. Document "Dr. Martin" in the Provider field.
8. Select the Request checkbox (Figure 4-178).

Coding & Billing

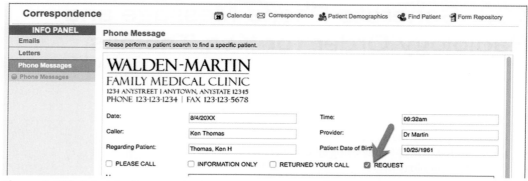

Figure 4-178 Select the Request checkbox before typing in the Message field.

9. Document the request for lumbar spine x-ray order in the Message field.
10. Document your name in the Completed By field and document today's date and time in the Date/Time field.
11. Click the Save to Patient Record button. Confirm the date and click OK.
12. Click the Form Repository icon.
13. Select Requisition from the Patient Forms section of the left Info Panel.
14. Select Radiology from the Requisition Type dropdown menu.
15. Click the Patient Search button to perform a patient search and assign the form to Ken Thomas.

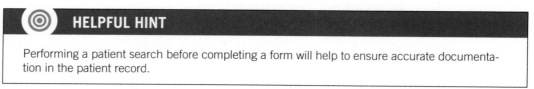

HELPFUL HINT

Performing a patient search before completing a form will help to ensure accurate documentation in the patient record.

16. Document this Monday's date in the Service Date field.
17. Document "James A. Martin, MD" in the Ordering Physician field.
18. Document "Low back pain" in the first Diagnosis field.
19. Place the cursor in the Diagnosis Code field to access the encoder. Accessing the encoder tool this way will auto-populate any selected codes where the cursor is placed.
20. Enter "Low back pain" in the Search field and select Diagnosis, ICD-10-CM from the dropdown menu.
21. Click the Search button.
22. Click the code M54.5 to expand this code and confirm that it is the most specific code available.
23. Click the yellow information icon to the left of the code to view the instructional notes, which mention the external cause of the code is also required for this diagnosis (Figure 4-179).
24. Click the code M54.5 for "Low back pain" that appears in the tree. This code will auto-populate in the ICD-10 field of the Add Problem window.
25. Document "Fall down embankment" in the second diagnosis field.
26. Place the cursor in the Diagnosis Code field to access the encoder. Accessing the encoder tool this way will auto-populate any selected codes where the cursor is placed.
27. Enter "Fall embankment" in the Search field and select External Cause, ICD-10-CM from the dropdown menu.
28. Click the Search button.
29. Click the code W17.81 to expand this code. Then, maximize the list of additional codes beneath this code by clicking the black triangle to the left of the code.
30. Select A for initial encounter (Figure 4-180). The code will auto-populate in the requisition form.
31. Select Spine under the X-ray column and document "Lumbar" in the corresponding field.
32. Select the Routine radio button at the bottom of the form to indicate that the exam is routine.
33. Click the Save to Patient Record button. Confirm the date and click OK.

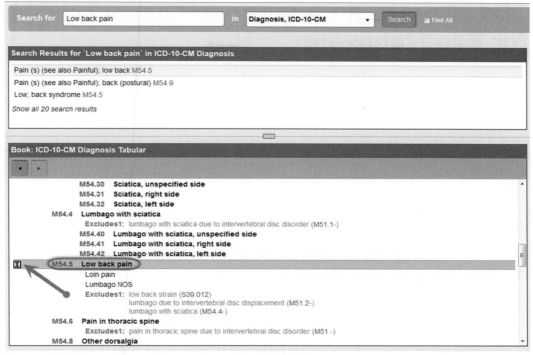

Figure 4-179 The yellow information icon to the left of the code.

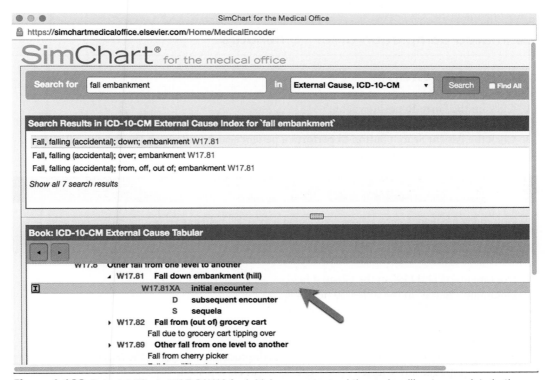

Figure 4-180 Select A [Code W17.81XA] for initial encounter and the code will auto-populate in the requisition form.

⊛ Now use the Back to Assignment link to complete the Post-Case Quiz found on the Info Panel for this assignment.

104. Create an Insurance Claim Tracer for Ella Rainwater

■ **Objectives**

- Complete an insurance claim tracer.

■ **Overview**

Amy, the medical coding specialist is reviewing outstanding claims from 11/15/2014. She notices that a claim for date of service 11/14/2014 on behalf of Ella Rainwater has yet to be approved. The claim was sent to Aetna. Her husband, Marcus Rainwater, is the insured on the account and the claim tracking number is MTH1119. The procedure performed is for a 12 lead ECG with interruption for the diagnosis of palpitations. The amount billed for the ECG is $89.00. Create an insurance claim tracer for Mrs. Rainwater.

■ **Competencies**

- Identify information required to file a third party claim, CAAHEP VIII.C-1b, ABHES 7-d
- Utilize software in the completion of HIM processes, AHIMA III.A-1, ABHES 7-b
- Utilize an EMR, CAAHEP VI.P-6, ABHES 7-b
- Interpret information on an insurance card, CAAHEP VIII.P-1

Estimated completion time: 15 minutes

Measurable Steps

1. Click on the Form Repository icon.
2. Select Insurance Claim Tracer from the Patient Forms section of the left Info Panel.
3. Click the Patient Search button to perform a patient search and assign the form to Ella Rainwater. Confirm the auto-populated details.

 HELPFUL HINT

Performing a patient search before completing a form will help to ensure accurate documentation in the patient record.

4. Document "MTH1119" in the Claim # field.
5. Document "Aetna" in the Billed To field.
6. Document "Amy" in the Contact Person field.
7. Document "Marcus Rainwater" in the Insured field.
8. Document "11/14/2014" in the Date(s) of Service column.
9. Place the cursor in the Procedure field to access the encoder. Accessing the encoder tool this way will auto-populate any selected codes where the cursor is placed.
10. Enter "ECG" in the Search field and select CPT Tabular from the dropdown menu.
11. Click the Search button.
12. Click the code 93000 for "Electrocardiogram, routine ECG with at least 12 leads, with interpretation and report". This code will auto-populate in the Procedure field (Figure 4-181).
13. Document "12 Lead ECG, with interpretation and report" in the Description field.
14. Place the cursor in the Diagnosis field to access the encoder. Accessing the encoder tool this way will auto-populate any selected codes where the cursor is placed.

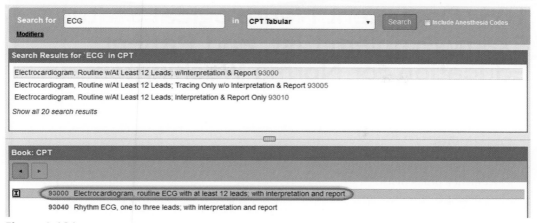

Figure 4-181 Populating the code in the Procedure field.

15. Enter "palpitations" in the Search field and select Diagnosis, ICD-10-CM from the dropdown menu.
16. Click the Search button.
17. Click the code R00.2 for "Palpitations (heart)" to expand this code and confirm that it is the most specific code available.
18. Click the code R00.2 for "Palpitations". This code will auto-populate in the Diagnosis field.
19. Document "11/14/14" in the Date Billed column.
20. Document "89.00" in the Amount column.
21. Document "89.00" in the Total field.
22. Click the Save to Patient Record button (Figure 4-182). Confirm the date and click OK.

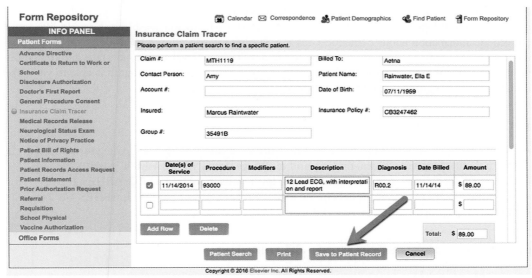

Figure 4-182 Click the Save to Patient Record button.

23. Click on the Find Patient icon.
24. Using the Patient Search fields, search for Ella Rainwater's patient record. Once you locate her in the List of Patients, confirm her date of birth.
25. Select the form from the Forms section of the Patient Dashboard. The form will open in a new window.

 Now use the Back to Assignment link to complete the Post-Case Quiz found on the Info Panel for this assignment.

105. Document Neurological Status Exam, Problem List, and Patient Education for Norma Washington

■ Objectives

- Document a neurological status exam.
- Document a problem list.
- Document patient education.

■ Overview

Norma Washington presents to the office complaining of memory loss that has progressively gotten worse over the past 2 months. Although her daughter usually accompanies her during doctor visits, Norma Washington is at the office alone today. Dr. Martin would like you to perform a neurological status exam on the patient. The medical assistant documents the following sections of the exam:

- Sequencing: Patient is not able to repeat exact statement. Document Incorrect. (Total 0)
- Time Orientation: Patient identified the correct date and day of week. Patient had an incorrect response for season. (Total 2)
- Drawing: Patient was unable to draw ladder with 6 rungs. Document Incorrect. (Total 0)
- Information: Patient is able to name the president and stars on the flag. (Total 2)
- Recall: Patient is unable to recall previous sentence elements. Document Incorrect. (Total 0)
- Total Exam Score: 4.

After consulting with the neurologist, Dr. Martin agrees with the assessment of Alzheimer's disease, early onset. Update the problem list using ICD-10 CM. Norma Washington would like some additional information about Alzheimer's disease. During the education intervention explanation and discussion, the medical assistant identifies the age/development level, emotional state, and time limitations as learning barriers. The medical assistant notes that Norma Washington is able to verbalize understanding. Document patient education for Norma Washington.

■ Competencies

- Analyze the documentation in the health record to ensure it supports the diagnosis and reflects the patient's progress, clinical finding, and discharge status, AHIMA I.B-1, ABHES 2-c, 7-b
- Differentiate between normal and abnormal test results, CAAHEP II.P-2, ABHES 2-c
- Document patient care accurately in the medical record, CAAHEP X.P-3, ABHES 4-a, 7-b
- Perform diagnostic coding, CAAHEP IX.P-2, ABHES 7-d

Estimated completion time: 35 minutes

Measurable Steps

1. Click on the Form Repository icon.
2. Select Neurological Status Exam from the left Info Panel.
3. Click the Patient Search button to assign the form to Norma Washington. Skip the Caregiver Questions section since no caregiver was present.
4. In the Sequencing section, select the No radio button to indicate that Norma Washington is not able to repeat the exact statement and document "0" in the Total field.
5. In the Time Orientation section, select the Correct radio buttons to indicate that Norma Washington identified the correct date and day of week and select the Incorrect radio button to indicate that Norma Washington did not identify the correct season. Document "2" in the Total field.

6. In the Drawing section, select the Incorrect radio button to indicate that Norma Washington was unable to draw the ladder with six rungs. Document "0" in the Total field.
7. In the Information section, select the Correct radio buttons to indicate that Norma Washington was able to name the president and state the number of stars on the American flag. Document "2" in the Total field (Figure 4-183).

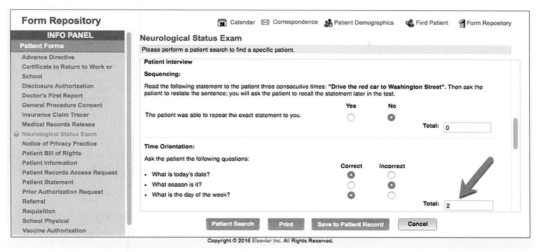

Figure 4-183 Document the answers to the questions in the Time Orientation section, and then document "2" in the Total field.

8. In the Recall section, select the Incorrect radio buttons to indicate that Norma Washington is unable repeat any of the words. Document "0" in the Total field.
9. Document "4" in the Total Exam Score field.
10. Click the Save to Patient Record button. Confirm the date and click OK.
11. Click on the Find Patient icon.
12. Using the Patient Search fields, search for Norma Washington's patient record. Once you locate her in the List of Patients, confirm her date of birth.

> ◎ **HELPFUL HINT**
>
> Confirming a patient's date of birth will help to ensure that you have located the correct patient record.

13. Select the radio button for Norma Washington and click the Select button.
14. Select Office Visit from the left Info Panel and click Add New.
15. In the Create New Encounter window, select Follow-Up/Established Visit from the Visit Type dropdown.
16. Select James A. Martin, MD from the Provider dropdown.
17. Click the Save button.
18. Select Problem List from the Record dropdown menu (Figure 4-184).
19. Click the Add Problem button to add "Alzheimer's disease" as a problem in the Diagnosis field of the Add Problem window.
20. In the Add Problem window, document "Alzheimer disease" in the Diagnosis field.
21. Select the ICD-10 Code radio button and place the cursor in the Diagnosis Code field to access the TruCode encoder. Accessing the encoder tool this way will auto-populate any selected codes where the cursor is placed.
22. Enter "Alzheimer's disease, early onset" in the Search field and select Diagnosis, ICD-10-CM from the dropdown menu.
23. Click the Search button.
24. Click the code G30.0 to expand this code and confirm that it is the most specific code available.

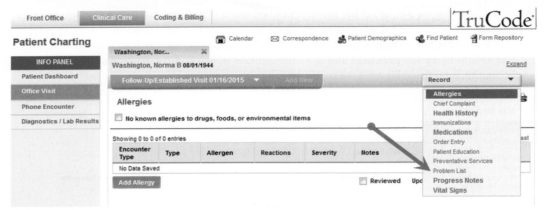

Figure 4-184 Problem List from the Record dropdown menu.

25. Click the code G30.0 for "Alzheimer's disease with early onset" that appears in the tree. This code will auto-populate in the ICD-10 field of the Add Problem window. Then click the code F02.80.
26. Document the current date in the Date Identified field.
27. Select the Active radio button in the Status field.
28. Click the Save button. The Problem List table will display the new problem (Figure 4-185).

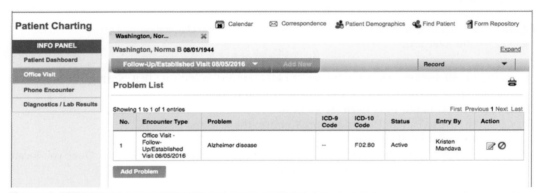

Figure 4-185 The Problem List will display the new problem.

29. Select Patient Education from the Record dropdown menu.
30. Select Diagnosis from the Category dropdown menu.
31. Select Nervous System from the Subcategory dropdown menu.
32. Select the Alzheimer's disease checkbox in the Teaching Topics field.
33. Select the Patient checkbox in the Persons Taught field.
34. Select Verbal Explanation and Discussion in the Teaching Methods field.
35. Select Age/Developmental Level, Emotional/Mental State, and Time Limitations in the Learning Barriers field.
36. Select Verbalizes Understanding in the Outcome field.
37. Click the Save button. This teaching topic will move from the New tab to the Saved tab.
38. Expand the accordion of the saved patient education category to view and print the handout.

⊛ Now use the Back to Assignment link to complete the Post-Case Quiz found on the Info Panel for this assignment.

Coding & Billing

106. Generate a Prior Authorization for Ken Thomas

■ **Objectives**

- Create a prior authorization for testing using the encoder.

■ **Overview**

Ken Thomas has been having some significant issues with the great toe of his left foot. Jean Burke, NP has diagnosed Ken Thomas with an ingrowing toenail. She is recommending that he have the toenail removed. Ken Thomas wants to be sure that his insurance carrier will pay for this procedure before he has it done. The procedure, nail removal w/matrix, would be performed at Walden-Martin Family Medical Clinic, 1234 Anystreet in Anytown, AL 12345-1234. Jean Burke would like it performed within the next two weeks. The procedure is not related to injury and the authorization number is AAX3638. The effective date is today and authorization will expire in 30 days. As the provider contact, generate a prior authorization request for this procedure.

■ **Competencies**

- Obtain precertification or preauthorization including documentation, CAAHEP VIII.P-3, ABHES 7-d
- Perform procedural coding, CAAHEP IX.P-1, ABHES 7-d
- Perform diagnostic coding, CAAHEP IX.P-2, ABHES 7-d
- Verify eligibility for managed care services, CAAHEP VIII.P-2, ABHES 7-d

Estimated completion time: 15 minutes

Measurable Steps

1. Click on the Form Repository icon.
2. Select Prior Authorization Request from the Patient Forms section of the left Info Panel.
3. Click the Patient Search button to perform a patient search and assign the form to Ken Thomas. Confirm the auto-populated details.

 HELPFUL HINT

Performing a patient search before completing a form will help to ensure accurate documentation in the patient record.

4. Document "Jean Burke, NP" in the Ordering Physician field.
5. Document your name in the Provider Contact Name field.
6. Document "Walden-Martin Family Medical Clinic 1234 Anystreet Anytown AL 12345-1234" in the Place of Service/Treatment and Address field.
7. Document "Nail removal with matrix" in the Service Requested field.
8. Document "1" in the Service Frequency field
9. Place the cursor in the Diagnosis/ICD Code field to access the encoder. Accessing the encoder this way will auto-populate any selected codes where the cursor is placed.
10. Enter "Ingrowing nail" in the Search field and select Diagnosis, ICD-10-CM from the dropdown menu.
11. Click the Search button.
12. Click the code L60.0 to expand this code and confirm that it is the most specific code available.

13. Click the code L60.0 for "Ingrowing nail" that appears in the tree. This code will auto-populate in the ICD-10 field of the Add Problem window (Figure 4-186).

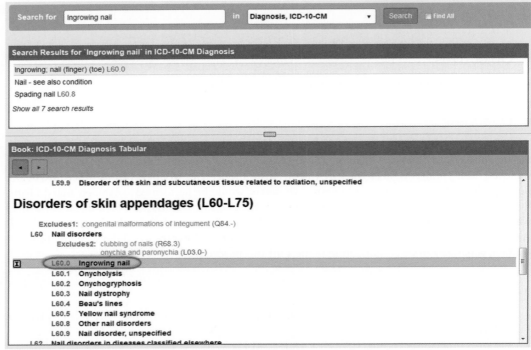

Figure 4-186 Populating the code in the Diagnosis field.

14. Place the cursor in the Procedure/CPT Code(s) field to access the encoder and click the TruCode icon to search for the CPT code.
15. Enter "Nail removal" in the Search field and select CPT Tabular from the dropdown menu.
16. Click the Search button.
17. Click the code 11750 for "Excision of nail and nail matrix, partial or complete, (eg, ingrown or deformed nail) for permanent removal". This code will auto-populate in the Procedure/CPT Code(s) field (Figure 4-187).

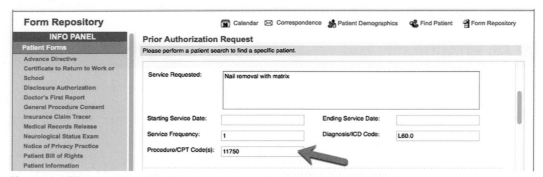

Figure 4-187 The CPT code will auto-populate in the Procedure/CPT(s) field.

18. Within the Prior Authorization Request form, click the No radio buttons to indicate that this procedure is not related to injury or Workers' Compensation.
19. Document "AAX3638" in the Authorization Number field, today's date in the Effective Date field, and the date 30 days from now in the Expiration Date field.
20. Click on the Save to Patient Record button. Confirm the date and click OK.
21. Click on the Find Patient icon.

22. Using the Patient Search fields, search for Ken Thomas's patient record. Once you locate him in the List of Patients, confirm his date of birth.
23. Select the radio button for Ken Thomas and click the Select button. Confirm the auto-populated details.
24. Select the form from the Forms section of the Patient Dashboard. The form will open in a new window.

 Now use the Back to Assignment link to complete the Post-Case Quiz found on the Info Panel for this assignment.

107. Update Medication Record and Problem List for Ken Thomas

■ Objectives

- Update the medication record.
- Update the problem list using an encoder.
- Document lab results.

■ Overview

Ken Thomas has recently started taking levothyroxine tablets once daily for hypothyroidism on July 17, 2014. Bloodwork performed on July 14, 2014 showed a TSH: 6.0 (Reference range 0.5-5.0). Update the medication list and problem list, then document the lab results in the Diagnostic/Lab Results tab.

■ Competencies

- Document patient care accurately in the medical record, CAAHEP X.P-3, ABHES 4-a
- Maintain laboratory test results using flow sheets, CAAHEP II.P-3, ABHES 4-a
- Maintain medication and immunization records, ABHES 4-a, 7-b
- Perform diagnostic coding, CAAHEP IX.P-2, ABHES 7-d
- Utilize an EMR, CAAHEP VI.P-6, ABHES 7-b

Estimated completion time: 20 minutes

Measurable Steps

1. Click on the Find Patient icon.
2. Using the Patient Search fields, search for Ken Thomas's patient record. Once you locate him in the List of Patients, confirm his date of birth.

 HELPFUL HINT

Confirming a patient's date of birth will help to ensure that you have located the correct patient record.

3. Select the radio button for Ken Thomas and click the Select button.
4. Select Office Visit from the left Info Panel.
5. In the Create New Encounter window, select Follow-Up/Established Visit from the Visit Type dropdown.
6. Click the Save button.
7. Select Problem List from the Record dropdown menu (Figure 4-188).
8. Click the Add Problem button to add "Hypothyroidism" as a problem in the Diagnosis field of the Add Problem window.
9. Select the ICD-10 Code radio button, place the cursor in the Diagnosis Code box to access the TruCode encoder.
10. Enter "Hypothyroidism" in the Search field and select Diagnosis, ICD-10-CM from the drop-down menu.
11. Click the Search button.
12. Click the code E03.9 to expand this code and confirm that it is the most specific code available (Figure 4-189).

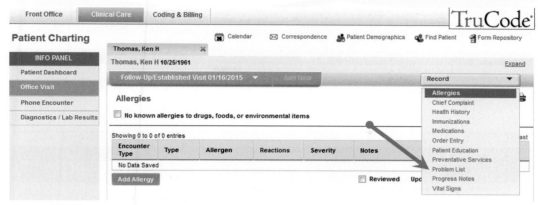

Figure 4-188 Problem List from the Record dropdown menu.

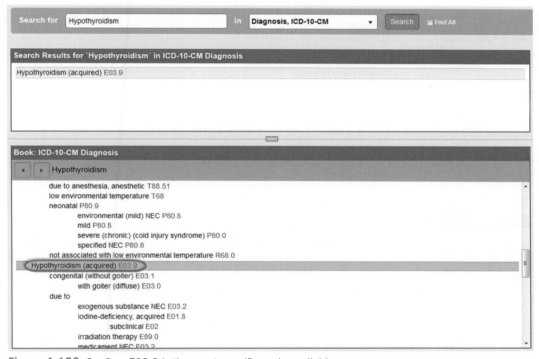

Figure 4-189 Confirm E03.9 is the most specific code available.

13. Click the code E03.9 for "Hypothyroidism, unspecified" that appears in the tree. This code will auto-populate in the ICD-10 field of the Add Problem window (Figure 4-190).
14. Document July 14, 2014 in the Date Identified field.
15. Select the Active radio button in the Status field.
16. Click the Save button. The Problem List table will display the new problem.
17. Select Medications from the Record dropdown menu.
18. Within the Prescription Medications tab, click the Add Medication button to add Levothyroxine to Ken Thomas's medications. An Add Medication window will appear.
19. Select Levothyroxine (T4) Tablet - (Synthroid, Unithroid) from the Medication dropdown menu or start typing the medication in the field.
20. Select 12.5 from the Strength dropdown.
21. Select Tablet from the Form dropdown.
22. Select Oral from the Route dropdown.
23. Select Daily from the Frequency dropdown.
24. Use the calendar picker to document "July 14, 2014" in the Start Date field.
25. Document "Hypothyroidism" in the Indication field.
26. Select the Active radio button in the Status field.

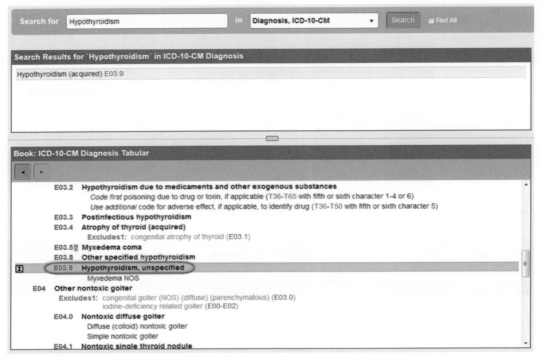

Figure 4-190 Populating the code in the ICD-10 field of the Add Problem window.

27. Click the Save button. The Medications table will display the new medication (Figure 4-191).

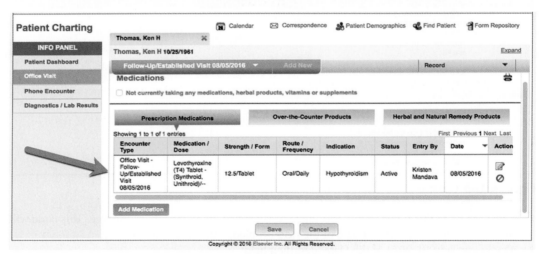

Figure 4-191 The Medications table will display the new medication.

28. Click Diagnostics/Lab Results in the left Info Panel.
29. Click the Add button below the Diagnostics/Lab Results table.
30. Use the calendar picker to document July 14, 2014 in the Date field.
31. Select Path/Lab from the Type dropdown menu.
32. Document results "TSH: 60 (Reference Range 0.5 - 5.0)" in the Notes field.
33. Click the Save button.

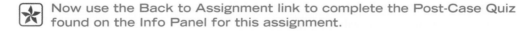 Now use the Back to Assignment link to complete the Post-Case Quiz found on the Info Panel for this assignment.

108. Generate Laboratory Orders for Ken Thomas

■ Objectives

- Generate laboratory orders.

■ Overview

Jean Burke, NP has ordered some laboratory testing for Ken Thomas. Due to his primary hypothyroidism, a TSH, T4 Free, and T3 Free should be completed in one month. The laboratory tests are not fasting and are routine. Generate a lab requisition.

■ Competencies

- Assist provider with a patient exam, CAAHEP I.P-9, ABHES 8-c, 8-d
- Coach patients regarding treatment plan, CAAHEP V.P-4d, ABHES 5-c, 8-h
- Identify critical information required for scheduling patient procedures, CAAHEP VI.C-3, ABHES 7-e
- Perform diagnostic coding, CAAHEP IX.P-2, ABHES 7-d

Estimated completion time: 20 minutes

Measurable Steps

1. Click on the Form Repository icon.
2. Select Requisition from the Patient Forms section of the left Info Panel.
3. Select Laboratory from the Requisition Type dropdown menu.
4. Click the Patient Search button to assign the form to Ken Thomas (Figure 4-192). Confirm the auto-populated patient demographics.

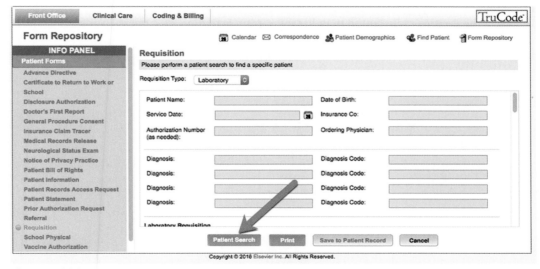

Figure 4-192 Click the Patient Search button to assign the form to Ken Thomas.

5. In the Diagnosis field, document "Primary Hypothyroidism".
6. Place the cursor in the Diagnosis Code field, click the TruCode icon to search for the ICD-10 code.
7. Enter "Primary Hypothyroidism" in the Search field and select Diagnosis, ICD-10-CM from the dropdown menu.
8. Click the Search button.
9. Click the code E03.9 to expand this code and confirm that it is the most specific node available (Figure 4-193).

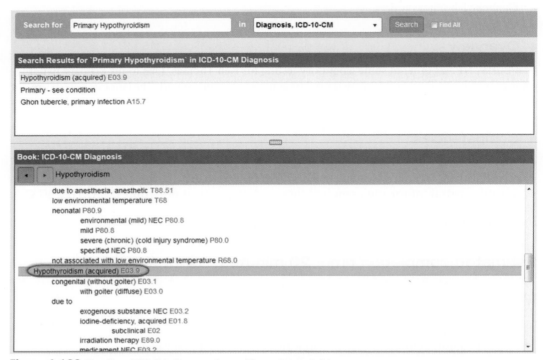

Figure 4-193 Confirm E03.9 is the most specific code available.

10. Click the code E03.9 for "Hypothyroidism, unspecified" that appears in the tree. The code will auto-populate in the Diagnosis Code field of the requisition form (Figure 4-194).
11. In the Laboratory field, select the checkbox for TSH, T3 Free, and T4 Free.
12. Select the Routine radio button to indicate the exam is routine. Document "Not fasting, due in one month" in the Patient Preparation field.
13. Click the Save to Patient Record button. Confirm the date and click OK.

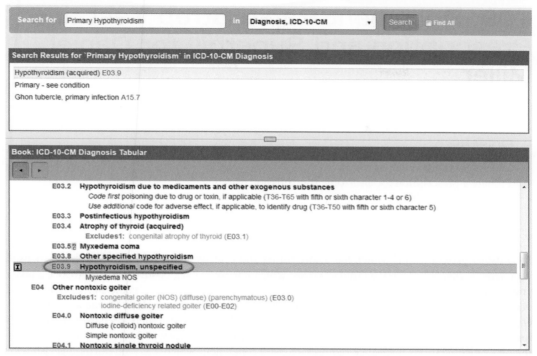

Figure 4-194 Populating the code in the Diagnosis Code field of the requisition form.

Now use the Back to Assignment link to complete the Post-Case Quiz found on the Info Panel for this assignment.

109. Document Rapid Strep Test and Prescription and Superbill for Daniel Miller

■ Objectives

- Document rapid strep test results.
- Prepare a prescription for electronic transmission.
- Complete a superbill.

■ Overview

Established patient Daniel Miller, has a sore throat and is at Walden-Martin for a problem-focused visit. Jean Burke, NP ordered a rapid strep test which has come back positive for streptococcal pharyngitis. The rapid strep was not sent for culture. As a result, Nurse Burke would like to start Daniel on Augmentin Suspension 200 mg/5 ml, by mouth twice daily for seven days. Create an urgent visit encounter and document the rapid strep performed during the visit. Then, prepare a prescription for Jean Burke's approval to send electronically to Anytown Pharmacy and complete a superbill for the office visit. Daniel's insurance requires a $25.00 copayment which was paid during his visit with a check.

■ Competencies

- Apply diagnosis/procedure codes according to current guidelines, AHIMA I.A-1, ABHES 7-d
- Describe the relationship between the anatomy and physiology of all body systems and medication used for treatment in each, AHIMA I.C-12, ABHES 2-a, 2-c, 6-a
- Explain the rationale for performing a procedure to the patient AHIMA III.A-2, ABHES 5-c, 5-h, 8-h
- Perform diagnostic coding, CAAHEP IX.P-2, ABHES 7-d
- Utilize an EMR, CAAHEP VI.P-6, ABHES 7-b

Estimated completion time: 35 minutes

Measurable Steps

1. Click on the Find Patient icon.
2. Using the Patient Search fields, search for Daniel Miller's patient record. Once you locate him in the List of Patients, confirm his date of birth.

 HELPFUL HINT

Confirming a patient's date of birth will help to ensure that you have located the correct patient record.

3. Select the radio button for Daniel Miller and click the Select button.
4. Select Office Visit from the left Info Panel.
5. In the Create New Encounter window, select Urgent Visit from the Visit Type dropdown.
6. Select Jean Burke, NP in the Provider dropdown.
7. Click the Save button.
8. Select Order Entry from the Record dropdown menu (Figure 4-195).
9. Click the Add button below the In-Office table to add an order.
10. In the Add Order window, select Rapid Strep Test from the Order dropdown menu.

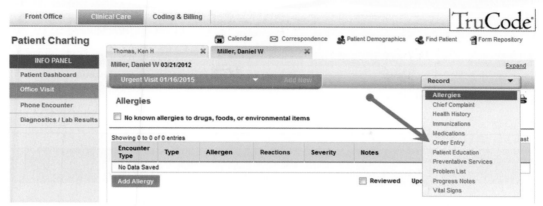

Figure 4-195 Order Entry from the Record dropdown menu.

11. Document Positive as the result. Document No in the Sent for Culture field (Figure 4-196). Click the Save button. The In-Office table will display the new order.

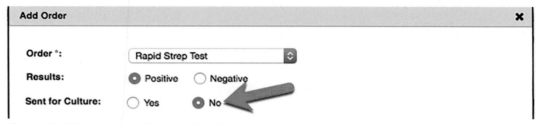

Figure 4-196 Document No in the Sent for Culture field.

12. Select the TruCode encoder button in the top right corner. The encoder tool will open in a new tab.
13. Enter "Streptococcal pharyngitis" in the Search field and select Diagnosis, ICD-10-CM from the dropdown menu.
14. Click the Search button.
15. Click the code J02.0 to expand this code and confirm that it is the most specific code available.
16. Copy the J02.0 code for "Streptococcal pharyngitis" that populates in the search results (Figure 4-197).
17. Click the Add button below the Out-of-Office table to add an order.
18. In the Add Order window, select Medication Prescription from the Order dropdown menu.
19. Indicate the provider by clicking in the box next to Jean Burke NP.
20. Paste the diagnosis from the encoder tool in the Diagnosis field.
21. Document "Augmentin Suspension" in the Drug field.
22. Document "Anytown Pharmacy" in the Pharmacy field.
23. Document "200 mg/5 ml" in the Strength field.
24. Document "suspension" in the Form field.
25. Document "oral" in the Route field.
26. Document "0" in the Refills field.
27. Document "Every 12 hours" in the Directions field.
28. Document "7" in the Days Supply field.
29. Select the Electronic transfer radio button and document the date in the Date field.
30. Click the Save button. The Out-of-Office table will display the new order.
31. Select Problem List from the Record dropdown menu.
32. Click the Add Problem button to add "Streptococcal pharyngitis" as a problem in the Diagnosis field of the Add Problem window.
33. Select the ICD-10 Code radio button and place the cursor in the text field to access the TruCode encoder. Accessing the encoder tool this way will auto-populate any selected codes where the cursor is placed.
34. Enter "Streptococcal pharyngitis" in the Search field and select ICD-10-CM from the dropdown menu.

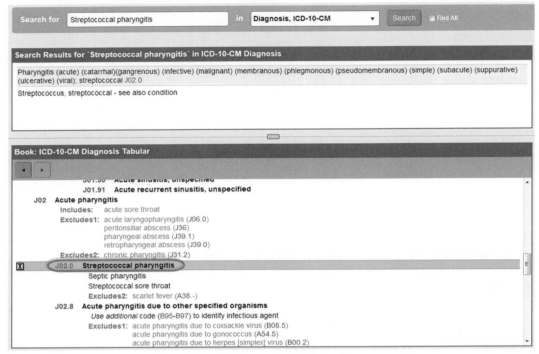

Figure 4-197 Copy the J02.0 code for "Streptococcal pharyngitis"

35. Click the Search button.
36. Click the code J02.0 to expand this code and confirm that it is the most specific code available.
37. Click the code J02.0 for "Streptococcal pharyngitis" that appears in the tree. This code will auto-populate in the ICD-10 field of the Add Problem window.
38. Select the Active radio button in the Status field.
39. Click the Save button. The problem list will display the new problem.
40. Select Medications from the Record dropdown menu.
41. On the Prescription Medications tab click the Add Medication button.
42. Select Amoxicillin/Clavulanate potassium Oral Suspension - (Augmentin ES Suspension, Augmentin Suspension) from the Medication dropdown menu.
43. Document "200 mg/5 ml" in the Strength field.
44. Select Suspension from the Form dropdown menu.
45. Select Oral from the Route dropdown menu.
46. Select Every 12 Hours from the Frequency dropdown menu.
47. Document the current date in the Start Date field.
48. Document "Streptococcal pharyngitis" in the Indication field.
49. Select the Active radio button in the Status field.
50. Click the Save button. The Medication window will display the new medication.
51. Click the Patient Dashboard.
52. After reviewing the details of the encounter, click the Superbill link below the Patient Dashboard.
53. Select the correct encounter from the Encounters Not Coded table and confirm the auto-populated details.
54. On page one of the superbill, select the ICD-10 radio button.
55. In the Rank 1 row of the Diagnoses box, place the cursor in the Diagnosis Code field to access the encoder.

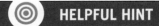

HELPFUL HINT

The View Progress Notes and View Fee Schedule links in the top right corner of the superbill provide information necessary in completing the superbill.

Coding & Billing

56. Enter "Streptococcal pharyngitis" in the Search field and select Diagnosis ICD-10-CM from the dropdown menu.
57. Click the Search button.
58. Click the code J02.0 to expand this code and confirm that it is the most specific code available.
59. Click the code J02.0 for "Streptocooccal pharyngitis" that appears in the tree. This code will auto-populate in the Rank 1 row of the Diagnoses box.
60. Document "1" in the Rank column for Problem Focused office visit. Select the View Fee Schedule link to obtain the charges and code.
61. Enter "32.00" in the fee column and "99212" in the Est column for the Problem-Focused Office visit.
62. Click the Save button and then go to page three of the superbill.
63. Document "2" in the Rank column for Strep, rapid. View the Fee Schedule to obtain the charges and code.
64. Enter "21.00" in the Fee column and "87880" in the Code column for Strep, rapid (Figure 4-198).

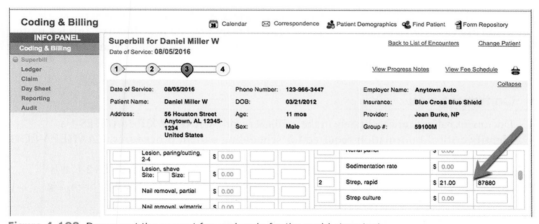

Figure 4-198 Document the correct fee and code for the rapid strep test.

65. Click the Save button and then go to page four of the superbill.
66. On page four, document "25.00" in the Copay field.
67. Confirm that the total in the Today's Charges field has populated correctly.
68. Document "28.00" in the Balance Due field.
69. Fill out additional fields as needed.
70. Select the I am ready to submit the Superbill checkbox at the bottom of the screen.
71. Select the Yes radio button to indicate that the signature is on file.
72. Document the date in the Date field.
73. Click the Submit Superbill button. A confirmation message will appear.

 Now use the Back to Assignment link to complete the Post-Case Quiz found on the Info Panel for this assignment.

110. Document Preventive Services and Generate an Order for Screening Mammogram for Celia Tapia

■ Objectives

- Generate a requisition.
- Update preventive services.

■ Overview

During Celia Tapia's wellness visit, Dr. Martin notices she is overdue for preventive services. Dr. Martin would like Celia Tapia to have a screening bilateral mammogram next Tuesday. This is a routine procedure. Generate the radiology order for the screening bilateral mammogram and update the preventive services record to include this procedure.

■ Competencies

- Document patient care accurately in the medical record, CAAHEP X.P-3, ABHES 4-a
- Identify critical information required for scheduling patient procedures, CAAHEP VI.C-3, ABHES 7-e
- Perform patient screening using established protocols, CAAHEP I.P-3, ABHES 2-b, 8-b
- Report relevant information concisely and accurately, CAAHEP V.P-11, ABHES 4-a, 7-g

Estimated completion time: 20 minutes

Measurable Steps

1. Click on the Form Repository icon.
2. Select Requisition from the left Info Panel.
3. Select Radiology from the Requisition Type dropdown menu.
4. Click the Patient Search button to assign the form to Celia Tapia. Confirm the auto-populated patient demographics.
5. In the Diagnosis field, document "Screening for Breast Neoplasm".
6. Place the cursor in the Diagnosis Code field to access the TruCode encoder. Accessing the encoder tool this way will auto-populate any selected codes where the cursor is placed.
7. Enter "Mammogram" in the Search field and select Diagnosis, ICD-10-CM from the dropdown menu.
8. Click the Search button.
9. Click the code Z12.39 for "Encounter for other screening for malignant neoplasm of breast" that appears in the tree (Figure 4-199).
10. This code will auto-populate in the requisition (Figure 4-200).
11. In the Women Imaging section, select the correct checkbox for Screening Mammogram.
12. Click the Save to Patient Record button. Confirm the date and click OK.
13. Click on the Find Patient icon.
14. Using the Patient Search fields, search for Celia Tapia's patient record. Once you locate her in the List of Patients, confirm her date of birth.

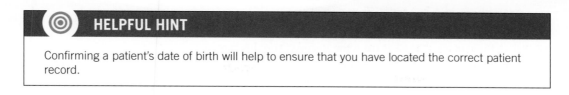
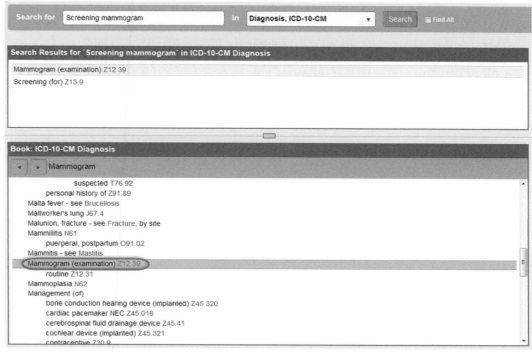

Figure 4-199 Click Z12.39 to view additional details about the code.

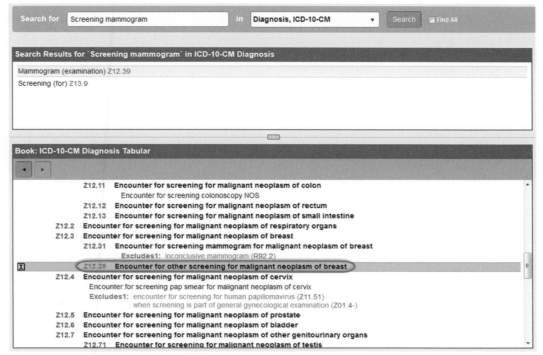

Figure 4-200 Populating the code in the Requisition.

15. Select the radio button for Celia Tapia and click the Select button.
16. Click the Wellness Exam in the Encounters area of the Patient Dashboard.
17. Select Preventative Services from the Record drop down menu.
18. Note any overdue notifications and click the Preventative Services Schedule link to determine which services are overdue.
19. Click the Add button in the Procedures section.
20. Select "Mammogram" in the Health Recommendation field.
21. Use the calendar picker to document the date in the Date Performed.
22. Document "Bilateral Screening Mammogram" in the Comments field and click the Save button. The preventative service you added will display in the Preventative Services table.

 Now use the Back to Assignment link to complete the Post-Case Quiz found on the Info Panel for this assignment.

Coding & Billing

Appendix
Showcasing Experience
and Portfolio Tips

Showcasing Experience

In order to begin your career as a medical assistant, you must communicate the skills learned in school to potential employers. Showcasing how your experience in SimChart for the Medical Office has helped you become familiar with EHR workflow will serve as a marketable asset when you begin your job search.

Resume

Highlighting the skills you have gained will make your resume look more attractive to a potential employer.

- List all software you are familiar with in the Skills section of your resume, including SimChart for the Medical Office.

In the Front Office module, you managed patient appointments using established protocols, set up an appointment matrix, completed forms, and created correspondence.

In the Clinical Care module, you charted patient information such as allergies, chief complaint, health history, immunizations, medications, order entry, patient education, preventative services, problem list, progress notes, and vital signs.

In the Coding & Billing module, you identified the correct codes to assign to a patient visit and completed documents such as the Superbill, Ledger, Claim, and Day Sheet.

Interview

You will probably be asked about your experience with an electronic health record during the interview process. A potential employer may use terms such as electronic health record, electronic medical record, EHR, EMR, or practice management software. All of these terms refer to documenting patient information in an electronic format.

- Discuss how the variety of activities you completed in SimChart for the Medical Office make you a valuable asset in any medical office.
- If a potential employer does not ask about your experiences during the interview process, volunteer this information at the end of the interview. The fact that you have extensive experience with an electronic health record product could be the deciding factor that gets you the job!

Portfolio Tips

A professional portfolio demonstrates learning evidence for skills. A potential employer should have an overview of an applicant's work after a quick portfolio review. A portfolio can make your resume stand out and ultimately help you earn the job. Every portfolio is unique, but these instructions are a good starting point.

Organization

Binders simplify the process of updating a portfolio by easily adding or removing documents. Starting with a Table of Contents provides a potential employer with the reference needed to quickly find areas of interest.

- Organize work samples in a 1-inch or 3-inch ringed binder.
- Use Dividers to separate binder sections.

Binder Sections

Campus Career Services can help you create or update a resume and cover letter, in addition to practice mock interviews. They can even forward your resume to potential employers.

- Include samples of diagnostic and procedural coding such as an exam or a sample case.
- Provide work products from insurance and reimbursement methods such as a complete CMS 1500 form, printed work within the 5010 of SimChart for the Medical Office, and/or a patient statement.
- Include SimChart for the Medical Office assignments or projects that demonstrate your medical office skills.
- Include work products from classes like Medical Terms, Basic Human Structure and Study of Disease to demonstrate your knowledge of the human body.
- Brag about any special recognition in an Awards or Achievements section.

These suggestions are a great starting point but are not required. Remember, Campus Career Services offers free assistance for resume, cover letter, and portfolio development.

Appendix

Glossary

ADJMT Adjustment found on the Ledger and Day Sheet. An adjustment is a change to a patient's account that is neither a charge for services nor a payment.

Annual Exam Patient visit that occurs yearly and includes a complete physical examination.

Assignment of Benefits Release a patient signs that gives the insurance carrier permission to pay the medical office directly instead of sending the payment to the patient.

Calendar The landing page upon entering the simulation used to review and manage appointments. Some fields throughout the simulation also utilize calendar pickers, which indicates that a date must be chosen.

Chief Complaint The reason a patient scheduled an appointment to see the physician. Although only one chief complaint can be assigned to an encounter, it could include several conditions such as sore throat, fever, and a headache. Only one Encounter type per day is allowed for a patient.

Claim Located in the Coding & Billing Info Panel, the 5010 CMS Claim is submitted electronically to the insurance carrier and generated for a specific encounter. The Claim contains information the insurance carrier needs to process the charges associated with the patient visit and make a payment to the medical office. It is important to note, however, that the print functionality within the electronic claim does generate a CMS 1500 form. The print functionality is available for students who wish to print work for instructors.

Clinical Care The second module in the simulation where all of the clinical charting for a patient occurs.

Coding & Billing The third module in the simulation featuring all of the necessary forms and documentation for coding, billing, and ultimately completing a patient encounter.

Comprehensive Visit First encounter type displayed in the Clinical Care Info Panel that includes Annual Exam, Follow-Up/Established Visit, New Patient Visit, Urgent Visit, and Wellness Exam.

Correspondence Icon located in the task bar at the top of the screen that directs students to email and letter templates for patient and office communication.

CPT Current Procedural Terminology used for procedural coding.

Day Sheet Form located in the Coding & Billing module, used to record services and charges associated with patient care.

Diagnostic/Lab Results Located in the Clinical Care Info Panel and used to record the results of diagnostic procedures and laboratory tests.

Encounter Patient visit. Students must select or create a new encounter before documenting in a patient record in order to tie documentation to a specific date and time. Encounter types include Comprehensive Visits, Office Visits, and Phone Consultations.

Established Patient A patient that has been seen in the medical office within the last three years.

Fee Schedule A list of the amounts charged for services and supplies in a medical office.

Find Patient Icon located in the task bar at the top of the screen which directs students to the Patient Search tool. Selecting a patient directs students to the Clinical Care module to begin documenting in the patient record.

Follow-Up/Established Visit Patient visit for a patient following up on a previously diagnosed condition or a patient who has been seen in the medical office within the last three years but is not coming in for an annual exam, urgent visit, or wellness exam.

Form Repository Icon located in the task bar at the top of the screen that contains all patient specific forms saved to the patient record. The repository also contains general Office Forms that are not saved to a patient record.

Front Office The first module in the application featuring all of the administrative functionality performed in a medical office.

Guarantor The individual legally responsible for the bill. A guarantor must be designated in the Patient Demographics section. The guarantor could be the patient or the patient's spouse or parent. See also: Insured.

ICD-9/ICD-10 International Classification of Diseases 9th or 10th revision. Used for diagnostic coding. SimChart for the Medical Office utilizes both ICD-9 and ICD-10.

Info Panel Located on the left side of the screen in all modules, the Info Panel is the primary source of navigation within the application. Options change depending on the selected module.

Insured The policy holder for the health insurance policy. The insured could be the patient, a spouse, or a parent. See also: Guarantor.

Ledger Located in the Coding & Billing module, the Ledger lists all of the transactions that have occurred for a guarantor, including transactions for all patients the guarantor is legally responsible for. All charges, payments, and adjustments are recorded in the Ledger.

Link Blue, underlined text that a user can click to navigate to another location or screen within SimChart for the Medical Office.

Module Tabs displayed just below the SimChart for the Medical Office logo at the top of the screen that act as the main navigational method within the medical office. The three modules are Front Office, Clinical Care, and Coding & Billing.

New Patient A patient who is seeing the physician for the first time or who has not been to the medical office within the last three years.

New Patient Visit Patient visit for a patient who is seeing the physician for the first time or who has not been to the medical office within the last three years.

Office Visit Second encounter type displayed in the Clinical Care Info Panel for a generalized patient visit including Annual Exam, Follow-Up/Established Visit, New Patient Visit, Urgent Visit, and Wellness Exam.

Patient Dashboard Located in the Clinical Care module, the Patient Dashboard provides a summary of the patient record, including a list of previous encounters.

Patient Demographics Icon located in the task bar at the top of the screen used to add a new patient or edit an established patient's information. Any updates to patient information should be completed within patient demographics, not the Patient Information form. Updated patient information entered in Patient Demographics will update the Patient Information form upon saving.

Phone Consultation Third encounter type displayed in the Clinical Care Info Panel that is used to document a patient phone call. Unlike Comprehensive and Office visits, a patient can have more than one of these encounter types in a business day.

Progress Notes The section of the patient record where new information for each patient visit is recorded using the SOAPE format. Refer to information documented in the Progress Note from within the Coding & Billing module if there is a question during the billing process regarding services provided and/or the diagnosis.

Record The Record dropdown menu displays chart sections of the patient record. Menu options change based on the encounter type selected, but most include allergies, chief complaint, health history, immunizations, medications, order entry, patient education, preventive services, problem list, progress notes, and vital signs.

Signature on File Used in the Coding & Billing module, 'Signature on File' indicates that the medical office has the patient's signature on file. This allows the release of information to an insurance carrier and usually includes the authorization for the assignment of benefits.

SOAPE Format used in the Progress Note to record new information for the patient visit. The information is recorded in the appropriate category: S for subjective, O for objective, A for assessment, P for plan, and E for evaluation.

Superbill Electronic form located in the Coding & Billing Info Panel that acts as the first step in completing the billing process for a patient visit. All services, diagnoses, patient payments, and supplies provided must be recorded on the Superbill.

Urgent Visit Patient visit type for a patient with a serious condition who must see the physician on the same day they request an appointment.

Wellness Exam Visit type for a patient who needs to see the doctor but is not sick. This visit type encompasses preventive services such as a colonoscopy, sigmoidoscopy, mammogram, or bone density study.

1. Schedule Appointment for Talibah Nasser
2. Schedule Appointment for Celia Tapia
3. Prepare Scheduling Matrix
4. Prepare Appointment Reminder Letter for Amma Patel
5. Prepare Certificate to Return to Work Form for Diego Lupez
6. Prepare Medical Records Release Form for Daniel Miller
7. Complete Incident Report for Celia Tapia
8. Complete Incident Report for Employee
9. Complete Incident Report for Medical Office Evacuation
10. Prepare Office Memorandum
11. Complete Office Inventory Form
12. Complete New Patient Registration for Malcom Little
13. Update Demographics and Complete Advance Directive Form for Amma Patel
14. Schedule Appointment and Prepare New Patient Forms for Al Neviaser
15. Schedule Appointment and Prepare New Patient Forms for Ella Rainwater
16. Schedule Appointment and Prepare Appointment Reminder Letter for Anna Richardson
17. Send Missed Appointment Email to Ella Rainwater
18. Complete New Patient Registration and Schedule Appointment for Lisa Rae
19. Prepare Referral Form for Ella Rainwater
20. Prepare Prior Authorization Request Form for Mora Siever
21. Schedule Appointment and Order X-Ray for Mora Siever
22. Schedule Appointment and Order Procedures for Aaron Jackson
23. Prepare Order and Medical Records Release Form for Norma Washington
24. Schedule Appointment and Update Problem List for Ella Rainwater
25. Upload Test Results and Prepare Lab Results Letter for Julia Berkley
26. Update Problem List and Document Vital Signs for Aaron Jackson
27. Update Problem List for Johnny Parker
28. Update Problem List for Anna Richardson
29. Update Problem List for Ella Rainwater
30. Document Allergies for Al Neviaser
31. Document Immunizations and Schedule Follow-up Appointment for Daniel Miller
32. Document Allergies and Medications for Daniel Miller
33. Document Immunizations for Al Neviaser
34. Document Medications for Al Neviaser
35. Document Immunizations and Medications for Diego Lupez
36. Document Health History for Ella Rainwater
37. Document Phone Encounter and Prepare Medication Refill for Casey Hernandez
38. Document Patient Education for Amma Patel
39. Document Patient Education for Casey Hernandez
40. Document Vital Signs for Amma Patel
41. Document Vital Signs for Ella Rainwater
42. Document Preventative Services for Amma Patel
43. Document Encounter and Schedule Appointment for Walter Biller
44. Document Order and Preventative Services for Diego Lupez
45. Document Progress Note and Order for Norma Washington
46. Document Allergies and Medications for Ella Rainwater
47. Document Lab Results, Preventative Services, and Order for Walter Biller
48. Document Preventative Services and Test Results for Diego Lupez
49. Document Immunizations and Order for Celia Tapia
50. Document Preventative Services for Diego Lupez
51. Document Progress Note and Order for Charles Johnson
52. Document Phone Encounter and Order for Charles Johnson
53. Document Phone Encounter for Ella Rainwater
54. Document Preventative Services and Immunizations for Ella Rainwater
55. Document Vital Signs, Allergies, Medications, and Order for Maude Crawford
56. Document Health History for Al Neviaser
57. Document Problem List, Chief Complaint, Medications, and Allergies for Carl Bowden